FIFTH EDITION

Clinical Methods and Practicum in Speech-Language Pathology

FIFTH EDITION

Clinical Methods and Practicum in Speech-Language Pathology

M. N. Hegde, Ph. D.

Deborah Davis, M.A.

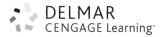

DELMAR
CENGAGE Learning

Australia • Brazil • Japan • Korea • Mexico • Singapore • Spain • United Kingdom • United States

DELMAR
CENGAGE Learning™

Clinical Methods and Practicum in Speech-Language Pathology, Fifth Edition

M.N. Hegde, Ph. D.
Deborah Davis, M.A.

Vice President, Career and Professional Editorial: Dave Garza

Director of Learning Solutions: Matthew Kane

Senior Acquisitions Editor: Sherry Dickinson

Managing Editor: Marah Bellegarde

Product Manager: Laura J. Wood

Editorial Assistant: Anthony Souza

Vice President, Career and Professional Marketing: Jennifer McAvey

Executive Marketing Manager: Wendy E. Mapstone

Senior Marketing Manager: Kristin McNary

Marketing Coordinator: Scott A. Chrysler

Production Director: Carolyn Miller

Production Manager: Andrew Crouth

Senior Art Director: David Arsenault

For product information and technology assistance, contact us at **Cengage Learning Customer & Sales Support, 1-800-354-9706**

For permission to use material from this text or product, submit all requests online at **www.cengage.com/permissions**. Further permissions questions can be e-mailed to **permissionrequest@cengage.com.**

Library of Congress Control Number: 2008943669

ISBN-13: 978-1-4354-6956-3

ISBN-10: 1-4354-6956-9

Delmar
5 Maxwell Drive
Clifton Park, NY 12065-2919
USA

Cengage Learning is a leading provider of customized learning solutions with office locations around the globe, including Singapore, the United Kingdom, Australia, Mexico, Brazil, and Japan. Locate your local office at: **international.cengage.com/region**

Cengage Learning products are represented in Canada by Nelson Education, Ltd.

For your lifelong learning solutions, visit **delmar.cengage.com**

Visit our corporate website at **www.cengage.com**

Printed in the United States of America
2 3 4 5 6 7 12 11 10 09

CONTENTS

Part II: Clinical Methods in Speech-Language Pathology

Appendices

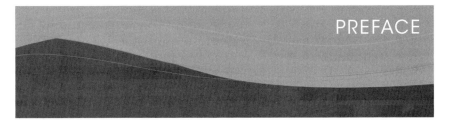

This text was written for students in speech-language pathology who are about to begin their clinical practicum. The text was also written for supervisors of clinical practicum who need a systematic body of information on the various structural, methodological, and ethical aspects of clinical practicum and its supervision. Our goal was to offer a single and comprehensive source of information that will help establish clear expectations for both student clinicians and clinical supervisors. By dividing the book into two major parts, we have covered both the structural and conceptual aspects of clinical practicum and the basic clinical methods of client management. We emphasize that the clinical practicum is a learning experience and that it involves clearly defined expectations, governed by ethical principles of clinical services, and requiring effective and efficient methods of treatment.

Students who read this book prior to starting their clinical practicum will be better prepared to meet the exciting and yet often challenging task of providing ethical and effective services to children and adults with various forms of communicative disorders. Student clinicians will gain an understanding of the structure of various clinical practicum sites; principles of ethical practices; conduct, behavior, and competencies expected of them; justifiable expectations of their clinical supervisors; and the many fundamental principles of assessment and intervention across a variety of disorders. Clinical supervisors, too, may find the book helpful in understanding their own roles and responsibilities better so that they can create a productive and exciting clinical practicum experience for student clinicians.

We have received excellent comments from instructors and reviewers for the earlier editions. Many positive and constructive comments have reinforced our belief that the book offers a single source of comprehensive information on clinical practicum and supervision. Such comments also have helped us in this revision.

For the fifth edition, we have updated: ASHA requirements or guidelines for certification and clinical practicum in speech-language pathology; the methods by which university departments are expected to track a student's progress in the program; clinical practicum sites, related agencies, and professional expectations; the use of *Response to Intervention*; and assessment of individuals with English as a second language. The clinical methods section of this edition includes new information on treatment targets for clients with swallowing disorders. We have added additional information on assessment and treatment of emergent literacy skills in preschool children. We have further revised or expanded the existing information on target behaviors and treatment strategies for voice disorders (including functional aphonia), childhood apraxia of speech, augmentative and alternative communication, traumatic brain injury, right hemisphere syndrome, dementia, stuttering, and other disorders of communication. The text includes several boxed sections that refer students to specific guidelines. Finally, a comprehensive appendix provides resources and examples for students' reference.

As in the previous editions, our motivation to revise and expand this book came from the students and their devotion to excel and help their clients, the clients and their amazing resilience and dedication to hard work, and the professionalism and expertise of paid and volunteer staff with whom we work. All have enriched our lives and taught us much about the practice of speech-language pathology.

We would like to thank the anonymous reviewers whose comments and suggestions have immensely helped us improve this revision. We are thankful to Sherry Dickinson, the Senior Acquisitions Editor, and Laura Wood, the Product Manager, at Delmar Cengage Learning for their sustained, courteous, and competent support in planning and completing this revision.

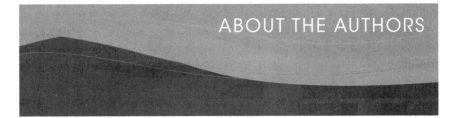

M. N. (Giri) Hegde, Ph. D., is Professor of Communication Sciences and Disorders at California State University, Fresno. He holds a master's degree in experimental psychology from the University of Mysore, India, a post master's diploma in medical (clinical) psychology from Bangalore University, India, and a doctoral degree in speech-language pathology from Southern Illinois University at Carbondale.

Dr. Hegde is a specialist in fluency disorders, language disorders, research methods, and treatment procedures in communicative disorders. He has made numerous presentations to national and international audiences on various basic and applied topics in communicative disorders and experimental and applied behavior analysis. With his deep and wide scholarship, Dr. Hegde has authored several highly regarded and widely used scientific and professional books, including *Treatment Procedures in Communicative Disorders, Clinical Research in Communicative Disorders, Introduction to Communicative Disorders, A Coursebook on Aphasia and Other Neurogenic Language Disorders, A Coursebook on Scientific and Professional Writing in Speech-Language Pathology, Hegde's PocketGuide to Communication Disorders, Hegde's PocketGuide to Treatment in Speech-Language Pathology, and Hegde's PocketGuide to Assessment in Speech-Language Pathology*. He has served on the editorial boards of scientific and professional journals and continues to serve as an editorial consultant to *Journal of Fluency Disorders,* the *American Journal of Speech-Language Pathology,* and the *Journal of Speech-Language Pathology—Applied Behavior Analysis.*

Dr. Hegde is a recipient of various honors, including the Outstanding Professor Award from California State University, Fresno, CSU Fresno Provost's Recognition for Outstanding Scholarship and Publication, Distinguished Alumnus Award from the Southern Illinois University Department of Communication Sciences and Disorders, and Outstanding Professional Achievement Award from District 5 of California Speech-Language-Hearing Association. Dr. Hegde is a Fellow of the American Speech-Language-Hearing Association.

A speech-language pathologist for over twenty years, **Deborah Davis, M.A.,** is a special education Program Manager with the Fresno County Office of Education. She oversees special education services for infants and preschoolers as well as services for children with autism and communication disabilities. Prior to accepting Program Manager responsibilities, Ms. Davis was Director of the Speech and Hearing Clinic at California State University, Fresno, where she supervised on- and off-campus practicum. Ms. Davis has worked extensively as an itinerant speech-language pathologist in the public schools and as a teacher in a classroom for children with communicative disorders. She also worked with the geriatric populations in skilled nursing facilities and home health. Ms. Davis received her bachelor's and master's degrees from California State University, Fresno, and is a Fellow of the California Speech-Language-Hearing Association.

Clinical Practicum

When you have completed a certain course in communicative disorders, your advisor may tell you that you are ready for clinical practicum. This means that you have acquired some basic knowledge about communication and its disorders. Yet, you may not know much about the practicum itself. Therefore, in Part I of the text, we have described the organization of clinical practicum, various rules and regulations you must follow, the relationship with your clinical supervisor, and some basic principles of working with clients. Read this part of the text carefully to understand what practicum is and how to prepare yourself for it.

In Part II of the text, we have described the basic clinical methods of treating clients with communicative disorders. We have given an overview of commonly used treatment techniques with an emphasis on working with families of your clients to achieve maintenance of treatment gains.

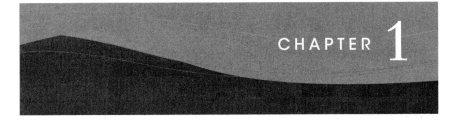

CHAPTER 1

Clinical Practicum in Speech-Language Pathology

Chapter Outline

- Clinical Practicum: An Overview
- General Preclinic Requirements
- ASHA Guidelines on Practicum
- Clinical Practicum as a Learning Experience

Speech-language pathology is a profession with scientific and academic bases. To be a speech-language pathologist, you need to gain both academic and scientific knowledge through coursework and practical experience in working with clients who have communicative disorders. Therefore, speech-language pathology degree programs at colleges and universities include two types of training.

The first type of training is offered through **academic coursework.** You learn about speech, language, communication, and communicative disorders by taking various academic courses. Some academic courses are a prerequisite to beginning clinical practicum and others may be taken in conjunction with clinical practicum. The academic portion of the training program provides you with an empirical as well as theoretical basis from which you can expand your knowledge and carefully analyze the validity of new ideas and trends in the assessment and treatment of communicative disorders. Your academic training also provides the foundation for clinical practicum.

The second type of training is offered through **clinical practicum.** Clinical practicum gives you the opportunity to apply and practice what you have learned in academic courses, under the guidance of your clinical mentor (supervisor). You will have diverse clinical experiences and may use these opportunities to help you determine an area, or areas (e.g., medical, pediatric, adult, etc.), in which you are most interested in pursuing more advanced study and employment. The combination of academic coursework and practicum provides you with well-rounded training in speech–language pathology and prepares you to pursue a variety of career options.

Occasionally, students try to rate the importance of academic classes versus practicum assignments. However, there is no comparison because each is equally important. Without a strong academic background, you would not know how to assess and treat people with communicative disorders. Without practicum, you would not learn the skills you must have to be a successful speech–language pathologist. Therefore, from the beginning, avoid making judgments in favor of one or the other and apply yourself fully and equally to your academic courses and practicum assignments.

Although reference may be made to academic coursework, this text emphasizes clinical practicum. If you have any questions regarding specific academic requirements, contact your advisor. Questions regarding clinical practicum requirements should be referred to your advisor, clinical supervisor, or clinic director.

Clinical Practicum: An Overview

Clinical practicum is an exciting component of your educational experience. You will have opportunities to work with a variety of professionals and clients, apply much of what you have learned in your academic courses, and expand on your knowledge of communication and its disorders. Your clinical practicum is a supervised experience in which you learn professional skills of assessing and treating people with communicative disorders. In some assignments you learn to work independently, and in other assignments you learn to work as a member of a team. Your clinical practicum experiences are designed to prepare you for your future role as a professional speech–language pathologist. Enrollment in clinical practicum is a required part of the curriculum in programs accredited by the **American Speech-Language-Hearing Association (ASHA).** Clinical practicum provides you with the necessary opportunities to apply and expand the information learned in academic courses. Your **enthusiasm, dedication,** and **hard work** are important variables that influence the degree to which you will benefit from your clinical assignments.

Students generally enroll in clinical practicum during their senior year as undergraduates or during their first semester as graduate students. Certain universities allow students to participate in clinical practicum earlier in the training program. In some cases, this early experience may be limited to observing graduate students providing clinical services and assisting with a client or two toward the end of the semester. For example, you may be assigned to observe a student clinician for a semester prior to being assigned your own clients. You will be involved gradually in the treatment process. You may be required to assist in charting responses, developing stimulus materials, and eventually working with a client for one or two sessions as the primary clinician. Your training program structures your activities to maximize your learning as well as your academic and clinical success.

As much as a university clinic's caseload allows, a beginning student clinician is assigned clients with less complex disorders. In most universities, student clinicians are assigned clients based on the academic courses they have completed. For example, during your first semester of graduate work, you may enroll in a course in articulation and be assigned clients with articulation disorders only. As you complete coursework on other disorders of communication, you may be assigned clients with those types of disorders.

Other universities take a more gestalt view of clinical experience and provide a student clinician with a variety of clients each term, based on the student's level of expertise and previous educational experience and the supervisor's expertise. For example, as a first-semester graduate student, you may take a seminar in articulation, a seminar in language, and a seminar in research methods. However, in your clinical practicum, you may be assigned a client with a fluency disorder based on your undergraduate class in fluency and the expertise of your clinical supervisor.

You will participate in clinical practicum assignments at the university clinic and various off-campus clinical sites. Many universities require student clinicians to complete a certain minimum number of clinical hours before they are assigned to off-campus practicum sites. Your clinical practicum may include hospital, school, or various other clinical sites.

As you progress through your clinical and academic programs, you are given more responsibility in planning, evaluating, and treating clients. As a beginning student clinician, you will not be expected to have all the answers; your clinical supervisor will help you find those answers. Although you will be supervised throughout your clinical practicum, as you gain clinical experience, you will be expected to perform more independently in most of your clinical responsibilities. Eventually, you will be expected to conduct most of your clinical duties with minimal supervisory input.

General Preclinic Requirements

In addition to a solid academic foundation, good writing skills are necessary for success in clinical practicum. Equally important is your ability to talk to people from all walks of life and of all ages. Finally, there are less tangible, personal characteristics without which you cannot successfully complete your clinical practicum; for example, you must be conscientious and reliable. You should be able to organize your schedule and allocate sufficient time to your clinical responsibilities. Your flexibility and nonjudgmental disposition will influence your clinical success. Although you may begin the term with a specific clinical assignment, your clinic assignment may be altered mid-term due to a client schedule change, supervisor change, or other uncontrollable variables. You should accept and adapt quickly to such changes. In addition, you may be assigned a client whom you dislike—perhaps you do not approve of the client's demeanor or lifestyle. Nonetheless, be flexible and find a way to work effectively with this person. You are always expected to be committed to providing the best quality of client care possible. You are not expected to enter clinical practicum with all the necessary skills, but you should be able to learn from your clinical experiences and the interactions with your supervisor.

Academic Requirements

Preclinic academic requirements are completed both at the undergraduate and graduate levels. At the **undergraduate level,** one of your first courses may be an introduction to communication sciences and disorders. Then you will probably take courses on phonetics; anatomy and physiology of speech, swallowing, and hearing mechanisms; speech science (perception and production of speech); and those courses related to normal acquisition of speech and language. Some clinical courses, especially those related to disorders of articulation, language, voice, fluency, and hearing, also may be taken at the undergraduate level.

Graduate courses provide you with more advanced information on all aspects of communication sciences and disorders and on assessment and treatment of various disorders. These courses are more research based than the undergraduate courses. Graduate courses build on the information offered at the undergraduate level and emphasize specialized information. For example, besides taking advanced courses in articulation and language, you also take courses in fluency, adult language disorders, craniofacial anomalies, augmentative communication, dysphagia (swallowing disorders), and motor speech disorders. At the graduate and postgraduate levels, an increasing number of universities offer courses in administration and supervision, including the supervision of **speech–language pathology assistants (SLPAs),** a trend reflecting ASHA's position on the use of qualified assistants.

Although *course requirements and sequences vary* from university to university, students are expected to have completed, as a minimum, introductory courses in normal and abnormal speech and language development and courses in speech and hearing science before beginning clinical practicum. You should discuss the specific requirements with your advisor well in advance of the time you plan to begin your clinical practicum.

General Writing Requirements

Accurately documenting and precisely reporting clinical information in writing are necessary skills in the practice of speech–language pathology. The approval for patient treatment by insurance companies; a doctor's decision to provide medical intervention; monetary reimbursement for your services; and your determination of the need for initiating, continuing, or discontinuing services are just a few of the areas that may be influenced by your documentation and reports. Therefore, part of your clinical practicum will include learning different reporting formats.

Student clinicians are required to write numerous clinical reports, treatment programs, lesson plans, and progress notes. You will discover that different clinical settings have varying writing requirements. Regardless of the specific requirements, you will be expected to have good basic writing skills at each of your assignments. In many instances, your reports may be read by other people, including clients' family members, physicians, teachers, and other speech-language pathologists. It is important that you develop your writing skills before enrolling in clinical practicum. Unless you have had a course on professional writing in communicative disorders, you are not expected to know the specific formats for reports and some of the technical terms before clinical enrollment, but you should be able to write clearly and concisely. You should be able to organize your thoughts coherently and write grammatically correct sentences. Your writing should be free from spelling errors and be clear and simple enough to be understood by the intended audience. With these skills, you should be able to adapt your writing to the different formats and styles expected at various sites.

Before you are awarded your graduate degree, you will be required to demonstrate professional writing skills sufficient for entry-level practice in speech-language pathology. If you are concerned about your general writing skills and your program does not offer a course on professional writing, discuss the problem with your advisor as early in your program as possible. Your advisor can assist you in overcoming your writing problems. You may need to take a writing course, or you may need additional practice in writing. You may practice professional writing skills in a book that is designed for self-teaching. One such book is by Hegde (2010), which gives exemplars of scientific and professional writing along with opportunities to practice writing skills. Take these and other steps that will prepare you for meeting clinical writing requirements.

Oral Communication Skills

Effective oral communication skills are essential to the practice of speech-language pathology. As a student clinician, *you will communicate with many clients with varied educational, socioeconomic, and cultural backgrounds.* You also will interact with many professionals. For example, you may discuss your clients' evaluation, treatment, and progress with physical therapists, physicians, nurses, teachers, audiologists, psychologists, and other speech-language pathologists.

Regardless of the client, professional, or family member you communicate with, you must speak so that that individual will understand you. With some clients you will need to use simple, brief language; with other clients you may use technical terms, advanced vocabulary, and you can present complex concepts. At times, to establish a shared basis of understanding, you may need to use some professional jargon along with an understandable definition. With certain individuals you may introduce the term *apraxia* and explain exactly what you are referring to when you use that term. With other individuals you may introduce the term *apraxia* and provide the common definition followed by an analogy that will assist them in understanding it. At another time you may refer to an "SST" (student study team) meeting and explain the meaning of that initialism. You should develop the flexibility to speak at whatever level the communicative situation requires. In all instances, you should *clearly and concisely articulate* information. You should learn to communicate in the way that maximizes comprehension for the listener. You will develop your communication competence as part of your graduate training; however, it is helpful to begin with a certain skill level. Your department or one of the other departments in your university may offer a counseling course that teaches specific interpersonal communication skills. Consider taking such a course and discuss this with your academic advisor.

Personal Characteristics

In addition to academic preparation and good written and oral communication skills, there are some personal characteristics that are required for successful clinical work. Responsible behavior is probably one of the most important characteristics.

Student clinicians are expected to **act responsibly** in all areas of clinical involvement, including preparation for treatment sessions, meeting with clients, report writing, and interactions with office staff and clinical supervisors. You will have deadlines for various clinical assignments, including scheduling of clients, completion of various reporting forms needed by clinic administrative staff, and submission of diagnostic reports, treatment plans, and lesson plans. Regardless of other academic or personal commitments, you must be well-prepared for all your diagnostic and treatment sessions.

As a graduate student, you will have many obligations and it will be important for you to organize your time. Typically, this means you must **establish priorities and prepare in advance.** You may have an examination scheduled and a new client to evaluate on the same day a major paper is due. Obviously, to accomplish all these well, you must allow for sufficient preparation time.

Student clinicians work with many people, and your ability to **maintain your professional boundaries while empathizing with your clients and their families** is essential. You must not become overly involved in your clients' personal lives or allow them to become overly involved in your personal life. However, you must combine your technical knowledge with care and regard to your clients' living situations and their personal concerns. For example, it probably would not be useful to expect clients living alone in private care facilities to be able to find people with whom to practice a speech assignment. However, knowing this, you might talk with cooperative nursing assistants and ask them to help your clients practice their speech. Many *external and internal factors* influence clients' progress. It will be important for you to know and understand the interactions among your clients' disabilities, living situations, and support systems and how they affect your clients' speech therapy.

Student clinicians should learn to work independently within their level of experience. For example, as a beginning clinician, you are expected to rely on your supervisor for assistance more than experienced clinicians do; however, you still must be prepared to research material independently and, with your supervisor's help, evaluate the efficacy of your clinical sessions, determine areas of needed change, and implement appropriate modifications that your supervisor suggests to you. You will be expected to demonstrate systematic *progress toward working independently*. See Chapter 4 for more on student clinician responsibilities.

Knowledge of the Profession and Related Agencies

In addition to your university's requirements, several agencies and professional organizations affect your training and career as a speech-language pathologist. As you prepare to enroll in clinical practicum, you should have at least a basic knowledge of the various accrediting and licensing agencies and regulations related to the profession of speech-language pathology. Two agencies affect your training and professional career the most: the ASHA and, if your state has a licensure law, the *Board of Examiners for Audiology and Speech-Language Pathology* (or other licensing agency in your state).

The American Speech-Language-Hearing Association (ASHA)

The ASHA is the national professional organization representing speech-language pathologists and audiologists. Students and student clinicians in departments of communication sciences and disorders or speech-language pathology will repeatedly hear references to ASHA and its various activities, guidelines, and requirements that affect the profession. Student clinicians will constantly be told of ASHA's requirements on how to complete their clinical practicum. Also, students will be expected to become members of ASHA's student organization, the **National Student Speech-Language-Hearing Association (NSSLHA).**

As you probably know, ASHA is a *scientific and professional organization* with a long history of contributions to communication sciences and disorders. This national organization is the major force that shapes our scientific and professional discipline. The organization acts as an advocate for individuals with communicative disorders and the professionals who provide services to these individuals and has nine goals (American Speech-Language-Hearing Association, 2008a).

The Goals of the American Speech-Language-Hearing Association

1. Encourage basic scientific study of the processes of individual human communication with special reference to speech, language, and hearing and related disorders;

2. Promote high standards and ethics for the academic and clinical preparation of individuals entering the discipline of human communication sciences and disorders;

(continues)

3. Promote the acquisition of new knowledge and skills for those within the discipline;

4. Promote investigation, prevention, and the diagnosis and treatment of disorders of human communication and related disorders;

5. Foster improvement of clinical services and intervention procedures concerning such disorders;

6. Stimulate exchange of information among persons and organizations, and disseminate such information;

7. Inform the public about communication sciences and disorders, related disorders, and the professionals who provide services;

8. Advocate on behalf of persons with communication and related disorders; and

9. Promote the individual and collective professional interests of the members of the Association.

Source: *Bylaws of the American Speech-Language-Hearing Association* by the American Speech-Language-Hearing Association, 1997–2008, Rockville, MD: Author.

ASHA works in various ways to help maintain high standards of clinical competence of speech-language pathologists and audiologists. Two governing bodies interact to identify and respond to priorities of the profession. The *Board of Directors* is comprised of 16 elected officers and the Executive Director of the Association. *The Advisory Council* (AC) consists of an Audiology Advisory Council and a Speech-Language Pathology Advisory Council. Each AC has 53 members including one elected member from every state, the District of Columbia, and other areas. Two members of the NSSLHA also are elected to serve on the AC. (American Speech-Language-Hearing Association, 2008a.) ASHA sponsors conferences and workshops to encourage continuing professional education. It collects and disseminates data related to research, clinical service delivery, education, and career opportunities. It has a policy on the scope of practice for speech-language pathologists and audiologists and has established accreditation and certification procedures that outline minimal standards of education and clinical service delivery. These standards are outlined in the form of academic and clinical preparation guidelines and include required compliance with the ASHA Code of Ethics. These standards are designed to protect consumers and the professionals who serve them.

ASHA Accreditation

University training programs that meet ASHA standards may receive accreditation from it. ASHA's **Council on Academic Accreditation in Audiology and Speech-Language Pathology (CAA)** accredits academic programs.

A university must request accreditation of its program. When it does this, the university may seek accreditation for its speech-language pathology program or audiology program, or both. ASHA will then send a team of trained professionals to evaluate the programs seeking accreditation. ASHA accredits only programs offering advanced degrees.

The evaluation team looks at the quality and number of faculty teaching the courses, the curriculum offered by the department, physical facilities and instructional equipment and laboratories, the library and other resources of the university, the administrative support, and such other factors that affect the education of future speech-language pathologists and audiologists.

The professionals evaluating clinical services offered by a department look at the qualifications and certification status of clinical supervisors, financial resources and management, adequacy of clinical facilities and equipment, and all other factors that affect the quality of clinical services offered to the public. The teams may schedule meetings to discuss the training program with current students as well as graduates of the program. After the site visit, the team submits a report to the ASHA board. Based on the report, a final decision on whether to accredit the program is made.

The CAA requirements directly influence you and your training program. First, if you are attending a program accredited by ASHA, you are assured that the department has met ASHA's standards. Second, you must have initiated and satisfactorily completed all of your graduate academic coursework and clinical practicum (in the area in which certification is sought) at a CAA-accredited program to be eligible for the Certificate of Clinical Competence.

ASHA Certification

ASHA certifies both audiologists and speech-language pathologists. The **Certificate of Clinical Competence** is more commonly referred to as the CCC (pronounced "sees"). The **Council for Clinical Certification (CFCC)** sets the standards for and awards the CCC to speech-language pathologists and audiologists who have successfully met ASHA's academic, clinical, and ethical standards (Lubinsky, 2003). Earning the CCC indicates that individuals have met a certain level of professional competence. Under ASHA's guidelines, individuals with their CCCs may supervise student clinicians, support personnel, and professionals who do not hold certification. When you complete a program of study and clinical experience approved by ASHA you may receive this certification. This certificate may be in audiology or speech-language pathology. Effective January 1, 2005, ASHA evaluates CCC applicants based on *outcome standards* that were designed to ensure that applicants have demonstrated specific academic knowledge and clinical skills.

To be eligible for certification in speech-language pathology, you must satisfy the following standards:

1. **Earn a graduate degree.** You must have earned a master's (MA or MS) or doctoral (SLPD or PhD) degree in the area in which you are applying for certification at an accredited institution of higher education. As you know, your graduate coursework and practicum must be initi-

ated and completed at a program accredited by ASHA's CAA in the area for which certification is sought. At least 75 semester hours must be completed in approved coursework related to speech-language pathology. A minimum of 36 of the 75 semester coursework hours must be at the graduate level. (American Speech-Language Hearing Association, 1997–2008.)

2. **Demonstrate knowledge and skills adequate for entry into professional practice.** Your training program will have been designed such that you acquire the knowledge and skills necessary to speak, listen, write, understand, and evaluate written clinical and research information at a level sufficient for clinical practice and professional interaction. Your training program also will have designed a method by which to document your acquisition of knowledge and skill necessary to practice the profession. Students who have nonstandard dialects, English accents, or have been educated outside of the United States will be required to perform at a level defined by ASHA. (See Chapter 6 for additional information.)

    In addition to specialized knowledge in speech-language pathology, you will be required to demonstrate knowledge of certain principles of biology, physical sciences, social and behavioral sciences, and mathematics. The coursework you take as part of your general undergraduate requirements may fulfill some of these requirements. In addition, you will demonstrate knowledge and skill to analyze, synthesize, evaluate, and apply information in the following areas:

    - Basic processes and principles of human communication and swallowing

    - Swallowing and communication disorders, including the disorders of fluency articulation, voice and resonance, receptive and expressive language, hearing, and assistive and augmentative technologies

    - Cognitive aspects of communication, including memory, attention, sequencing, and problem solving

    - Social and behavioral aspects of language (e.g., working with children with autism or other challenging behaviors)

    - Prevention, assessment, and intervention for communication and swallowing disorders

    - Ethical conduct

    - Research and evidence-based practice

    - Current professional issues including professional certification, credentials, licensure and other professional regulations and recognitions

    You and your academic department are responsible to document that you have acquired the knowledge and skills necessary to practice the profession.

This documentation may be done on the **Knowledge and Skills Acquisition form (KASA)** that ASHA has designed and recommended; however, programs may also develop and use their own forms. Academic departments have an established procedure to track and record each student's progress in acquiring the necessary knowledge and skill. Your academic advisor and clinic supervisor (along with the department chair and clinic director) may monitor your progress and help you document how and when you have met specific requirements. This documentation should be continuous and current. Each semester, when you meet with your academic advisor, you may update your KASA form.

3. **Complete clinical practicum.** A minimum of 400 supervised clinical practicum hours must be completed in specific areas of observation, evaluation, and intervention. Twenty-five hours are obtained in observation, and the remaining hours are obtained during direct client contact. At least 325 of the clinical practicum hours must be completed at the graduate level. Your program of study will be designed to meet all of ASHA's outcomes for knowledge and skills. To achieve these outcomes, you will work with clients of different ages and cultures and who present with various disorders. These clinical skill outcomes are defined under the areas of evaluation, intervention, and interaction and personal qualities and are discussed in greater detail later in this chapter.

4. **Pass formative and summative assessments.** As you progress through your graduate program, you will be required to demonstrate your knowledge and skills in a variety of ways. Formative assessments will include oral, written, and clinical measures. After you have completed your degree program, you will be required to pass the *ASHA Boards* or approved summative assessment known as the *Praxis Examination*. The examination is a comprehensive assessment of an individual's knowledge in speech-language pathology or audiology. Although the *Praxis* can be taken any time before you complete your *Speech-Language Pathology Clinical Fellowship (SLPCF)* year, many individuals take the test soon after they have completed their academic courses or taken their final comprehensive examinations at the university. Studying for a comprehensive examination also helps students prepare for the *Praxis*. There are books available and review courses offered on studying for the *Praxis* (Payne, 2001; Roseberry-McKibbin & Hegde, 2006). The *Speech-Language Pathology test* is administered as part of a Specialty Area Test of the *Praxis II®: Subject Assessments* by the Educational Testing Service (ETS). It consists of objective questions and can usually be taken through your university's testing office. Also, the ETS has a site on the World Wide Web. You can obtain information from this Web site and from your university testing center.

5. **Complete an SLPCF.** The purpose of the SLPCF is to help you transition from student clinician to independent professional. During your SLPCF you will learn many skills specific to service delivery in your employment

setting and improve and hone the skills you learned as a student clinician. The SLPCF consists of paid (or volunteer) experience mentored by a professional holding current ASHA certification in speech-language pathology. The SLPCF is not part of a university clinical training program. Although your mentor will regularly assess your work, no grades are given at the end because your SLPCF is outside the scope of a university program. As a general rule, your university and former professors are not involved in your SLPCF. Typically, after you graduate, you will obtain employment as a speech-language pathologist. Often, your employer can supply SLPCF mentoring. In fact, during your preemployment interviews, it is a good practice to ask if SLPCF mentoring will be provided and by whom. However, you and your mentor need not work in the same setting. You may request a qualified speech-language pathologist from outside your work setting to mentor your SLPCF. Once you begin work and have a SLPCF mentor, you may begin your SLPCF. Within 4 weeks of beginning your SLPCF you will meet with your mentor and write desired outcomes and performance levels on the *SLPCF Report Form*. Once you have completed your clinical fellowship, you will send the SLPCF Report Form, the *Speech-Language Pathology Clinical Fellowships Skills Inventory*, and the *Employer's Verification Form* to the CFCC. The SLPCF can be completed in 36 weeks of full-time work (at least 30 hours per week) or up to 72 weeks of part-time work (15–19 hours per week). Less than 15 hours of work per week does not meet ASHA's SLPCF requirements (American Speech-Language Hearing Association, 1997–2008).

6. **Know and adhere to the ASHA Code of Ethics.** The ASHA Code of Ethics is vital to the practice of speech-language pathology. It presents guidelines and standards for the protection of clients and clinicians. All individuals (students and graduates) seeking ASHA certification must agree to abide by the ASHA Code of Ethics. Chapter 3 contains a more detailed discussion of the Code of Ethics.

7. **Submit your application for certification and pay your membership fee.** ASHA publishes a *Membership and Certification Handbook* that contains application forms as well as detailed information regarding academic, practicum, SLPCF, and membership requirements. The latest version of the *Membership and Certification Handbook* is available for download at ASHA's Web site. Also, your training program will provide guidance in completing the KASA form and other documents that may be required in the membership application. If you have been an NSSLHA member, you may be eligible to receive a discounted application fee. This information is also detailed in the *Membership and Certification Handbook*.

8. **Demonstrate continuous professional development.** After you receive your ASHA certification, you will continue your professional growth. ASHA requires that speech-language pathologists renewing their certification obtain at least 30 contact hours of continuing education within a

3-year period. You may accumulate ASHA **continuing education units (CEUs)** by participating in workshops, conferences, independent study of journal articles, internships, and other activities offered by approved providers. You may also obtain CEUs by taking certain university coursework or through appropriate employer-sponsored inservices. However, for membership renewal purposes, your CEUs must be obtained within a 3-year period beginning from the time you received your CCC. Therefore, the workshops you attend while preparing to become a speech-language pathologist will not count toward later CEU credit.

Although the CCC does not confer any legal status, it is nationally recognized as a requisite for practice in most employment settings, excluding public schools. As you now know, the CCC indicates that you have met minimum proficiency standards set by ASHA to practice speech-language pathology, and it sometimes assists you in establishing credibility with new patients and associates. Many state licensure requirements are based on the CCC requirements, and holding the CCC may make it easier for you to obtain a license in certain states.

Speech-language pathologists benefit from an agreement negotiated by ASHA, the Canadian Association of Speech-Language Pathologists and Audiologists (CASLPA), the Royal College of Speech and Language Therapists (RCSLT) in the United Kingdom, and the Speech Pathology Association of Australia Limited. This agreement, which was effective January 1, 2005, provides reciprocal recognition among professional organizations in the United States, Canada, United Kingdom, and Australia; promotes common standards of clinical competence; and simplifies the process for mutual recognition of credentials among participating organizations.

State Licensure Board

Depending on where you live and in what setting you practice, you also may need to meet state licensure and credentialing requirements. In states that have a licensure law, ASHA's CCC is not sufficient to practice speech-language pathology or audiology. For example, regardless of their certification, credentials, or degrees, private practice speech-language pathologists in many states must be licensed by the state before they can provide clinical services.

Licensure is regulated by a state government agency (e.g., Board of Examiners for Audiology and Speech Pathology). The large majority of states in the United States now have licensure requirements for speech-language pathologists. With the exception of only a few states, the state licensure requirements are compatible with those of the CCC. Many states also have licensure reciprocity with the CCC. Sometimes exempt from licensure requirements are speech-language pathologists providing services in the public schools or federal government agencies.

Your university will coordinate your training so that you meet the minimum requirements of the state licensure board as well as ASHA certification requirements. However, if you are planning to move to another state after you graduate, you should contact the licensure board of that state to ensure you will have met their licensure requirements. You can obtain information on different states' practice requirements by accessing ASHA's Web site at http://www.asha.org. Specific licensure information can be obtained from the *National Council of State Boards of Examiners for Speech-Language Pathology and Audiology* (NCSB). You can locate their Web site at http://www.ncsb.info/home.

Department of Education

The speech–language pathologist who plans to work in the public schools may need to obtain an educational **credential** or certificate from the state's department of education. A credential is a document that verifies that you have met certain requirements and have obtained certain competencies. In many states, to practice speech–language services in the schools, the clinician need not have the state licensure or ASHA's CCC, but many clinicians have them anyway because the credentials indicate a certain level of commitment to the profession and its standards of excellence. A majority of states require a master's degree and a credential to practice speech–language pathology in the public schools. Reauthorized in November 2004, the *Individuals with Disabilities Education Act* (IDEA), one of several amendments to P.L. 94–142, is a federal law that defines professional qualifications for individuals working in the schools. Prior to IDEA 2004, the law required speech–language pathologists working in the schools meet their state's standard for speech–language pathologists working in nonpublic school settings. This is referred to as "highest state standards" in your educational practicum. IDEA 2004 eliminated this standard and aligned qualifications with state-approved or state-recognized certification or licensing for public school employment. In certain states a speech–language pathologist working in the public schools legally may not need to meet the same standards as speech–language pathologists working in other settings. However, ASHA strongly endorses the requirements for speech–language pathologists to hold the highest state standards regardless of their employment setting. (Chapter 5 contains more information on IDEA regulations.) Educational and practicum requirements of most educational credentials are similar to those of CCC and state licensure. However, each state may have some unique requirement for the educational credential.

In addition to the coursework required for the master's degree, a student seeking a school credential often needs to take courses related to public school speech, language, and hearing programs. Additional courses related to public school education also may be required. A student internship in the school setting is a typical credentialing requirement.

Several states offer more than one educational credential for speech–language pathologists. One credential may allow you to teach a class with students who are communicatively handicapped. In these special classes, you may teach academic courses, physical education, art, and music, while emphasizing intervention for each child's communicative needs. Another credential may allow you to offer clinical services on an individual or small-group basis to children with communicative disorders. Many of these services are provided in a private speech therapy room. However, as appropriate, speech and language services are provided in the classroom itself, with emphasis on integration into the class curriculum. Each state has its own educational credential laws for speech–language pathologists.

Because of this diversity and unique educational requirements for state public school credentials, you must consult on this with your advisor early in your clinical training. As you continue your training program, you will become more familiar with the various requirements in your state.

The National Student Speech-Language-Hearing Association (NSSLHA)

The NSSLHA is a national organization affiliated with ASHA. Its main purpose is to help students in speech–language pathology and audiology programs get involved with their future profession. An excellent source of professional information in your department might be the local chapter of the NSSLHA. *Local chapters* of NSSLHA are run by students with the help of a faculty advisor.

Your local chapter is an association of *supportive fellow students* who organize fundraising activities, social events, and professional workshops and seminars. You should, therefore, become a member of the local chapter of NSSLHA early in your undergraduate program. This membership will help you keep current with all aspects of your profession.

NSSLHA membership dues are a fraction of the ASHA dues, and yet you receive many of the same benefits offered to full dues-paying professional members of ASHA. Members of NSSLHA receive all ASHA journals. These journals are a valuable source of scientific and professional information you cannot do without. As a graduate student, you will appreciate having your own collection of journals, which you frequently will be asked to read. NSSLHA also publishes its own journal, which is distributed to its members free of charge. NSSLHA members are eligible to attend certain state and national conferences at reduced rates. Besides, NSSLHA gives students the opportunity to begin developing a social and professional affiliation with individuals having similar interests.

ASHA Special Interest Divisions

ASHA's special interest divisions (SIDs) are subgroups of ASHA composed of individuals who want to *focus on specific areas of interest*. For an additional fee, ASHA members may join certain SIDs. These divisions include such areas as Administration and Supervision, Neurophysiology and Neurogenic Speech and Language Disorders, Speech Science and Orofacial Disorders, and Language Learning and Education. In 2008, there were 16 SIDs. Division members network among other professionals with similar interests. The SIDs publish newsletters, sponsor continuing education, offer specialty certification, and influence the scope of practice for their division areas.

State Speech-Language and Hearing Associations

Many states have speech–language and hearing associations. These associations provide *local support* for speech–language pathologists, audiologists, and individuals with communicative disorders. The state organizations often sponsor workshops and conferences, help disseminate information, and, in conjunction with ASHA, develop professional guidelines. Involvement at the state level allows you to be active in state legislation, organization of state and local conferences, and networking with other professionals in your vicinity. Often members of state organizations also are ASHA members.

Related Professional Organizations

Although ASHA represents the profession of speech-language pathology as a whole, there are many specialty areas in the practice of speech-language pathology. Speech-language pathologists specializing in a certain area of service delivery, such as augmentative communication, may belong to ASHA and other related organizations. Examples of related professional organizations are the United States Society for Augmentative and Alternative Communication, American Academy of Private Practice in Speech-Language Pathology and Audiology, Society of Hospital Directors of Communicative Disorders Programs, and Academy of Neurologic Communication Disorders and Sciences. Names and addresses of some related professional organizations are published on the ASHA Web site.

ASHA Guidelines on Practicum

To ensure that students receive a broad but comprehensive training program, ASHA has established guidelines on clinical practicum. You satisfy the clinical practicum and internship requirements by earning the required number of clinical clock hours under the supervision of an ASHA-certified speech-language pathologist or audiologist. ASHA mandates requirements for both students and supervisors. This section of the text emphasizes the requirements for students.

Clinical Observation

Clinical observation offers students an introduction to the clinical process. It allows you to begin your preparation for clinical practicum by observing the work of more experienced clinicians. Observation is your opportunity to find out how what you have learned through your academic coursework is applied in a clinic. By observing other clinicians, you begin to understand the assessment and treatment process. To maximize learning and meet ASHA's observation requirements, observe the following:

1. **A minimum of 25 clock hours.** ASHA requires students to obtain a minimum of 25 clock hours of supervised clinical observation as part of their clinical practicum. Although the 25 hours are a minimum requirement, students often observe for a greater number of hours. Completion of the 25 observation hours is not a prerequisite for direct client contact; however, to enhance learning and ease your transition to active clinical involvement, you may want to observe as many evaluation and treatment sessions as possible.

2. **Live or videotaped sessions within the scope of practice of speech-language pathology.** Most students will observe live clinical sessions. However, observation of videotaped sessions or of live sessions on closed-circuit television monitors is also acceptable.

3. **A variety of clinical sessions.** Observation hours may be obtained for treatment and evaluation of individuals with communicative or swallowing disorders. Observations may be of children or of adults. Also, you may want to observe some clients over a period of time to note the progression of treatment while you sample a variety of other clients and disorders. Regardless of the required distribution of observation hours, the 25 hours are a minimum requirement, and additional observation hours are strongly advised.

4. **Under supervision by an ASHA-certified professional.** You may observe professionals and other student clinicians. All observations must be under the supervision of an ASHA-certified professional. Your supervisors and the clinic director will examine the observation log and reports to verify your observation hours. Observations may be made simultaneously with the supervisor, or the student observer may submit reports to the supervisor for review and approval.

5. **With a purpose.** Determine what you want to learn from each observation. This will help you concentrate on certain events that occur during the clinical session and give you direction when you begin your direct client practicum. It is important to critically evaluate what you observe. It is not sufficient to just "watch" a clinical session and expect to gain much useful knowledge. Your supervisor will help you note the many variables that influence service delivery. To maximize the observation experience, you should take notes and describe specific components of a session. If possible, and with the supervisor's approval, you should review the client's file or discuss the session with the clinician prior to observing.

Questions a Student Should Be Able to Answer after Completing an Observation

1. What type and severity of communicative disorder did the client exhibit?

2. What were the objectives of the session?

3. What were the target behaviors?

4. How did the clinician greet the client?

(continues)

5. How was the session structured?

6. How did the clinician close the session and dismiss the client?

7. How was the room arranged?

8. How were the client and the clinician seated in relation to each other?

9. What types of materials and activities were used?

10. What strategies did the clinician use to teach the target behaviors?

11. What types of cues were used (e.g., visual, tactile, etc.)?

12. What types of reinforcers were used and on what schedule?

13. How were undesirable behaviors decreased?

14. How were responses charted?

15. What activities seemed to be most effective?

16. What activities seemed to be least effective?

17. If you were the clinician, what changes might you make for the next session?

Responsibilities of Student Observers

Remember, as a student observer you are a representative of your university and are expected to demonstrate responsible and ethical behavior. When observing at both on- and off-campus sites, you should comply with the following guidelines:

1. **Arrive on time for observations.** Regardless of how unobtrusive you try to be, if you arrive late for a scheduled observation you may disrupt the evaluation or treatment session. You also will not have a chance to discuss the client with the clinician prior to the session. If you do not know how the sessions started, you may have trouble understanding what you observe. Arriving late for a scheduled observation is irresponsible behavior. Clinical supervisors may not allow late arrivals to observe a session.

2. **Introduce yourself and request permission to observe.** Clinical supervisors are responsible for their clients' rights to privacy and for ensuring that you derive the greatest benefit from your observations. Although the observation may have been scheduled previously, there may be reasons to disallow a particular observation. For example, the client may have, for whatever reason, decided against being observed; the clinical supervisor may have determined that the observation area was too crowded or that the observation would not be beneficial for you or the client.

3. **Observe the entire clinical session.** This is necessary to obtain the greatest benefit from your observation. Each treatment and evaluation session contains certain sequenced events and procedures. If you arrive late or leave early, you get only a glimpse of the clinical process, and, hence, you do not get the total picture. You may observe some isolated techniques while missing out on the rationale, antecedents, or consequences of certain techniques.

4. **Always respect the client's right to confidentiality.** All client information is confidential. As a student you will discuss with or report to others on your observations. These follow-up discussions or reports, or both, will help enhance your learning. However, be careful to protect each client's privacy. Never discuss clients in public areas. If you have a report to make regarding your observation, you may refer to the person observed as "the client," "the individual," or, in some cases, you may use an alias for the client's name.

5. **Privately discuss a client with the clinician or the supervisor.** Discuss the client only when confidentiality is ensured. Do not discuss the client when there are other people who may overhear your conversation.

6. **Do not interrupt the session or waste the clinician's time.** Clinicians need time to prepare for their sessions and the few minutes they have between clients are important for them. Ask appropriate questions when the clinician has time to respond, but do not converse about unrelated topics. Arriving on time for your observations and observing entire sessions should help provide opportunities for you to talk with the clinician.

7. **Do not remove clinical files from the clinic area.** In most cases, you will be able to review a client's file to obtain background information. While reviewing the files, do not write in them or remove anything from the files. Take only notes that are helpful to your observation (e.g., medical history, therapy history, and so on). Once again, remember that all client information is confidential. Do not discuss with others any personal or clinical information you read in client files. Read Chapter 3 for more specific information on client confidentiality.

8. **Increase your observation skills.** To accomplish this, phonetically transcribe utterances, chart correct and incorrect productions, and take note of test results. This practice may help sharpen your observational skills as well as increase your recording skills. The more you learn during your observations, the more skills and confidence you will have to bring to your first practicum experience. The time you spend observing is for your benefit, so use it profitably.

9. **Complete an observation report form for each client.** Do this as soon as an observational session ends. Request the clinical supervisor to sign the observation report. Without a signature, observation hours are not

valid. Observation reports should be turned in to the clinic director or clinical supervisor. These reports will be used to substantiate your observation hours before your admittance to clinical practicum. Each university requires different reports and documentation. Follow the specific guidelines of your training program.

10. **Present yourself as a professional.** There will be clients, family members of the client, and other professionals at your observation site. You need to dress and behave like a professional. Therefore, follow the clinic dress code. Professional attire is considered appropriate dress. If you have doubts as to whether something is appropriate to wear, do not wear it. Communicate appropriately with the clinician, clinical supervisor, other student observers, clients, and clients' family members. Others, especially clients and their families, may easily misinterpret careless comments. Avoid judgmental remarks and unnecessary questions.

Various clinical sites may have additional rules and procedures. It is your responsibility to know the guidelines for observers at your site. It is also your responsibility to follow ASHA's Code of Ethics (American Speech-Language-Hearing Association, 2003a). The Code of Ethics is described in Chapter 3.

Clinical Practicum

After you have completed your training program's requirements, you are qualified to begin working directly with clients. Clinical practicum clock hours are earned for *screening, evaluation, and treatment* of communicative and swallowing disorders. Some hours may also be earned from clinical staffings. You will gain experience with children and adults, practice in a variety of settings, and work with clients from diverse cultural and linguistic backgrounds. You will have some experience with audiologic patients; of course, most of your experience will be in speech-language pathology. To ensure quality training of speech-language pathologists and audiologists, ASHA has developed minimum requirements for students and supervisors.

Supervision Requirements of Clinical Practicum

1. **The clinical supervisor must hold a current CCC in speech-language pathology or audiology.** Many states have licensure and credential requirements that clinical supervisors must also meet.

2. **Supervision may be provided only in areas in which the supervisor is qualified.** Speech-language pathologists may supervise all aspects

of speech-language pathology service delivery, including evaluation and management. They also may supervise aural habilitation and rehabilitation services and audiologic screenings (nondiagnostic) for the initial identification of communicative disorders or as part of a speech or language evaluation. Audiologists may supervise all audiological services and aural habilitation and rehabilitation services. They also may supervise speech and language screenings for the initial identification of communicative disorders. Under no circumstances should individuals supervise clients they believe they are not qualified or prepared to supervise.

3. **A minimum of 25% of a student's total contact with any client must be supervised.** This rule must be followed regardless of a student clinician's level of experience. Additional supervision may be provided with beginning student clinicians and with more complex clients.

4. **A clinical supervisor must be available to consult with the student.** The supervisor must hold a current CCC and be available for consultation during all service delivery.

5. **The clinical supervisor should provide direct observation, instruction, and feedback.** Supervision also may include activities such as indirect observation via closed circuit television or videotapes, review of written reports, and conferences with the student clinician.

Number of Clinical Clock Hours Required

Effective January 1, 2005, individuals submitting applications for the CCC in Speech-Language Pathology must comply with the academic and clinical standards approved by ASHA's Council on Professional Standards in October 2000. These standards require students to complete a minimum of 400 clock hours that include the following:

1. **A minimum of 25 supervised clinical observation hours.** Hours must be earned by observing activities within the scope of practice of speech-language pathology. Many of these hours will be completed prior to beginning direct client contact; however, it is not required that all 25 hours be completed prior to working directly with clients. The university training program or its affiliates must supervise the observation hours.

2. **A minimum of 375 direct client contact practicum clock hours.** A total of 325 of these hours must be earned at the graduate level in the area in which the certificate is sought (audiology or speech-language pathology) at a program accredited by the CAA. The direct client contact hours in speech-language pathology may include working with clients with disorders of voice, fluency, articulation, dysphagia, or language.

3. **Clinical practice with clients representing diverse demographics.** Clock hours must be earned with children and adults from culturally or linguistically different backgrounds. Also, the clock hours must reflect experiences with a variety of types and severities of disorders and differences with clients representing ages across the lifespan. To obtain these diverse experiences you may complete your practicum in several settings. For instance, your practicum may include assignment at an acute care hospital, a public school, and your university clinic.

4. **Adequate depth and breadth of supervised clinical experiences to be able to perform evaluation, prevention, and screening activities** including the following:

   • *Perform screening and prevention activities.* You will learn to use standardized and nonstandardized methods to screen for communicative or swallowing disorders. For example, if you are completing practicum in a medical setting, you may learn to perform a bedside swallowing evaluation to determine if a client needs to be referred for a videofluroscopy. If you are working with young children, you may screen their speech to determine if articulation errors are developmentally appropriate or if a complete evaluation is required. In the case of certain infants who are at risk for developing communicative disorders, you may design a home language stimulation program to prevent or reduce the magnitude of the disorder.

   • *Obtain case history information from a variety of sources.* Much of your case history information will come from your client's family. Chapter 5 provides guidelines for interviewing and obtaining a client's history. In addition, you will obtain information from reports by other professionals. You may request copies of written reports or you may have information that was shared verbally. Refer to Chapter 3 to learn more about respecting and maintaining client confidentiality.

   • *Choose and administer appropriate evaluation procedures as well as adapt testing procedures to meet a client's needs.* There are many published instruments to assist in the evaluation of communicative disorders. In addition, there is much information that you can obtain from nonstandardized measures including behavioral observations. You will learn to select and use the methods correct for your client.

   • *Make a diagnosis and recommendations.* As you gather speech, language, or swallowing data, you will form an opinion regarding your client's diagnosis and make appropriate recommendations based on your diagnosis. For example, a client may be referred to your clinic because a teacher noticed the client stuttering. After a complete evaluation, you determine that the dysfluencies are not due to what is typically thought of as stuttering, but reflect a word finding problem. Your recommendation would reflect language-based intervention rather than fluency intervention.

- *Document and report information verbally, or in writing, or both.* You will learn to perform any documentation or reporting required for your evaluation. It is likely that each of your practicum sites will have different paperwork and reporting requirements. Learning a variety of styles will help you adapt more quickly when you graduate and begin working independently.

- ***Refer clients if other services are needed.*** You may not always recommend speech-language pathology services for each client you evaluate. You will learn to identify the clients who will benefit from your services and which clients require different services. Certain clients may require services in addition to (or instead of) what speech-language pathologists provide. You will learn to identify when a client needs to be referred for other services and where in your community these services can be obtained.

5. **Sufficient depth and breadth of supervised clinical experiences to develop and provide effective treatment.** You will acquire the necessary skills to perform the following activities:

  - *Develop and write appropriate intervention plans and measurable goals.* Your intervention plans will vary depending on your clinical practicum setting. For example, in the school setting, your intervention plan will follow the format of the individualized education program (IEP; see Chapter 5 for additional information). In the university clinic, your intervention plan will align with those required at the clinic or by your clinic supervisor. In any case, your plans will reflect the specific needs of your client and contain measurable goals that your client will be able to achieve. Chapter 5 contains specific information for writing goals and objectives.

  - *Provide intervention.* Your intervention may include direct service to the client or training family members or other individuals to work with the client. In some instances, you will begin providing individual intervention and progress to training the client and others to assist with intervention, generalization, and maintenance. In other instances, you may begin by training family members to provide intervention. For example, when working with certain infants and toddlers, the primary interventionist may be a family member and the speech-language pathologist is the parents' "coach" or consultant.

  - *Use appropriate materials and equipment for prevention and intervention.* There are an enormous number of products on the market that are designed for intervention. It is not necessary to spend a great deal of money to have the necessary materials for effective intervention, but it is imperative that you are able to select appropriate materials and equipment. As part of your clinical practicum, you will learn to create some of your materials, to identify and locate materials that you need to purchase, and to use items found within your client's environment. You will not be expected to purchase large, expensive items. For example, your training program or practicum site will provide you with access to the more expensive assistive technology equipment required for certain clients. If a client needs to use a "low-tech" communication system, such as a picture exchange system or a simple communication board, you may be involved in creating the necessary items.

- *Collect data to measure your client's performance.* You will learn various methods to obtain information about your client's speech, language, or swallowing behaviors and to analyze the information that you acquire. Regardless of the data collection method you choose to use, the easiest way to collect data is to first have well-written goals that contain behaviors that can be measured. (Refer to Chapter 7 for more information on choosing target behaviors.)

- *Modify intervention as necessary.* Rarely does intervention follow a prescribed course. That is one of the reasons ASHA requires a graduate degree for speech-language pathology certification. Your interaction with your client and your data collection will help you to identify when your intervention plan, strategies, or materials need to be altered. You will learn to identify what and how your intervention activities need to be changed.

- *Document and report information in writing, or verbally, or both.* Each professional site will have different documentation and reporting requirements. You will learn to complete any of the record-keeping and reporting requirements at each of your practicum sites.

6. **Personal qualities and interactions** that demonstrate the ability to do the following:

- *Communicate effectively* with individuals with different values, communication modes, and cultural, linguistic, and socioeconomic backgrounds. As a speech-language pathologist you will be required to interact with many people. Family members, teachers, physicians, and other allied professionals may play integral roles in the services that you provide. Therefore, it is important that you communicate effectively with a variety of individuals.

- *Collaborate with other professionals.* You will learn to work with other professionals to provide optimal services and case management for your clients. Nurses, physicians, occupational therapists, psychologists, and teachers are just a few of the professionals with whom you may interact. Chapter 5 lists and describes many of the professionals with whom you will work.

- *Counsel clients, family members, and caregivers* regarding communication and swallowing disorders. In all settings, it will be necessary for you to educate others about your clients' disorders. For example, if you are working with a client who has a special diet due to swallowing difficulties, you will discuss the client's strengths and limitations with the family and teach the family how to manage the client's diet, what type and frequency of clinical and medical follow-up is necessary, and what to expect (prognosis) with the type of difficulty the client exhibits. In another case, you may be working with a young child who exhibits behavior problems because of difficulty communicating his or her needs. You will educate the family about how the communication deficit affects the child's behavior, teach the family how to facilitate communication and enhance appropriate behavior, and discuss available community and professional resources available. In both of these examples, to achieve the most successful outcomes for your clients and their families, you will need to listen carefully and learn fully about not only the needs of the clients but also about the needs and the dynamics of the families.

- *Adhere to the ASHA Code of Ethics and other professional standards of your site.* For example, to protect client confidentiality and to allow correct data reporting, you may be required to maintain client files in a certain order and in a certain location. You will always be required to follow ASHA's Code of Ethics. You will also learn and adhere to other guidelines such as ASHA's Scope of Practice and universal health precautions.

What to Count as Clinical Clock Hours

Sometimes there is confusion on what types of activities can be counted as clinical clock hours and what category the clock hours should be counted under. Use the following guidelines in recording your clock hours.

1. **Count clock hours earned in conjunction with a class assignment and during clinical practicum.** For example, if as part of a class assignment in a course on aphasia, you are required to evaluate a client with aphasia, you may earn diagnostic clock hours even when not enrolled in clinical practicum. However, to earn those hours, your practicum assignment must be preapproved and you must be supervised by an individual who holds a CCC in speech-language pathology.

2. **Count clock hours spent on screening and assessments of communication and swallowing disorders.** Typically, the student clinician may screen individuals at local preschools, area public and private schools, health fairs, and the university clinic. Speech, language, and swallowing screenings may be performed at facilities serving the elderly. Evaluations will likely be part of your experience at any clinical site. Evaluation hours may be earned while you are enrolled in a section of the clinic designated solely for diagnostics. Formal reevaluations may also be counted. For example, you also may acquire diagnostic hours as part of the assessment of your clients at the beginning of a treatment period. Readministering

specific tests or other assessment procedures at the end of treatment to document the status of the client also may be counted as evaluation hours. However, *administering probes during the treatment period should not be counted as evaluation hours.* Time spent administering probes should be counted with treatment hours.

3. **Count clock hours spent counseling clients or counseling or training family members.** Such counseling, of course, is closely related to the swallowing or communicative disorder of a client. For example, providing treatment for a client with a diagnosis of aphasia might include not only direct language intervention with a client but also sharing information with the client's family. It might be necessary for you to explain to the family members what aphasia means and how they can help the client regain some of the lost communicative behaviors. Or, your articulation treatment for a preschool child might include a home training program. In that case, you need to train the parents to ensure that they are able to carry out the home assignments.

4. **Count clock hours spent in obtaining or giving assessment and treatment information.** You can count the time you spend taking a case history and interviewing the client, or the client's family, or both. You can also count the time you spend discussing your diagnosis and recommendations with the client or client's family.

5. **Count clock hours spent during treatment and evaluation of a variety of disorders.** You will work with clients of varying ages who exhibit different communicative and swallowing disorders. In your medical practicum site you will gain much experience in evaluating and treating swallowing disorders. You will also evaluate and treat clients with such disorders as aphasia, dysarthria, and other neurological disorders. Working with school-age clients, you will evaluate and treat disorders of fluency, articulation, voice, and language. You may work with infants and toddlers who have speech, language, or swallowing and feeding problems secondary to genetic syndromes or other risk factors. Each site will offer different learning opportunities, so learn as much as you can at each site.

6. **Count time spent on certain clinically related activities.** These include activities performed to prevent communicative disorders or to develop, maintain, or maximize communication skills. For example, in certain settings the team of professionals providing rehabilitation services for a client may meet to discuss the client's treatment, progress, prognosis for further gains, and recommendations for future treatment. Also, you may be in a setting where you will train certain staff members to communicate more effectively with your client and to assist your client in communicating more effectively with the staff.

7. **Do not count preparation time as clinical clock hours.** Although you will spend much time in gathering materials or ideas, writing reports

and lesson plans, scoring tests, or transcribing language samples, you cannot count clock hours spent on these activities.

Remember that most clinical practicum clock hours are earned for direct client contact time only. Your clinical supervisor will answer any questions you have regarding how to count, record, or report your clinical hours.

Payment for Clinical Services

Before 1995 students were not allowed to be paid for their clinical practicum. However, in 1995, the Legislative Council approved Resolution LC 12-95, repealing the restriction on pay for practicum. According to ASHA guidelines, student clinicians may have a paid clinical practicum. Financial incentives may be in the form of wages, stipends, grants, or scholarships. Although some sites pay students, many do not. A university may have restrictions on students receiving pay for their clinical practicum, in which case its policies supersede those of ASHA's. Regardless of whether the sites provide students monetary reimbursement, each site must adhere to ASHA's guidelines on student practicum and supervision. Your advisor and the financial aid office at your university can give you information on financial assistance available to you.

Clinical Practicum as a Learning Experience

Clinical practicum is designed to give you an exceptional learning experience. It gives you an opportunity to gain experience with a wide variety of individuals with communicative and swallowing disorders. Under the supervision of qualified speech-language pathologists, you learn to evaluate and treat clients with fluency, voice, language, articulation, and swallowing disorders of various severity and etiological factors. You will gain experience in many different clinical settings, including acute care hospitals, rehabilitation facilities, psychiatric hospitals, skilled nursing facilities, private practices, and public schools.

Initially, you may be somewhat apprehensive about beginning your practicum. This is a normal response, but you will discover that clinical practicum is exciting and rewarding as you gain more experience and confidence. You are encouraged to experience as many types of clients and clinical settings as you can.

Be assured that you are a student and are not expected to perform like an experienced professional. What is expected of you is that you act responsibly within the guidelines of ASHA and those of your training program and that you demonstrate consistent progress in each of your practicum assignments. Speech-language pathology is exciting partly because there is always something new to learn.

Now you have a general idea of the personal and academic requirements for a successful clinical practicum. You also know ASHA's requirements for types of practicum hours and clinical settings in which to acquire them. This is your chance to apply information learned in academic classes and explore some of the challenging and exciting possibilities the profession of speech-language pathology has to offer.

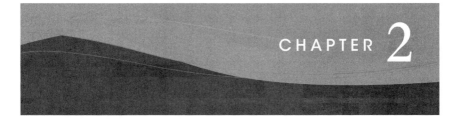

CHAPTER 2

Organization of Clinical Practicum

Chapter Outline

- On-Campus Clinical Practicum
- Off-Campus Clinical Practicum Sites
- Clinical Internships
- General Administrative Procedures
- Clinical Supplies, Materials, and Equipment

Clinical practicum is organized on a hierarchy of clinical experiences and expectations. Typically, clinical practicum begins at a university clinic, where beginning student clinicians are assigned two or more clients. As student clinicians gain experience, become more confident, and are able to make more independent decisions, their client caseload may be increased and varied. The student clinicians then may be assigned to off-campus clinical settings for clinical internships.

Distance learning programs may have clinical practicum requirements designed specifically for students in that program. Those requirements must meet ASHA's minimum requirements. Students enrolled in distance learning programs take academic classes through such methods as the Internet and videotaped or televised courses. Distance learners often are not on the host campus from where the courses are offered. However, their clinical practicum is done in a more traditional manner. An ASHA-certified supervisor must be available.

Regardless of the type of program you are enrolled in, you may begin your clinical practicum after you have completed the required hours of supervised clinical observation, prerequisite coursework, and other departmental requirements. Many clinical practicum settings, including some international practicum sites, are available for the speech–language pathology student clinician. The clinical sites are described in detail after an overview of commonly available practicum sites.

Commonly Available Clinical Practicum Sites

- *University clinic.* For most students, the practicum experience begins at the university speech, language, and hearing clinic. Experience in on-campus clinics prepare the students for off-campus experiences.

- *Public schools.* Most, if not all, students gain some practicum experience in public schools to gain the state department of education credential to work with children in educational settings. University departments of communicative disorders may require the completion of a clinical practicum in an educational setting.

- *Hospitals.* Many students, even if not required by their academic department, complete a clinical practicum in a medical facility to gain specialized skills in assessing and treating communication disorders associated with various medical conditions.

- *Skilled nursing facilities.* Practicum experiences may be gained in skilled nursing facilities, where patients requiring convalescent care may be treated and attended to.

- *Rehabilitation facilities.* For individuals who are disabled and requiring extensive rehabilitation, there are rehabilitation facilities that offer opportunities to learn specialized methods of restoring or improving communication. Therefore, rehabilitation facilities also offer good clinical practicum opportunities to students.

- *Psychiatric hospitals or clinics.* State or privately operated psychiatric hospitals and clinics offer opportunities to learn assessment and treatment procedures for communication disorders associated with mental or behavioral disorders.

- *Preschool agencies.* Experience in assessing and treating children in the age range of 3 to 5 may be gained in preschool settings.

- *Prisons.* Adult prisons and juvenile detention facilities also offer clinical practicum experiences.

- *Private practice.* Expanding opportunities for clinical practicum are available in many private clinics and with privately contracted service providers.

On-Campus Clinical Practicum

University Clinic

The university clinic strives to provide high-quality clinical services in conjunction with appropriate educational experiences for student clinicians. Typically, the clinic is designed and equipped to facilitate clinical training and promote clinical research. As a student clinician you may be involved in research activities or provide direct client services, or both.

Prerequisites

As pointed out earlier, prerequisites for clinical practicum include *completion of a designated number of supervised observation hours and certain preclinic academic courses.* Your university may have additional requisites such as a health clearance, acceptance into the graduate or clinical practicum program, faculty recommendations, and so on. Beginning student clinicians are not expected to work without guidance from a supervisor. However, they are expected to apply information learned in academic coursework, implement supervisor recommendations, ask questions, and, as the semester progresses, expand on supervisor suggestions. These, together with your clinical performance, are some of the behaviors your supervisor will use to judge your ability to succeed in future clinic assignments.

Supervision

Regular observation and supervision are integral components of your university clinic assignment. The university teaching faculty, full-time supervisory faculty, part-time supervisory staff, or a combination of the three may provide supervision at the university clinic. You may have one supervisor per term, or you may have more than one supervisor, based on the departmental policy and clinical schedule. Most departments tend to assign a single supervisor to beginning clinicians. All supervision in ASHA-accredited programs will be in compliance with the ASHA guidelines on supervision. The amount of supervision provided also may be adjusted upward depending on your level of clinical experience, your clinical skill level, the complexity of your client's disorder, or a combination of these factors.

University clinical facilities are arranged to maximize observation of sessions with minimal distractions. Many clinics are equipped with observation windows for viewing and with an audio system for listening. Student clinicians providing clinical services at a university clinic should be prepared for frequent observations by supervisors, family members of clients, and other students. Although some beginning student clinicians find it unsettling, it is not unusual for supervisors to enter the treatment room to observe a session or to demonstrate a specific treatment technique. Your sessions also may be videotaped for later observation or class demonstration. Once you get over the embarrassment of seeing yourself on video, self-evaluating your clinical session by reviewing a recording of a session is an excellent learning tool. A camera also may record your sessions for a closed-circuit television monitor. This allows supervisors to view clinical interactions from a central location without interfering with the evaluation or therapy sessions.

Your supervisor frequently evaluates your clinical skills to ensure that you are acquiring the necessary knowledge and abilities. You may get both written and verbal feedback. You may have weekly meetings with your clinical supervisor, weekly staffing, or discussions after each clinical session. At the minimum, you will receive a written final evaluation; most departments provide written midterm evaluations as well. If your progress in the clinical practicum is unsatisfactory, you will be notified and counseled regarding your continued participation in the program. If you feel you are not getting sufficient feedback from your supervisor, prepare appropriate questions, make an appointment, and meet with him or her to discuss your questions and concerns.

Clinic Schedules

Typically, a university clinic is operated on an 8 a.m. to 5 p.m. weekday schedule. Some universities also have evening hours to accommodate individuals who cannot attend the clinic during regular business hours. Some university clinics provide services only during the academic year. This schedule is not optimal because it disrupts services offered to clients who often need sustained and continuous treatment. To provide more continuous services, some clinics operate 12 months of the year, with professional staff providing services during the intersessions.

Clients receiving speech-language pathology services usually are scheduled for two to three sessions per week, with each session lasting 30 to 60 minutes. Evaluation sessions are sometimes scheduled for larger blocks of time. Most clients are scheduled for individual treatment sessions; however, some clients may be scheduled for group sessions. Generally, you will be allotted 5 to 10 minutes between clients to organize your materials. It is important to be prepared for your sessions in advance; the few minutes between clients is obviously not the time for planning assessment or treatment activities. This is the time for you to finish with one client and greet the next client in the clinic waiting room.

At the beginning of the semester, you will receive your clinical assignment. You will be given your clinic schedule, and your supervisor or clinic director will assign you clients. At many universities, the student clinician is responsible for telephoning the client and confirming the client's clinic schedule.

Routinely check with the clinic administrative assistant to verify clinic appointments and note any changes in your clinic schedule. Each university has different methods for scheduling clients and communicating the scheduling to student clinicians. To avoid confusion, missed appointments, or last-minute preparations, adhere to the procedures of your university.

Prior to meeting your client, you must review the client's clinical file, develop a plan for the first meeting with your client, and discuss the plan with your clinical supervisor. You should also discuss any evaluation plans with your supervisor and notify him or her of the time the evaluation is scheduled. For additional information on working with clients, refer to Chapter 5.

Types of Clients

A wide range of ages and communicative disorders are represented in the university clinic's caseload. The university caseload is influenced by demographic factors and the availability of other speech-language pathology services in the community. For example, if there is a large rehabilitation agency in the area, the clinic may enroll fewer clients with diagnoses of aphasia; if there is a pediatric hospital offering speech and hearing services, the clinic may serve a limited number of children. Economic factors also affect the types of clients typically seen at the university clinic. Compared to private practices or hospitals, a university clinic often has a reduced-fee scale and, because of this, may attract clients with limited incomes or no insurance coverage.

Other factors influencing the university client caseload are the expertise of faculty members, specialty clinics, and the department's relationship with allied health professionals. For instance, if your department has faculty members well known for their expertise in fluency disorders or if your program offers specialized services for individuals with autism, the clinic may attract a large number of clients with these disorders. In addition, if your university is affiliated with a medical center, your clinic may provide outpatient or follow-up services for its clients.

Report Writing and Record Keeping

University clinics have varying policies and terminology regarding writing assignments. Most universities require some type of written description of how you plan to help remediate your clients' disorders. This may be in the form of **daily lesson plans, weekly lesson plans,** or **semester treatment plans.** You may be required to submit typed plans, handwritten plans, or computer-generated plans. Whatever the format, your supervisor will review all your plans. Throughout the term, you will be required to **regularly document your clients' progress** and any changes in your treatment plans. At the end of the term, you will be required to write a **final summary** or progress report. The final summary should describe the client's status at the beginning of treatment, the treatment goals, the treatment procedures, and the progress made by the client.

Your clinical supervisor will give you instructions regarding the format and timelines for all written work. Report writing and record keeping are discussed in greater detail in Chapter 5.

Off-Campus Clinical Practicum Sites

Off-campus practicum sites vary from region to region and from university to university. Common off-campus practicum sites include public schools, hospitals, skilled nursing facilities, rehabilitation agencies, psychiatric hospitals, preschool programs, correctional facilities, and private speech and hearing centers. Less common clinical practicum experiences may be available through partnerships between your training program and international organizations. Check ASHA's Web site or talk with your clinic director for information on international practicum opportunities.

As you know, the first semester (or quarter) of clinical practicum typically is completed in a university speech and hearing clinic. Depending on the policy of your academic department, you may begin off-campus practicum anytime after your first term of clinical practicum, although some university departments require up to three semesters of clinical practicum on campus, performed directly under the supervision of the faculty. An ASHA-certified speech-language pathologist who works at an approved external site, with consultation provided by the university supervisor, usually supervises off-campus practicum. All off-campus sites must comply with ASHA's regulations on the frequency and type of supervision.

Student clinicians usually are required to follow the holiday schedule of the off-campus site instead of that of the university. Student clinicians also must comply with the site's requirements regarding professional responsibility and conduct. University grading policy and the department's criteria of acceptable performance dictate the grading. However, the site supervisor evaluates the student's performance and suggests a grade. The off-campus supervisor's judgment of the student's performance greatly influences a student's final grade.

Public Schools

Typically to work in the public schools, a *credential* (or certificate) issued by the state's department of education is required. A credential is a document that indicates that certain competencies have been met and authorizes the individual holding it to provide services according to its parameters. For example, you might earn a credential authorizing you to provide individual speech and language services in the schools or teach in a classroom, or both. In many states, to obtain a credential or certificate to work as a speech-language pathologist in the public schools, student clinicians must complete a practicum experience in a school setting.

A university seminar may accompany the school clinical practicum assignment. Although the practicum provides experience in assessing and treating children who are communicatively handicapped in the school, a seminar held at the university provides a forum for discussing issues and exchanging ideas. In such a seminar, historical and current issues affecting the school speech-language pathologist and the organization and administration of speech-language pathology programs in the public schools may be discussed. Also, seminars offer student clinicians an opportunity to share their practicum experiences with fellow students and the university faculty and exchange ideas.

Prerequisites

The prerequisites to internship in the public school depend on the university and state credential requirements. Although it may be helpful for beginning your public school practicum, you need not have experience working with groups. However, you will need to have completed coursework relative to childhood speech and language disorders, and you will need to have worked with children of different ages and disorders. Prior to enrolling in your public school clinical practicum, you may be required to enroll in your university *credential program*. To verify that you have met the prerequisites to begin a public school practicum, the credential program's personnel review your records, required test results, grade-point average, and so on. Certain states may require you to pass a competency examination. In conjunction with the credential application, individuals may be required to obtain a character and identification clearance that includes submission of fingerprint identification cards to the Department of Justice (DOJ). In addition, credential applicants must show evidence of having passed a recent tuberculosis (TB) test. Review your school's prerequisites with your advisor.

Supervision

The student clinician completes an *internship* assignment (popularly known as student teaching) under the supervision of a school speech-language pathologist who is ASHA certified and who meets the state's credential requirements. Supervision is provided in accordance with ASHA guidelines. The supervisor is available to guide your decision making and answer questions; however, you are expected to be at a more independent level than you were during your first practicum experiences. In addition to regular feedback, generally, the supervising speech-language pathologists give student clinicians a midterm and a final evaluation that are aligned with university grading policy. A supervisor from the university training program coordinates this arrangement and may periodically meet with the student and supervisor or communicate with them by telephone or e-mail.

School Internship Schedules

School internships generally are full-day assignments, 3 to 5 days a week, perhaps in conjunction with a weekly seminar. The school day usually is from 8 a.m. to 3 p.m., but you should be prepared to spend additional time for writing reports, planning sessions, attending meetings, and preparing materials.

Although basic diagnostic and treatment principles do not vary from those appropriate in other clinical settings, several scheduling and service delivery models may be unique to the school setting. For example, your previous experience in working with children may have followed only the clinical model, and school-based speech services may be provided through different service delivery models. To compound scheduling issues, many students with mild to severe disabilities are *fully included* in a regular education class (McCormick, Loeb, & Schiefelbusch, 2003; Sands, French, & Kozleski, 2000; Meyen, Vergason, & Whelan, 1996). That is, they receive instruction in a regular education classroom with peers of their age. This setting is referred to as an inclusive setting. Typically, support is provided to fully included students by different educational specialists, who provide services in the classroom or make suggestions to the teacher, or both. Other schools and parents may determine that separate special education classes better meet the needs of their students.

Regardless of the format followed at your school setting, you should have the option of providing a *continuum of services*. In the school setting, these services may be either direct or indirect.

Direct services are services in which the speech-language pathologist works with a student individually or with other students. These services may be provided by following the traditional clinical format in which a clinician works with individual children or children in small groups. In the **pull-out model,** children are served in the speech-language pathologist's office or a clinical room set aside for this purpose. Students generally attend treatment sessions one to two times per week. Treatment may include some stimulus material unrelated to classroom curriculum; however, it is essential for school curriculum to be incorporated into treatment when it is appropriate to the student's speech or language needs. Also, functional treatment goals and objectives reflecting educational benchmarks are written. This model commonly is referred to as the pull-out model because students are taken out of their classes to receive speech-language services.

You also may provide direct speech-language services in the student's class on a one-to-one or small-group basis. This is sometimes referred to as **pull-in services** (Merritt & Culatta, 1998). In this case, you may provide treatment for one or more students in a separate area of the classroom while the rest of the class continues other activities. When classroom instruction is divided into *learning stations,* you may treat children at one of the stations. The classroom teacher and aide may be responsible for two other learning stations, and another station may be for independent study. Students rotate from one station to the next, typically spending 10 to 15 minutes at each station. This type of scheduling may be common in kindergarten and special day classes. *Special day classes* are classrooms where education is provided to students with specific educational needs by teachers who have specialized training to meet those students' academic needs. Generally, students are in the special day class for much of the day but participate in regular education for designated times during portions of the day.

A different model of whole-class intervention is more commonly used at the secondary level. In this model, the school speech-language pathologist teaches one period of the day and students attend the class as they would their mathematics or history classes. This may be a **language laboratory** or a **language and speech class.** In some schools, this class may fulfill the students' requirements for English language.

Direct speech-language services in the schools also may be provided within a **collaborative instruction model.** In this model, the speech-language pathologist and classroom teacher coordinate their lessons and work together to provide students with appropriate learning opportunities. Collaborative models have been identified in various ways.

Collaborative Intervention Models

- *Supportive learning* allows the primary instructor to teach a lesson while the coinstructor provides supplementary teaching or activities. In one lesson, the speech-language pathologist may teach a lesson with the classroom teacher offering supportive activities. In another lesson, the teaching roles may be reversed, with the classroom teacher instructing the class and the speech-language pathologist providing supplementary and supportive activities. In this model, you might present language lessons to all the students in the class. During the lesson, you also will work on the speech and language objectives of the students enrolled on your caseload. Occasionally, you may teach a subject, such as mathematics, to demonstrate to the teacher how changing the language in a lesson can benefit children with language disorders.

- *Team teaching* is a model in which the teacher and speech-language pathologist share in the responsibilities of planning and teaching a lesson. Typically, the lesson is divided into segments, with each professional teaching certain parts of the lesson.

- *Complementary instruction* is similar to team teaching. The speech-language pathologist and teacher instruct a lesson together. The teacher focuses on such content areas as science, social studies, math, and so on. The speech-language pathologist teaches such language-related skills as mapping of ideas, selecting main ideas, outlining, and taking notes (Merritt & Culatta, 1998).

Sufficient planning time is critical to the success of collaborative instruction. When you develop your schedule, you must allow time not only for teaching a lesson but also for planning with the teacher. In the collaborative instruction model, the speech-language pathologist and classroom teacher discuss the needs of the class and the specific needs of the students enrolled for speech or language services. The speech-language pathologist models an appropriate language and learning environment for students with communicative disorders. The teacher and speech-language pathologist share effective methods of teaching and obtain new ideas by observing each other. In addition, students with communicative disorders receive services in a natural communicative setting that emphasizes classroom curriculum and assists with generalization of skills. Chapter 5 contains additional information on working collaboratively with the classroom teacher, parents, and other professionals.

Indirect speech-language pathology services are another service delivery option used in the public schools. **Indirect** services are provided under a **consultative model** in which the speech-language pathologist works with the student's parents, teachers, or other professionals to address the needs of the student. In this model, the speech-language pathologist is a consultant who does not directly treat the child. You may assist the teacher by providing suggestions for working with certain students who are not on your caseload. In other cases, you may determine that certain students who were receiving treatment for a language disorder no longer require direct services. You discuss with the teachers and parents ways to modify communication to maximize a student's performance. The students remain on your caseload for a few months as you monitor their progress. During this monitoring stage, you may make suggestions to the parents and teachers. In some instances, you may determine that a student should be reenrolled for direct services.

All of these models have a place in the delivery of speech-language pathology services. However, each should be viewed on a continuum of need. Some students require intensive, direct services for most of the time they are under your care. Some who need intensive, direct care to begin with may be switched over to a less intense indirect care. Others require less direct intervention from the beginning and benefit from modification of teaching strategies. A few who did benefit to an extent with indirect services may need a more direct service later. Therefore, you must view each student's needs separately. Your public school practicum is an opportunity to learn when and how to effectively implement the various service delivery models while supporting the students' academic needs.

Scheduling sessions, as you might imagine from the variety of service delivery options, can be difficult. A new experience in the public school setting is that you also may be required to serve a large number of students. At the university speech and hearing clinic, you may be used to working with two to three clients per term. In your school practicum, it is likely that you will be asked to gradually assume a caseload of a full-time clinician. You usually will see each student at least once a week. States have differing guidelines on the caseload size for a school-based speech-language pathologist. ASHA recommends that states establish caseload size based on *workload* versus a specific number of students (American Speech-Language-Hearing Association, 2002a). However, most states utilize a numerical measure to guide caseloads resulting in some schools with speech-language pathology caseloads of 40 students and other schools with as high as 80 students (American Speech-Language-Hearing Association, 2002a). A large caseload limits the speech-language pathologist's effectiveness; however, a reduced and manageable caseload size is a goal that is yet to be realized in all of the nation's public schools.

Group treatment sessions may be a new kind of clinical experience you may have in a public school setting. Because of the large number of students, public school speech-language pathologists typically serve students in small groups. Often, the number in each group depends on the total caseload of the clinician. The larger the caseload, the bigger the group size.

Options for Grouping Children

- *Homogeneous grouping* refers to the practice of grouping together students with similar disorders.

- *Heterogeneous grouping* refers to the practice of grouping together students who exhibit different disorders. This type of grouping may allow one student to model for another student. For example, a child with a language disorder may provide an excellent model for production of /r/. The child who mispronounces /r/ may model different language structures. Given the choice of grouping children of widely different ages (e.g., 5- to 12-year-olds) and those of different disorders, it may be better to group according to age, so that the students share certain comprehension and attention levels. Grouping children with no consideration for their target behaviors or functional levels may not be productive.

In addition to scheduling specific students, you must allow time in your day to communicate and collaborate with other professionals such as the classroom teacher, school psychologist, reading and writing (literacy) specialist, and school nurse. Also, have specific blocks of time allocated for testing students, writing reports, making telephone calls, and meeting with parents. More specific information regarding scheduling of clients is discussed in Chapter 5.

Types of Clients

As one might expect from the wide range of ages offered services in the public schools, the caseload for student clinicians participating in clinical practicum in that setting can be varied enough to satisfy almost anyone's professional interests. In addition to the different age groups, children with a wide range of disabilities are served in public schools. Depending on the school assignment, your caseload could include children who have a single articulation error to those with multiple errors resulting in unintelligible speech. You will work with many children exhibiting speech and language disorders of unknown etiology. You also will play a role in the prevention of reading and writing difficulties and, when warranted, in providing direct services to enhance literacy skills in children (American Speech-Language-Hearing Association, 2001a, 2001b, 2001c). With the national emphasis on literacy, the speech-language pathologist's role in helping children acquire pre-reading, reading, and writing skills has gained much importance. You may work as a member of a team to determine how language and learning disorders affect the children's acquisition of literacy skills and, when found necessary, provide direct literacy services to children and offer indirect services to parents (see Chapter 7 for literacy intervention targets). You also might work with students with multiple physical and sensory disabilities. Children who have speech or language disorders associated with autism, traumatic brain injury, cerebral palsy, emotional disorders, cognitive handicaps, hearing impairment, cleft palate, or any number of medically related disorders also are served in public schools. In many of these cases, you will not work just with the children. In providing effective treatment, you may work collaboratively with the family, teacher and other professionals who deliver additional services to the same children. You will discover that your school internship gives you the opportunity to work with children exhibiting a variety of disorders. A caseload at a kindergarten through sixth-grade school may consist of students with fluency, language, articulation, and voice disorders. There are also schools that specialize in serving a specific population. For example, a residential school for children who are deaf may focus on oral communication and another may focus on sign language for communicating. Regardless of the type of communication disorder with which a student initially presents, you will be required to analyze how that disorder affects the student's academic, social, or vocational performance (Moore-Brown & Montgomery, 2005).

Federal and State Laws

Speech-language pathology services in the public schools are designed to meet the needs of all individuals who are communicatively handicapped and eligible for school services as mandated by federal legislation. The *Education of All Handicapped Children Act (EHA), Public Law 94–142* (P.L. 94–142) was passed on November 25, 1975, and provided for educational services for all handicapped children (Dublinske & Healey, 1978). Although several amendments to the EHA have been made over the years, it remains the cornerstone for special education services. The discretionary programs of the EHA were reauthorized in 1990. At that time, the name was changed to IDEA. Congress reauthorized IDEA in November 2004 and the President signed it into law in December 2004. The law became effective in July 2005.

The EHA Amendments of 1986, P.L. 99-457, established funds for states to provide services for children from birth through 2 years of age who have disabilities. Services to the families of these children also were included in P.L. 99-457 and are continued under the 2004 reauthorization mandates. In addition, the 1986 EHA Amendments included legislation (Part B of EHA) on personnel standards. Part B of P.L. 99-457 required state education agencies to develop and maintain personnel standards based on the highest requirements in the state. For speech-language pathologists, including school speech-language pathologists, in many states this standard is the master's degree. As noted in Chapter 1, the requirement for highest state standards for school-based speech-language pathologists was eliminated as part of reauthorization of the IDEA. However, ASHA continues to strongly endorse highest state standards for school-based speech-language pathologists and supports the highest standards for all speech-language pathologists, regardless of the setting in which they work.

The school speech-language pathology services are governed by several other federal laws and guidelines. State laws and regulations on special education also affect speech-language pathology services provided in the public schools. School speech-language pathologists must know and follow all guidelines affecting their school sites.

Mandated School-Based Speech-Language Pathology Services

1. *Identification* of students with speech or language disorders through such activities as whole–class or individual screenings

2. *Assessment* of speech and language

3. *Treatment* of students with identified communicative disorders

4. *Consultation* with parents, teachers, and others regarding communicative disorders

5. *Referral* to other professionals for service necessary for the remediation of a communicative disorder (Dublinske & Healey, 1978)

In addition, school-based speech-language pathologists may work with children with swallowing and feeding disorders and work closely with teachers in assessing and treating reading and writing disorders.

The *eligibility criteria* for public school students to receive speech-language pathology services differ from those used in most university clinics. There are both federal and state eligibility guidelines regulating admission to a school speech-language program. These guidelines do not always coincide with the commonly accepted practices in speech-language pathology. For example, in California, a child who only has a single articulation error may not be eligible to receive services through the public school until 7 or 8 years of age (California State Department of Education, 1989), whereas the same child might receive treatment at a much younger age at a university clinic. The determination of eligibility for special education, including speech-language pathology services, changed with implementation of IDEA 2004 and the introduction into the schools of the term **Response to Intervention (RtI)**. The concept of special education shifted from being a "place" to a "service." The emphasis on simply administering tests and placing children into special education changed to emphasizing child outcomes and the prevention or reduction of learning disabilities through the RtI process. The RtI process is a multilevel approach that includes early identification of children struggling to learn, scientifically based interventions in addition to the general education curriculum, frequent and objective monitoring of children's learning and rate of learning, and decisions for general and special education, types of services, and intensity of interventions based on the data obtained in the RtI process. When you participate in your school-based internship, your supervisor will provide you with the eligibility guidelines that are specific to the setting.

Report Writing and Record Keeping

In addition to providing assessment and remediation services, school speech-language pathologists have many administrative duties of report writing and record keeping. You will learn to organize and maintain records for all of the students on your caseload according to each of their **individualized education programs (IEPs).**

The IEP is a *contract between the parents and the school* that outlines a child's current level of performance, needs, objectives, and intervention that will be provided. Because students receive speech and language treatment in the public schools to maximize their educational opportunities as much as possible, your speech and language objectives should be tied to educational benchmarks. The IEP is one of the cornerstones of service delivery in the public schools and is discussed in greater detail in Chapter 5. In addition to learning more about the IEP and how to write one, you will learn other new terms in your school practicum. Appendix A contains a list of acronyms and abbreviations used frequently in the educational setting.

Working with Parents and Professionals

As a student intern in the public schools, you may schedule and conduct meetings with parents and other professionals. You will learn to communicate effectively and work cooperatively with them to enhance your students' learning. Some schools employ SLPAs to assist the speech–language pathologists. ASHA has several guidelines on standards for SLPAs and their supervision (American Speech-Language-Hearing Association, 2002b, 2004a). These are discussed in greater detail in Chapter 5. As a student intern, you will not evaluate an SLPA. Nonetheless, as part of your practicum, your supervisor may ask you to select certain activities that the SLPA could appropriately complete according to ASHA's guidelines or you may be asked to train the SLPA to perform certain activities. This will help you gain experience in determining ways to most effectively provide services, complete paperwork, and organize materials as well as enhance your ability to communicate ideas and instructions. Collaboration with other professionals is an important component of your school-based treatment experience. (Chapter 5 contains additional information on this area.) On occasion you may work closely with or refer your students to school nurses, physicians, audiologists, occupational therapists, assistive technology specialists, social workers, psychologists, principals, or special and regular education teachers. You also may be called to provide staff and parent inservices. Because you may have only a limited amount of time with each student, you must learn to maximize your effectiveness through appropriate collaboration.

Hospitals

Hospital speech-language pathology covers a gamut of services. When completing a clinical practicum in a hospital setting, you may work with patients in the acute care phase, subacute care facility, inpatient rehabilitation units, outpatient departments, or at the home of the patient under the home health care provisions. You will learn new skills and vocabulary that are specific to medical settings. You will learn about associations and organizations that affect services in the medical setting. For example, you will hear about the **Joint Commission on Accreditation of Healthcare Organizations (JCAHO).** The JCAHO is a regulatory agency that sets standards for patient care and accredits many hospitals. Similar to ASHA's accreditation activities, JCAHO periodically reviews accredited hospitals to validate that they are meeting its set standards. As does ASHA, JCAHO and its regulations will influence different aspects of your clinical practicum.

The activities of your practicum will depend both on the organization of the hospital and the requirements of your individual practicum assignment.

The following sections are only an overview of some of the experiences you may gain in a hospital setting. In a comprehensive medical setting, you will encounter a wide range of stimulating and challenging learning opportunities.

Prerequisites

Ideally, before you begin your clinical practicum at a hospital, you will have completed academic courses in *aphasia, voice, dysphagia* (swallowing problems), *motor speech disorders* (dysarthrias and apraxia), and *traumatic brain injury*; refreshed your knowledge of anatomy and physiology of speech and hearing mechanisms; and have some experience in assessing and treating clients with communicative disorders associated with medical conditions. Because you can expect a large percentage of patients with swallowing disorders to be on a hospital-based speech-language pathologist's caseload, you will want to complete a course in dysphagia.

Supervision

As a student intern, you gradually will assume the responsibilities of the staff speech-language pathologist under the supervision of a licensed and certified speech-language pathologist on the hospital staff. The staff clinician who supervises in a hospital must follow the ASHA guidelines. Supervision may increase to 100% for patients with complex or unusual disorders. For example, for patients with swallowing disorders, a student clinician may provide limited evaluation and treatment and only after extensive training and with close supervision. The clinic director or a university supervisor will coordinate this internship, routinely communicating with your supervisor at the hospital.

Hospital Schedules

Hospital-based speech-language pathologists typically work an 8-hour day, 5 days per week. Speech-language pathologists may be required to work a variable schedule depending on patient and staffing needs. In some cases, their day begins at 8 a.m. and ends at 5 p.m. In other cases, to cover swallowing treatment during the patients' breakfast or dinner, the day may begin earlier or later. In other cases, the speech-language pathologist may need to work on Saturdays to meet treatment and fee guidelines. In addition, speech-language pathologists may travel between hospital sites to ensure that they are generating sufficient "billable" time. Rotating schedules are used in many hospitals. The hospital clinician may be assigned a rotating schedule that includes home health services or alternating weekends, or both. For example, the clinician may work 4 months in the hospital, 4 months with home health, and 4 months with outpatients. The speech-language pathologist may also be required to work some weekends to cover the required 6-day-per-week treatments. In addition to hospital-based clinicians, private agencies or individual speech-language pathologists contracting for these services may provide in-home speech services.

Unlike programs in the public schools, treatment in hospital settings is typically offered in individual sessions. The clinician most often works with a patient in the patient's room, the clinician's office, or individual treatment rooms. Bedside evaluation and treatment are sometimes provided for patients with more acute medical conditions. For example, a patient just recovering from a cerebrovascular accident (CVA) or traumatic brain injury may not be medically stable enough to leave his or her hospital room. It still may be necessary for you to perform an assessment to determine the patient's communicative status and need for intervention. In medical settings, speech–language pathology consultation is becoming more frequent as a model of care. The patient's decreased length of stay (due to decreased medical reimbursement to acute care hospitals, among other factors) causes assessment and intervention to concentrate on a patient's immediate needs and safe discharge to other settings. Once you have received a doctor's order to see patients, those who are hospitalized may receive speech and language services 5 or 6 days per week. Outpatients are usually seen less frequently and may be seen in the office or as part of home health services.

Hospital patients may be seen more frequently than those attending university clinics, but they may receive services for a shorter duration. Because of health care costs, most hospitals discharge patients as soon as possible, with due regard to the patient's well-being. Consequently, you may think that you are just beginning to know a patient or observe some progress when that individual is discharged from the hospital. In fact, hospital-based speech–language pathology services are increasingly concerned with discharge planning rather than individual therapy.

Videofluorographic and bedside evaluation of the swallowing mechanism is a large part of the job for many hospital-based speech–language pathologists. **Videofluorographic evaluation** is an objective procedure in which the client's swallowing mechanism is recorded on a moving picture (that is, video). The speech–language pathologist gives the patient foods or beverages containing radiopaque (barium) material. The radiologist records images of the patient's swallow using a fluoroscopy camera. During and following the examination, the speech–language pathologist can examine the patient's ability to safely swallow foods of various textures. Student clinicians often observe and assist with this procedure but rarely perform the evaluation independently.

The **bedside evaluation** is less objective and more controversial regarding the validity of the results. During the bedside swallowing evaluation, the speech–language pathologist notes the patient's medical and swallowing history, oral secretion and awareness levels, general cognitive level, nutritional status, motor control, presence of normal and abnormal reflexes, oral sensory level, and ability to safely eat selected foods. Your internship in the hospital will give you experience working with many patients with swallowing disorders.

Types of Patients

The speech–language pathologist providing services in the acute care setting is responsible for the speech and language evaluation and treatment of patients with many medical conditions. In various hospital settings, you will encounter patients with *neurological diseases* and *traumatic brain injury (TBI)*, those recovering from a

CVA, and those facing or recovering from a laryngectomy. The large majority of your caseload, however, will involve *evaluation and treatment of dysphagia*. Also, and more frequently in the rehabilitation or outpatient setting than in the acute care setting, you may be involved in assessing the need for and training in the use of augmentative communication equipment.

In most hospital and rehabilitation facilities, patients of all ages may be served. An exception is a pediatric setting in which student clinicians work exclusively with children.

The speech-language pathology department is an integral part of a hospital's rehabilitation services. A speech-language pathologist serves as a member of a **multidisciplinary team** and provides assessment and intervention for patients admitted for rehabilitation services. The multidisciplinary team is a group of professionals and family members who work together to determine and provide optimal patient management. In the hospitals, some team members you may work with include a nurse, physician, physical therapist, occupational therapist, family caregiver, and social worker. For additional information on allied health professionals and working on a team, refer to Chapter 5.

Some patients are transferred to the rehabilitation department after discharge from the acute care setting. Other patients are discharged from the hospital for convalescence and may later be readmitted when they become candidates for rehabilitation.

In a *hospital rehabilitation setting*, you may have the opportunity to work with patients over a longer period of time than you will with most of the patients in acute care settings. You will establish both short-term and long-range communicative objectives for your patients and help them to regain their independent living skills.

Individuals are sometimes discharged from the hospital acute care or rehabilitation setting before they have completed their speech or language treatment. These individuals may be served in the hospital outpatient setting or in their homes via home health services. Patients who are too ill to travel to the clinic outpatient facilities are seen in their homes.

Home health service may be provided to individuals after they are discharged from the hospital. As a home care provider, you may travel extensively because assessment and treatment are provided in patients' homes. Service delivery in the home enables you to evaluate patients' functional communication skills within their natural environments. In the homes, you also can assess the interactional patterns between the patient and his or her family and provide treatment in the natural environment. The speech-language pathologist is one of several home care providers, which include nurses, physical therapists, and occupational therapists.

Treatment may be enhanced by *working with the patient and his or her family in their home*, but there are several factors you must consider. Because you are working in an individual's home, you must be aware of cultural or traditional characteristics of the home. For example, members of a family may remove their shoes before entering the home; other families do not readily accept strangers into their homes. You also must be aware of safety factors such as the type of neighborhood a home is located in (e.g., high crime area), the presence of an aggressive and unfriendly dog in the home, the possibility of substance abuse in the home, and the overall safety of the home. Also, while in a patient's home, there are many distractions from other family members, doorbells, and ringing telephones.

As is the case with speech-language pathologists working in the schools, hospital-based speech-language pathologists and their services are regulated by several agencies, including the federal government. The sort of clients on your caseload and the frequency, duration, and type of service largely may be influenced by private insurance company policies and the federal government's Medicare program.

Report Writing and Record Keeping

As you will find in all your practicum assignments, the speech-language pathologist in the hospital is responsible for carefully documenting assessment results, treatment plans, and patient progress. In addition, you will learn to complete different insurance and Medicare forms. You will hear reference to, and learn how to use, various health care codes including *Current Procedural Terminology* (CPT), *Healthcare Common Procedure Coding System* (HCPCS), and *International Classification of Diseases, 9th edition, Clinical Modification* (ICD-9-CM). In many cases, accurate and appropriate documentation will determine if your hospital receives reimbursement for your services from an insurance company. You will frequently hear and read the acronym **FIMs,** which means **functional independence measures.** FIMs are similar to the objectives you will have learned to write in your initial clinic experiences; however, FIMs are written with the emphasis on a patient's ability to perform functional tasks (e.g., tell when he or she is ill) with as little assistance as possible. One of the frequently utilized means of communication among professionals in hospitals is through notations in the patients' charts. These progress notes are commonly known as **SOAP notes** (subjective, objective, assessment, plan). Refer to Chapter 5 for additional information regarding progress notes. Your supervisor will assist you with the specific requirements at your hospital practicum site.

When reading your patients' charts, you will encounter many abbreviations, symbols, and acronyms with which you may be unfamiliar. Some of the commonly used medical abbreviations and symbols are listed in Appendix B.

Working with Families and Professionals

Counseling the hospital patient and the patient's family concerning the communicative disorder is a major responsibility of speech-language pathologists. Through counseling and consultation, the speech-language pathologist educates the family and the patient about the communicative disorder and assists them in learning to deal with the disorder during the rehabilitation process. To deliver the best care for your patients, you will work with other professionals, including physical therapists, nurses, social workers, occupational therapists, and physicians. (The specific roles of these professionals are discussed in Chapter 5.) As you know, together with the speech-language pathologist, these professionals often serve as part of a multidisciplinary team. The assessment and treatment decisions you make are likely to involve other team members. In addition to multidisciplinary teams, many hospitals are promoting **transdisciplinary teams.** Transdisciplinary teams are composed of different professionals and paraprofessionals who may provide some services for another team member. For example, if one of your patient's goals is to communicate when in discomfort, the nurse may work on this goal during nursing activities.

Multiskilling is similar to the idea of transdisciplinary teams. In multiskilling, you might be trained to take a patient's temperature and blood pressure during management of a swallowing disorder. Generally, multiskilling is not popular with most hospital personnel but is being offered as a cost-saving alternative by some insurance and research groups. ASHA has published a position on the use of multiskilled personnel that you should read before you begin a medical internship (American Speech-Language-Hearing Association, 1997).

In *hospital rounds*, you and other care providers meet with the physician in charge and share information about the patient or ask questions about the results of the various assessments and treatments. Rounds may be performed in the patient's room or in a separate conference room. You will participate in rounds and learn how each team member contributes to the overall care and rehabilitation of the patient.

Skilled Nursing Facilities

Skilled nursing facilities (SNF) or long-term care facilities (LTC) are designed to provide services for individuals requiring convalescent care for many medical reasons. These services are provided following discharge from the hospital and before the patients return home. The SNF (commonly pronounced "sniff") also provides services for individuals who need long-term medical care. Generally, patient services in the SNF are similar to those in a hospital.

Nursing care in the SNF involves regularly monitoring the patients' vital signs (such as temperature, pulse, respiration) and giving medications and other types of medical care. These patients also may receive services from other professionals such as a physical therapist, speech-language pathologist, occupational therapist, recreational therapist, and social worker.

Prerequisites

As in other medical practicum settings, it would be ideal for you to have completed *courses in aphasia, voice, dysphagia, TBI, and neurologically based speech disorders* (dysarthria and apraxia) before beginning practicum in a SNF. A course in gerontology is highly desirable. Also, knowledge of the SNF's general structure, function, and clinical and administrative procedures is helpful, although much of this is acquired during the practicum.

Supervision

Many SNFs do not employ their own speech-language pathologists. Instead, they contract with private practices to provide services such as speech-language pathology, physical therapy, and occupational therapy. Therefore, although your supervisor is responsible for service delivery at the SNF, he or she may not be an employee of the site. Supervision is provided by the on-site speech-language pathologist. The university supervisor monitors the practicum experience by routinely consulting with the supervisor and the student. The university supervisor also may make periodic site visits.

Schedules

Individual treatment sessions are common in SNFs, although some group sessions may be held. Group sessions are helpful in promoting social communication skills in an environment where social interactions sometimes are limited. Group sessions also are used to monitor patients' swallowing abilities as they progress to independent eating. In a SNF, you will soon find that many patients fatigue quickly, so the length of both the evaluation and treatment sessions depends on the patients' health.

Typically, work in the SNF is 5 days a week for 8 hours each day. For certain patients, speech-language pathology services are provided 6 days a week. In those cases, you may work some Saturdays. To manage patients' swallowing, speech-language pathologists sometimes begin at 6:30 a.m. or arrive later and work until 7 p.m. If you are treating a patient for a swallowing disorder, you may often work with him or her during meals. For example, to work with patients during their breakfast, you may arrive early, work with them through lunch, take your own lunch break, and leave at 4 or 4:30 p.m. As with most clinical practicum assignments, you follow the schedule of your clinical supervisor unless other arrangements are agreed on.

Types of Patients

In the SNF, student clinicians work primarily with elderly patients. The communicative disorders of the patients you work with often are associated with *CVAs, head injury, carcinomas of the head and neck, hearing loss, and a variety of neurological diseases* (e.g., Alzheimer's disease, Huntington's disease, and Parkinson's disease) that may lead to dementia.

Although speech-language pathology services in a SNF include assessment and treatment of communicative disorders, the majority of the caseload is with patients who have dysphagia. However, because of liability issues and different degrees of training, student clinicians may be involved on a limited basis with the evaluation and treatment of patients with swallowing disorders.

Report Writing and Record Keeping

Basically, report writing and documentation of treatment sessions in the form of progress notes are similar to those in the hospital setting. In the SNF you may be involved in telephoning physicians for orders to evaluate or treat an individual. You also may be directly involved in billing private and federal insurance and in appealing decisions of third-party payers (e.g., insurance companies) that deny payment for services. As in all cases, your documentation and report writing should be accurate and appropriate to the patient and the clinical setting.

Working with Families and Professionals

In addition to direct patient contact, the speech-language pathologist provides *indirect services through consultation* with the SNF staff. A significant part of this indirect service is to educate the staff (nurses and aides) regarding communicative and swallowing disorders. You may train the staff to help identify and refer patients who appear to have communicative disorders. You need to train both the staff and the patient's family on ways to optimize communication with the patient. The patient's family can be invaluable in accurately evaluating and treating the patient. In addition to providing patient history, family members also may be actively involved with carryover of some treatment activities.

For your patients who have swallowing disorders, you will work closely with the dietitian and nursing staff. You will ensure that your patients have the correct diet and that there are staff trained to appropriately and safely feed them.

Rehabilitation Facilities

Rehabilitation facilities provide comprehensive services to individuals disabled by an accident or illness. The goal of rehabilitation is to maximize recovery and minimize any residual dysfunction.

Rehabilitation facilities may be a part of community hospital services or a private agency. There are also an increasing number of rehabilitation hospitals that specialize in treating persons with disabilities. Both inpatient and outpatient services are provided by the members of a multidisciplinary team. The speech-language pathologist is an important member of the rehabilitation team. You will find participating in practicum at a rehabilitation site an interesting and rewarding learning experience.

Prerequisites

To derive the greatest benefit from your practicum experience in a rehabilitation facility, you should have completed coursework in aphasia, dysphagia, neurological speech disorders, and voice.

Supervision

As in other medical settings, direct supervision of student clinicians is provided by a staff speech-language pathologist with coordination of the clinical practicum by the university supervisor. Again, supervision must meet ASHA's minimum standards for supervision of student clinicians.

Schedules

Patients served in rehabilitation facilities receive intensive treatment, sometimes two times a day, 5 to 6 days a week. Usually, treatment is offered between 8 a.m. and 5 p.m.; however, this schedule may vary depending on the needs of the patient. As in other medical settings, if you are treating a patient for a swallowing disorder, your treatment may cover mealtime.

Types of Patients

A large percentage of the population served in a rehabilitation facility includes patients who have suffered head injuries resulting from automobile or motorcycle accidents. Head injuries may be called traumatic brain injury (TBI), closed head injury (CHI), or acquired brain injury (ABI). Communicative disorders of this population include dysarthria and a variety of pragmatic language disorders (Hegde, 2006). In addition, patients with TBI also may exhibit such cognitive problems as impaired attention, orientation, and memory. In rehabilitation settings, it is not unusual for speech-language pathologists to have patients with dysphagia or cognitive disorders on their caseload.

Patients recovering from CVA with associated speech and language disorders often are seen in rehabilitation facilities. Patients recovering from a CVA typically exhibit aphasia, although independent and coexisting problems may include apraxia, dysarthria, dysphagia, and cognitive disorders.

In addition to providing services for individuals recovering from head injury or stroke, some rehabilitation facilities serve individuals with orthopedic handicaps. For example, children with cerebral palsy benefit from several rehabilitative services such as physical therapy, speech and language treatment, and vocational therapy.

The clinician may be involved in *assisting the patient with relearning daily living activities* and functional communication and memory skills. The clinician also may teach the use of assistive communicative devices to patients with poor prognosis for verbal communication.

Report Writing and Record Keeping

Documentation requirements in a rehabilitation facility are similar to those of many hospitals. Follow the requirements of your site.

Working with Families and Professionals

The rehabilitation team often includes a physiatrist, physical therapist, speech-language pathologist, occupational therapist, nurse, neuropsychologist, and social worker. A **physiatrist** is a physician trained in rehabilitative medicine and often serves as the team leader. There is close communication among team members whose services are interrelated. For example, based on information obtained during patient staffing, the speech-language pathologist may find that a specific patient cannot reach across midline. During speech therapy, the clinician carefully places pictures the patient is required to point to within the patient's reach. In another instance, the physical therapist consults with the speech-language pathologist and discovers that a patient who has been nonverbal during physical therapy sessions is able to produce single-word utterances; consequently, the physical therapist prompts the patient to respond to questions verbally during treatment sessions.

The rehabilitation team also works closely with the patient's family. The family members take an active part in rehabilitating the patient. A psychologist or social worker may counsel family members to help them deal with the emotional adjustments required. The speech-language pathologist also counsels the family members and works with them to reestablish a patient's communicative skills.

Psychiatric Hospitals

Psychiatric facilities often are state operated and designed to serve *individuals who are mentally handicapped or developmentally disabled*. Most of these facilities offer speech and hearing services. Although residential care is part of psychiatric hospitals, outpatient services also are available. In recent years, there has been an increased emphasis on mainstreaming those who are mentally ill or have developmental disabilities. You may work closely with the client's family, teachers, or employers. You may work in more or less restrictive facilities, including state psychiatric hospitals, outpatient clinics, or schools.

Clinical practicum in a psychiatric setting offers you an opportunity to work with unique cases. You will interact with many different professionals. You will learn to work as a member of a multidisciplinary team, to resolve many behavioral issues, and to evaluate and treat individuals with communicative disorders associated with mental illness or developmental disability, or both.

Prerequisites

In addition to a strong background in speech and language disorders, student clinicians preparing for an internship in a psychiatric hospital will want to have a good understanding of principles of behavior management. A course in abnormal or clinical psychology in which different forms of psychiatric disorders are reviewed is useful. Some sites also may use assistive technology. At these sites, computer literacy and a course in augmentative communication are useful as well.

Supervision

As is the case in many off-campus placements, a staff speech-language pathologist of the psychiatric facility will supervise your practicum in accordance with ASHA guidelines. To coordinate your practicum assignment, the university supervisor communicates regularly with the off-campus supervisor. Because of the emphasis on mainstreaming and serving clients in their natural environment, your clinical practicum at the psychiatric hospital may include accompanying clients to locations away from the hospital. If you leave the hospital with a client for treatment, your supervisor will always accompany you.

Schedules

The frequency and length of treatment sessions will vary, depending on the needs of the patient, the specific setting the patient is seen in, and the financial resources of the patient and the agency. The length of a session also is dependent on the amount of time the patient can effectively be involved in treatment. Some psychiatric patients benefit from a 45-minute treatment session, whereas other patients may need a shorter session because of limited attention span.

Types of Clients

In psychiatric facilities, the speech–language pathologist provides services to both children and adults. In addition to working with individuals with speech or language disorders, the clinician may work with patients who have behavioral disorders as well. Frequently, the speech–language pathologist is requested to evaluate a patient's communicative disorder that might be contributing to his or her problem behavior. The speech–language pathologist may work as a member of a team (which may include a psychiatrist, clinical psychologist, social worker, etc.) to design treatment programs for psychiatric patients, including those diagnosed with schizophrenia.

Report Writing and Record Keeping

Documentation of assessment and treatment sessions is important; however, each facility's requirements are different. Generally, as with other sites, you will be required to write clear, comprehensive assessment reports and regularly chart the results of treatment sessions. If you are at a site that a government agency operates, you may be required to complete specific forms for that agency. Your supervisor will explain the report writing and record-keeping requirements at your site.

Working with Families and Professionals

Teamwork is typical in psychiatric settings. Therefore, the speech–language pathologist often works as a member of a multidisciplinary team, which may consist of a psychiatric nurse, psychologist, social worker, psychiatrist, and other professionals.

Because of the attempts to integrate individuals who are mentally ill or developmentally disabled back into their communities, clinicians may see them in different settings. Depending on the setting, you may work closely with a client's family, teacher, or employer.

Preschool Agencies

Preschool programs typically serve children ages 3 to 5 years. However, preschools now are expanding to include infants and toddlers. Although many preschools are privately operated, the primary agencies offering the services of a speech-language pathologist are government programs such as Head Start, state preschools, economic opportunity programs, and local school districts. To be most effective, services should be provided in a natural environment. This could be in the home or school but should represent an environment familiar to the child.

Prerequisites

To work in a preschool setting, you should have a good understanding of normal and disordered speech and language development, infant speech perception and production, and techniques of early intervention. A general knowledge of child development is helpful.

Supervision

The speech-language pathologist responsible for serving the children on site provides supervision. Since the passage of P.L. 94-142 and its later amendments, public schools are providing many preschool services for children with special needs. In many communities, clinicians providing speech and language services to preschool children in the public school setting are employees of the school district. In other communities, usually because of limited financial or personnel resources, the school district contracts with a private practice to provide mandated services for preschool children with speech-language disorders. Regardless of who the service provider is, he or she will supervise you according to ASHA guidelines on supervision of clinical practicum.

Preschool Schedules

In public schools and Head Start programs, the speech-language pathologist most frequently works as an itinerant clinician who travels from one location to another. The population served at each preschool setting is relatively small. Consequently, you will find that the itinerant speech-language pathologist providing services to such sites travels extensively, sometimes going to two or more sites per day.

You will have the opportunity to work with several service delivery models practiced in preschools. Preschool children are served individually or in small groups. Children with disorders of articulation, voice, or fluency are usually seen individually. Those with disorders of language are seen individually or in small groups. With the exception of early services to children with *Autism Spectrum Disorders (ASD),* the trend in preschools is to serve children with language disorders in group settings. Often, language activities may be integrated with other social and educational activities. This enables a child to experience more natural communicative interactions. Such integrated activities may promote generalization and maintenance. Initially, most children with ASD benefit from individual intervention. As children with ASD gain greater communication skills, they may be integrated into various group settings to promote social skills and generalized production of learned behaviors.

Types of Clients

Preschool programs serve children who have severe handicaps to those who are nondisabled, so you will have the opportunity to work with a wide spectrum of children. The more severe the physical and sensory disabilities of the children, the greater are their communicative problems. With children who are severely disabled, you will see the entire range of communicative disorders. In some preschools you may work with children using augmentative communication devices. In other preschools you may work with children who primarily have articulation or language delays. In many settings, you will include assessment and intervention for preliteracy skills acquisition. ASHA strongly endorses the role of the speech-language pathologist in developing reading and writing skills as they relate to language development. With the increasing demand for services for young children diagnosed with ASD, it is likely that you will be working with preschoolers with this disorder. Children with ASD often are first referred to speech-language pathologists because of impaired or limited communication skills; therefore, your services may include assessment, treatment, and such case management activities as referring to and co-ordinating services with other agencies as well as helping families receive available supportive services.

Report Writing and Record Keeping

Some children progress slowly, whereas others progress at a rapid rate. In all cases, documentation of treatment and its results is essential. Your clinical supervisor will outline the requirements of documentation and report writing at your practicum site.

Working with Families and Professionals

In preschools, you will learn to provide consultative services for the children's parents and teachers. You will learn to train preschool teachers and their assistants on ways to maximize your clients' communication and to reinforce your clients' emerging speech and language skills. Ideally, you also will work closely with the parents of preschool children. Often, initially, it is difficult for parents to accept that their child has communication disorders. In working with parents of preschoolers, you will use the skills you have acquired in previous practicum experiences and in any counseling courses you have taken.

Your work with parents of preschoolers involves training them in conducting home treatment programs when necessary. Training parents to work regularly with their child to teach target behaviors and to routinely provide language expansion activities is a major part of your work. Once a parent realizes that his or her child has a communication disorder and you are there to help the child, the parent may become one of your greatest assets.

Prisons

Prisons are a growing industry in the United States and a large number of prisoners have communicative disorders. Speech-language pathology services may be provided in adult prisons and are mandated services in juvenile facilities.

Prerequisites

In addition to a strong background in speech and language disorders, the student preparing to work in a correctional facility will want to have an understanding of criminal behavior and may want to take a class in criminal justice. Before beginning your internship you will be required to pass a security clearance. Also, you may be required to pass a training course that focuses on how to interact with prisoners, how to dress, and how to behave in an emergency.

Supervision

Typically, a correctional facility staff speech-language pathologist will provide supervision. In some juvenile facilities, the speech-language pathologist may be an employee of the area school district. Your supervision will be in accordance with all ASHA guidelines and will be coordinated by your university. Although not part of your practicum supervision, you may be observed by correctional authorities as part of their regular monitoring activities.

Prison Schedules

Schedules will vary depending on the facility. Typically, services will be provided between 8 a.m. and 5 p.m., Monday through Friday. At adult facilities, the frequency and duration of services will depend on the needs and availability of your client. For example, you may be seeing a client twice a week for 45 minutes each time. However, there may be times when your client is unavailable because of a personal discipline or prison lock-down. Prison lock-down means that all prisoners are locked in their cells because of a security concern.

In a juvenile facility, your services will be regulated by your client's IEP. Refer to the section on public school services and Chapter 5 for more information about IEPs. Also, services will be influenced by your client's personal discipline, facility lock-down, and duration of his or her sentence.

Types of Clients

In correctional institutions, you will see clients with disorders of articulation, voice, fluency, and language. Some clients may have only one disability or may have multiple disabilities. Some clients may have limited education and some may have behavioral disorders. However, prisons have strict rules for earning certain "benefits" and often prisoners are motivated and happy to work with you. If you work in a juvenile facility, you will see clients who have IEPs. For additional information on IEPs, see Chapter 5.

Report Writing and Record Keeping

Accurate and thorough report writing and record keeping are essential components of this setting. Your supervisor will give you complete information on the facility's requirements.

Working with Families and Professionals

Depending on the facility you are working in, you may have little contact with your clients' families. However, you may work with the facility's nurse, teachers, or correctional officers. These professionals may assist you in providing effective intervention for your clients. You will find that having to work in a locked facility and relying on each other for your safety helps build a close professional community.

Private Practice

Across the nation, private practices in speech-language pathology are rapidly growing. You might think that private practitioners provide speech-language pathology services only in their office to clients in individual treatment sessions. However, this scenario is only a small part of the picture. Besides working with clients in their office, private practitioners may contract to provide speech-language pathology services for other private agencies. For example, private practitioners may serve skilled nursing facilities, home health care agencies, hospitals without speech and hearing departments, psychiatric facilities, and private preschools. They also may contract to serve children in local public schools.

Some private clinics may *specialize*. For example, one private practice may specialize in pediatric services, with another perhaps serving adults only. Yet another private clinic may have expertise in treating patients with laryngectomy. There also are extensive private practices that hire large numbers of speech-language pathologists who contract to offer services to patients in skilled nursing facilities and home health care agencies.

Prerequisites

Students planning a practicum assignment in a private practice need a broad educational background. Clients may range from infants to elderly individuals. The entire range of communicative disorders may be treated in private settings.

Because the private practitioner depends on favorable public relations, you will need to have, or quickly develop, good interpersonal skills. You will not only develop your skills in assessing and treating communicative disorders, but you will also gain insight into the business aspects of your profession. You will learn about marketing your services to the public and getting reimbursed by insurance companies and such government programs as Medicare.

Supervision

Your opportunities to work with clients in private clinics may be somewhat limited because most expect and request services from an experienced, licensed, and certified professional regardless of the amount of supervision available for a student clinician. Still, there are many opportunities for working under the supervision of a speech-language pathologist providing contractual service to other agencies. Also, a speech-language pathologist with sufficient staff resources may provide additional services through a student clinician for a client who needs more frequent treatment but cannot afford it. Your supervisor will work closely with you to ensure maintenance of a practice's reputation of quality service. Minimally, all supervision will comply with ASHA's requirements for clinical practicum.

Clinic Schedules

Schedules will vary depending on the type of service delivery in which the private practice is involved. If you are working in a SNF, your schedule will resemble that already described. If you are working with clients in the private practice office, your schedule will be influenced by the times clients are available for appointments. Although many practices operate on an 8 a.m. to 5 p.m. schedule, often certain days are reserved for appointments outside of regular business hours (e.g., 6 p.m. to 9 p.m.). Typically, treatment is scheduled for 30-minute sessions two to three times per week. The duration and frequency of treatment are based on each client's needs and financial resources.

Types of Clients

Clients may range from infants through adults. Disorders can cover the gamut of communication difficulties. Severity may spread across the continuum from very mild to severe. Of course, if you are assigned to a private practice that specializes in a certain disorder, you will mostly see clients with that disorder.

Report Writing and Record Keeping

Similar to all practicum assignments, documentation of assessment and treatment is important, and, depending on the private practice, writing and record-keeping requirements will vary. Chapter 5 provides general report-writing guidelines. In addition to report writing, you may be more directly involved in billing for your services. Your supervisor will assist you in learning the requirements for your practicum site.

Working with Families and Other Professionals

One advantage to working with clients in private practice is that they have sought out your services and are in your office because they want to be. Therefore, it is sometimes easier to maintain family involvement with your clients' treatment. On occasion, however, because of the cost of private speech and language services, some families expect the speech-language pathologist to provide a quick cure for a client. On other occasions, it may be necessary to immediately include family members in a client's treatment because the client's finances or insurance allows only a limited number of appointments for speech-language pathology services.

Regardless of the situation, you will learn to communicate effectively and to work closely with various family members. Communication with other professionals may be written or verbal. Again, depending on the services the private practice you are assigned to provides, you will interact with different professionals. For example, if you are working in a rehabilitation setting or SNF, you will collaborate with different members of the facility's staff (e.g., physical therapist, occupation therapist, social worker, nurse, and physician) to maximize your clients' treatment.

Other Clinical Settings

There are many other clinical practicum settings that have not been discussed in this chapter. Among these are the speech-language pathology services provided at *adult day health care centers, veterans' administration hospitals, public clinics, and private practices.* The range of settings in which you might complete your clinical practicum may be limited by demographic factors and your university's resources. More frequently, however, the range is limited only by your own initiative. If you wish to gain practicum experience in a new setting, discuss your interest with your supervisor, clinical director, or academic advisor.

Clinical Internships

Clinical internships may be *part-time* or *full-time.* Though a part of clinical practicum, internships provide comprehensive, on-the-job experience for more advanced students. Also, an internship typically is completed in an off-campus clinical site. The qualifications of the student clinician and the requirements of the clinical site determine the type of internships available. Students enrolled in distance learning programs may have clinical practicum programs designed specifically for that program.

Part-Time Internships

Part-time internships can be divided into two sections, *intermittent* and *daily.* Intermittent part-time internships allow you to participate in clinical practicum at a given site on a periodic basis. For example, you might receive a practicum assignment at a skilled nursing facility for 2 hours a day, 2 days a week. Other intermittent internships may allow your hours to vary from week to week. Daily part-time internships are much closer to the requirements of a full-time internship. You are assigned a clinical site for a specified number of hours and are required to participate in practicum each day of the work week.

Part-time internships allow you to schedule your work and academic classes around clinical practicum. Some part-time practicum may be so limited that you will not learn much about the setting and the clients served there. However, in the early stages of clinical practicum, many student clinicians need additional time to assimilate and integrate new information and experiences. For these students, part-time internships are ideal.

Full-Time Internships

Full-time internships require you to participate in a clinical practicum with the number of hours, workdays, and holidays parallel to those of the clinical-site staff. If you are participating in a full-time practicum assignment at an elementary school, you might be there from 8 a.m. to 3:30 p.m., Monday through Friday, for a specific number of weeks or total number of hours. If you were assigned to a hospital practicum site as a full-time intern, you probably would be required to arrive at 8 a.m. and work until 5 p.m., Monday through Friday, for a certain number of weeks or until you earn a specific number of clinical hours.

Full-time internships and even daily part-time internships provide a more *comprehensive practicum* experience than do intermittent assignments. In full-time internships, you may experience more of the professional and interpersonal aspects of an assigned setting. In addition to direct patient contact, you also may be included in rounds or staffing and be more closely involved with allied professionals. You may attend or even provide staff development (training) inservices. A full-time internship allows you to experience the daily routines and pressures associated with a particular setting and to obtain a better understanding of the personal as well as professional requirements of the work setting. Part-time internships rarely provide you with this opportunity because you are not on-site long enough.

Because full-time internships are intensive and allow minimal time for class work, they often are reserved for student clinicians in their final term of graduate work or for summer practicum assignments. However, if you wish to take up a full-time internship sooner, discuss it with your advisor.

General Administrative Procedures

A primary goal of speech-language pathology training programs is to provide valuable practicum experience for student clinicians while offering and maintaining high-quality clinical services. Many administrative procedures are necessary to meet this goal.

Facilities and Equipment

The university must ensure that both on-site and off-site facilities are adequate and appropriate for clinical practicum. The university speech and hearing clinic should maintain a current inventory of evaluation instruments and supplies, provide a professional and safe environment in which to provide clinical services, and offer adequate supervision and guidance to students from qualified supervisors.

To maintain quality clinical services, the clinic also should use some method of quality review and improvement. This should include measurable goals and outcome indicators. The quality review and improvement process might include such activities as surveys of client satisfaction, review of calibration logs, and review of clinic documentation.

Before placing students in off-campus practicum sites, the university clinic director evaluates the sites for their appropriateness. The clinic director verifies the qualifications and certification status of on-site supervisors, the types and number of clients served at the setting, and the number of clock hours students could obtain. The director may visit the facilities to ensure they are safe and adequately maintained. If you have any concerns about on-campus or off-campus facilities, discuss them with your clinic director.

Supervisor Qualifications

Your academic department verifies supervisors' qualifications to ensure they have met accreditation and university standards. ASHA requires that clinical supervisors hold the ASHA CCC, which requires a master's degree in speech-language pathology or audiology from an ASHA-accredited program. In states that have a licensure law, the license to practice speech-language pathology or audiology also is required of all supervisors. Supervisors must effectively share information and assist students in developing clinical skills. The university clinic staff maintains and reviews supervisor records as frequently as a clinic assignment is made.

At the end of each clinical assignment, students have the opportunity to evaluate their supervisors. These evaluations are usually anonymous. In addition, the university periodically performs peer reviews. Constructive and specific feedback can help the clinical supervisor acquire more effective clinical teaching skills.

Clinic Fees

In conjunction with the university, the department faculty develops a fee scale for clinical services provided at the university speech and hearing clinic, which is often not for profit. Funds generated in fees are used to defray the costs of clinic materials, supplies, and equipment. Fees are implemented on a fixed or sliding scale and may be waived for clients unable to afford payment.

You may inform your clients about the clinic's fee schedule, but you have neither the responsibility nor the authority to reduce or waive fees. Clients or parents who ask questions about fees, waivers, payment plans, and so forth should be referred to the clinic office.

Scheduling Practicum Assignments

Scheduling and assignment of practicum experiences are made on the basis of a student's experience, the student's clinical clock hour needs, the student's specific area of interest, availability of practicum sites, the number of clients seeking services, and the availability of clinical supervisors. Because of these and other variables to be considered in making clinical practicum assignments, you may not always get the kind of assignments you desire. However, the better the communication between you and the clinic director (or other individual in charge of scheduling), the greater the likelihood of you having a successful practicum experience. Therefore, follow the format your university uses in registering for practicum each term and for expressing your practicum needs ahead of time.

Student Records

Prior to being admitted into clinical practicum, students' records are reviewed to find out if they meet the academic requirements for clinical practicum. Although ASHA provides minimum guidelines for student performance, individual universities may have additional requirements the students must meet.

The clinic staff maintains records of student clinicians. These records are reviewed periodically to ensure that they meet both the university and ASHA guidelines for clinical practicum, including the types of patients served and number of clinical hours earned. It is important that you accurately communicate through the forms your department uses the clock hours you have earned and the clinical experiences you have completed. ASHA requires you to maintain a record of your academic and clinic experiences. Your university department is likely to use ASHA's *Knowledge and Skills Acquisition Form* (KASA) for this purpose. Your university may require additional documentation. Appendix C contains a sample page of the KASA form.

The training director (or the department chair) ensures that an evaluation of your performance is written at the end of each clinical assignment. The supervisor discusses your evaluation with you and places a copy of the evaluation in your file. The evaluation of your clinical skills and the corresponding grade will influence your future practicum assignments. If your clinical skills are weak, your continued participation in clinical practicum may be a matter for discussion. If you disagree with an evaluation of your practicum, you should discuss your concerns with your supervisor. If necessary, follow established procedures students must use to protest evaluations.

Clinical Supplies, Materials, and Equipment

While you are in clinical practicum you will use a variety of supplies, materials, and equipment. The university clinic and many off-campus sites provide most of these items. However, you also will be required to purchase some materials, equipment, and supplies. You will want to begin building your own inventory of materials and supplies throughout your clinical practicum, regardless of the amount of materials and equipment available to you.

Clinic *supplies are consumable* items. These include tongue depressors, gauze, cotton swabs, gloves, finger cots, tissue, and disinfectant. Carefully follow your clinic's protocol regarding disposal of these items. Most sites designate specific containers in which to dispose supplies used in oral examinations and materials that have come in contact with saliva or blood during evaluation or treatment sessions.

Clinical *materials also are consumable or expendable* items. Typically included in this category are tests, test response forms, and such treatment materials as articulation cards, language programs, and books.

Your clinic library or media center may have a wide variety of tests for the evaluation of communicative disorders. Tests are generally arranged in alphabetical order or organized by the type of disorder the test is designed to evaluate. Follow the checkout procedures outlined at your university or clinical site. The same test will be used over and over again by many other individuals, so handle it carefully. Tests are expensive so the less money that has to be spent to replace worn-out or lost tests, the more money the clinic will have available to upgrade materials, equipment, and facilities.

As you progress in your clinical practicum you may want or may be required to take the opportunity to use many assessment instruments. Instead of continually administering the same test across clients, experiment. Learn and administer new tests. Find out which tests evaluate what they purport to evaluate, which tests are standardized for specific populations, and which speech and language behaviors might be better evaluated through analysis of speech samples. After you graduate you will select your own tests. Therefore, take time to learn to objectively evaluate most of the published tests made available to you at a practicum site.

Test response forms also are considered clinic supplies because they are consumable. Response forms are expensive, especially when they must be supplied to 20 to 40 student clinicians per semester. Use the response forms judiciously. Do not request or take more forms than you need. Some university clinics provide student clinicians with only one response form per semester for each client and require the student to pay for any additional forms needed because of incorrect scoring or response form loss. It is not appropriate to photocopy response forms for clinical use, unless the publisher specifically gives permission to reproduce them.

In addition to numerous tests, your clinic will have a supply of treatment materials. The type and quantity of materials differ across campuses and clinical sites. Generally available are a selection of articulation cards depicting pictures designed to evoke corresponding phonemes in a variety of word positions. Also, you frequently will have access to picture or photo decks representing many vocabulary and language concepts. Comprehensive language programs and books also may be available. Your clinic may supply different types of toys for use with younger clients. There is an abundance of commercial items available, although often the theoretical basis of the faculty and clinic staff influences the types of materials made available to the student clinician.

Treatment materials are the most individual or personalized of items used in clinical practicum. Therefore, it is not unusual for student clinicians to develop their materials. You can develop your materials by drawing pictures, using computer graphics, using pictures from books or magazines, creating charting forms, accumulating lists of words, phrases, and sentences designed to teach phonemes or language behaviors, and developing an activity file of various treatment techniques and ideas.

Many student clinicians find it functional, as well as beneficial, to allow their clients to create some of their treatment materials. With the assistance of a parent, a young client might be asked to cut pictures out of a magazine and bring them to the treatment session to put into a speech book. Another client might be asked to bring in newspaper articles to discuss during a treatment session. You may ask clients with good drawing skills to draw picture cards for use in their treatment sessions and home practice assignments.

In the school setting, clinicians increasingly are using curriculum materials as treatment materials. Clinicians in other settings may emphasize naturally occurring activities or events to evoke speech and language behaviors. Using functional and naturally occurring treatment materials can help you in promoting generalization and maintenance of target behaviors. Personalized materials the student clinician creates usually meet a specific need and are, consequently, functional; best of all, they are never checked out by another clinician.

Clinical *equipment is nonexpendable*. It is something that is used, one would hope, over a long period of time. Clinical equipment generally is much more expensive than supplies and materials. Examples of clinical equipment include audiometers, computers, audio and videotape recorders, sound level meters, auditory trainers, and augmentative communication devices. Less expensive items such as flashlights, stethoscopes, dental mirrors, and therapy mirrors also are in this category.

Again, note that the longer the life of the equipment, the more your clinic can invest in new equipment rather than simply replacing those that have been lost or broken. Handle the clinic equipment carefully. If you have questions about the appropriate way to use an instrument, ask your supervisor for assistance. Be careful when checking out or returning equipment. If equipment is broken or parts are missing when you check it out, notify the clinic administrative assistant or your supervisor so that the equipment can be repaired. When you return equipment, replace it correctly and carefully in its container or storage space.

In this age of rapidly advancing technology, there is an ever-increasing amount of equipment available for the speech-language pathologist. Some of the equipment is priced within the budget of student clinicians, so you may want to purchase a few items to add to your personal inventory. When deciding on the purchase of a piece of equipment, determine if it is something that you will use frequently or if it is something for which there is no substitute. For example, a flashlight is inexpensive, you will use it frequently, and there is not a better substitute for it. An audiometer, however, is expensive, you may or may not use it regularly, but there is not a substitute for it, unless referrals for audiological testing are easily made. On the other hand, an augmentative communication device may be used for a single client, is generally expensive, and, rather than carrying an inventory of augmentative equipment, the client may be referred to a clinic specializing in augmentative communication.

The supplies, materials, and equipment that you need often are dependent on your clinical practicum site. It is to your advantage to work with a variety of materials and equipment in many different clinical settings.

Now that you know some of the different clinical sites and practicum experiences available, you can begin planning your clinical program with your advisor. The clinical practicum portion of your training may be important in choosing the setting in which you want to work after graduation.

CHAPTER 3

The Conduct of the Student Clinician

Chapter Outline

- General Professional Behavior
- ASHA Code of Ethics
- Other Codes and Regulations

In addition to scientific knowledge and clinical competence, ethical behavior and professional demeanor are essential characteristics of the well-respected speech-language pathologist. Training in speech-language pathology includes the acquisition of knowledge about communication and its disorders, together with professional skills in assessing and treating those disorders. However, an equally important part of training is not formally discussed in most textbooks or classes: the acquisition of certain standards of behavior considered professionally appropriate. Professional behavior and the various codes and regulations governing this behavior are discussed in this chapter.

General Professional Behavior

Certain behaviors are traditionally accepted as professionally appropriate and governed by peer influence. Other behaviors are clearly defined and regulated by codes of ethics or other written rules. Throughout your enrollment in clinical practicum, you will have many opportunities to represent the profession of speech-language pathology, the university department and its clinic, and the university at large. You will interact with numerous clients, care providers, professionals, and related agencies in the community. You represent speech-language pathologists to people with whom you interact. The profession will be judged by your behavior, and you will begin to establish a reputation that you may build on as your professional career progresses. Therefore, you must demonstrate appropriate and acceptable professional behavior. *Honesty, integrity, respect for others, and a desire to help* are behavioral qualities admired in all people. They are especially important for professional people.

ASHA provides various guidelines to clarify your professional role, behavior, and responsibilities. Equally important, these documents help uphold high standards of service and protect your clients. These guidelines outline certain standards of care and include the ASHA Code of Ethics, ASHA's *Preferred Practice Patterns, Scope of Practice, Technical Reports, Guidelines, Position Statements,* and the *Consumer Bill of Rights.*

In addition to specific rules outlined by ASHA in its Code of Ethics and various reports, general rules of professional behavior include *punctuality* in meeting clinical appointments and clinic deadlines; *working cooperatively* with office staff, supervisors, and other student clinicians; *assuming responsibility* for clinic equipment and clinic facilities; being *well-prepared* for each clinical session; and *maintaining appropriate dress and demeanor*. Professional demeanor is one of the initial factors on which a student clinician is evaluated. *Professional demeanor* is a vague term but refers to such behaviors as appearing confident in your abilities, communicating clearly and appropriately with clients and supervisors, presenting yourself as a mature adult, following prescribed rules, and effectively utilizing clinical time.

Confidence in your ability to help your client is an important characteristic to develop. At the university clinic, you will work with many clients with varied backgrounds. You will probably be nervous when you first talk with your clients, but it is important that you make a good impression. You will often be the first clinic person to contact a client. Your initial meeting with a client sets the stage for future clinical relationships and may influence the client's willingness to pursue treatment. It is important for the client to see you as a self-confident and well-trained person. The client must believe that you are capable of providing quality clinical services. Also, your clients must believe they are important to you and trust that you will do all you can to help them. A large part of this trust is developed as you initially establish rapport with your clients.

There are many significant and insignificant factors that will influence your clients' opinion of your abilities. The degrees you have earned probably have the least influence. The way you dress, wear your hair, make eye contact, and shake hands are sometimes overlooked behaviors that will have much influence on your clients' desire to work with you. Again, much of the clients' initial impressions will be based on your professional demeanor.

Your professional demeanor and clinical ability will also affect other students. At off-campus practicum sites, you are a representative of the university. Administrators, supervisors, and medical, health, and allied health professionals may have little knowledge of the university and its training program. Based on your exemplary professional behavior or lack of it, a practicum site may continue to offer or withdraw its offer to provide practicum experiences for other student clinicians. Although student clinicians beginning off-campus practicum should be as well-prepared for the assignment as possible, no student is expected to know all of the procedures and regulations of a site. However, each student is expected to perform appropriately and professionally. You should *meet the deadlines, maintain regular attendance, work cooperatively with the site staff, learn new procedures, and follow the guidelines related to clinical practicum* in a particular setting.

Even if you do not have advance knowledge of some of the special rules and regulations of the off-campus site where you will complete your clinical internship, you should know the ASHA Code of Ethics. During your on-campus practicum, you also are expected to know and adhere to the ASHA Code of Ethics and various policies and procedures. Before you begin any clinical practicum assignment, you should reread ASHA's Code of Ethics.

ASHA Code of Ethics

The ASHA Code of Ethics (American Speech-Language-Hearing Association, 2003a) *gives guidelines of professional behavior* for individuals providing clinical services in speech-language pathology or audiology. ASHA members who hold the Certificate of Clinical Competence must adhere to the Code of Ethics. In addition, applicants for membership and individuals completing their Clinical Fellowship are required to adhere to the Code of Ethics. There is no legal basis for enforcement of the Code of Ethics, except in states that have adopted it as part of licensure requirements. However, a professional violating the Code of Ethics may lose his or her ASHA certification or membership in ASHA, or both.

As a student clinician and in the future as a speech-language pathologist, you will be faced with many pressures that will demand ethical judgments. Such factors as shortages of speech-language pathologists, increased demands to show profits, and wider scopes of practice can affect your service delivery. As a student, your supervisor will assist you in making the appropriate decision based on ASHA's Code of Ethics and other guidelines. As a professional, you will make your own decisions based on your judgment and knowledge of ethical practices. Throughout your professional career, you will refer to ASHA's Code of Ethics, guidelines, and position statements to make ethical professional decisions. In addition to learning the various guidelines on professional conduct early on, evaluate your own personal values. If your value system is not consistent with the value system professed by ASHA, you may want to pursue a different career.

The *Board of Ethics of ASHA is responsible for interpreting, administering, and enforcing* the Code of Ethics. To maintain ASHA certification, you are required to uphold and abide by the Code of Ethics. Also, many employers require that their employees providing speech-language pathology services hold current ASHA certification. Consequently, the Code of Ethics and the Board of Ethics have a significant impact on the profession.

All students participating in clinical practicum are required to comply with the ASHA Code of Ethics. The code helps you in developing ethically responsible professional behaviors. The information outlined in the Code of Ethics not only helps you answer questions related to professional and clinical issues but also to understand the rationale for certain clinic procedures.

The entire code, as well as its revisions, is published periodically in *The ASHA Leader*. Also, you may read the code on the ASHA Web site. The following discussion emphasizes specific areas of the code; however, you should read and understand the complete Code of Ethics, provided in Appendix D.

The ASHA Code of Ethics, revised January 1, 2003, is *composed of a Preamble, four Principles of Ethics, and numerous Rules of Ethics*. The Preamble briefly summarizes ASHA's philosophy of service delivery, provides an introduction to components of the Code of Ethics, and lists individuals who are governed by the code. The Principles of Ethics outlines basic ethical behavior. Subdivided under each Principle of Ethics, the Rules of Ethics describe more specifically acceptable professional behavior. Obviously, ASHA cannot foresee all instances in which a moral or ethical judgment must be made. Therefore, the Code of Ethics is designed as a guide of minimally acceptable behavior. The four Principles of Ethics are discussed in the following sections.

Principle of Ethics I

> Individuals shall honor their responsibility to hold paramount the welfare of persons they serve professionally or participants in research and scholarly activities and shall treat animals involved in research in a humane manner.

Principle I of the Code of Ethics is straightforward and not easily misinterpreted. Foremost are *client welfare and the welfare of individuals or animals involved in research*. Your training program will have guidelines on protecting research participants. Your academic department will likely have a Human Subjects Protection Committee (formally known as the Institutional Review Board), which is responsible for reviewing all research proposals to ensure that the participants are treated according to the university and federal government regulations. Also, you will adhere to any additional rules outlined by ASHA's Code of Ethics. When evaluating or treating clients, the difficult part for beginning student clinicians is determining what is best for the person being served. If you have a question about the legitimacy, efficacy, or ethics of a particular clinical situation, discuss it with your clinical supervisor. Remember that there are many unproven treatment strategies and invalid assessment instruments on the market. Recall from your research course the methods to evaluate treatment and assessment instruments to determine their efficacy. If you have a concern about the safety of a procedure, do not use it until you discuss your concerns with your supervisor. Familiarize yourself with what ASHA considers are some of the factors involved in protecting your clients' welfare.

Preparation

ASHA's Code of Ethics mandates that *services be provided competently*. In training programs, both the student clinicians and clinical supervisors must be competent. To be competent, one must be well prepared. At university clinics, student clinicians commonly are required to complete coursework in a specific communicative disorder before they are assigned a client with that disorder. Compliance with this policy helps ensure that student clinicians are academically prepared to work with clients with a specific disorder. To be prepared for specific clinical sessions, you should spend time in advance reviewing academic information related to your clients' disorders, your clients' records, and assessment materials, including standardized tests you plan to use. Also, you will need to gather treatment materials, forms for charting specific behaviors, and other supplies and equipment. Writing lesson plans, treatment plans, and clinical reports also should be part of this preparation. Ensure that you have appropriate knowledge, experience, and supervision before working with a patient with a swallowing disorder, tracheotomy, laryngectomy, or other serious medical complication.

Current ASHA certification is one of the criteria of minimal clinical competence defined by ASHA. Therefore, your clinical supervisors will have the Certificate of Clinical Competence in the areas in which they provide clinical supervision. Your speech-language pathology supervisor will have the knowledge and skills necessary to provide clinical services for your clients. Minimally, you will have a general background in a specific disorder before you are assigned a client with that disorder. However, you may be required to do additional research to effectively serve your client. During training, your supervisor will refer you to appropriate sources if you are unable to independently find the information you need. After your formal training and throughout your professional career, you should continue your education and research by being current in your practice and by continuously refining your skills.

ASHA also addresses client welfare and clinical competence by prohibiting service delivery by individuals whose services are hampered by substance abuse or physical or mental health problems. Obviously, such individuals are not appropriately prepared for effective service delivery. ASHA directs those individuals to seek assistance and to not provide service in the affected area. Find someone to help you whether or not you decide to continue your education in speech-language pathology if you have a substance abuse problem or are concerned about a mental or physical health condition. Discussions with your clinic supervisors, clinic director, department head, or other faculty will be confidential. They may be able to help you find appropriate services. Acknowledging and addressing certain problems will not necessarily preclude you from clinical practicum. However, as in the case of academic preparation, your supervisor may decide when you are physically and emotionally prepared to work with clients.

Remember, *maintaining professional competence is a continuing process*. It does not end with the completion of your formal professional education.

Referral

You will not always be able to provide all the services your clients need. Therefore, the requirement that you *provide only the services that you are qualified to provide* means that you should sometimes refer clients to other professionals. Also, some of your clients may need services in addition to those of speech-language pathology. For example, you may have a client recovering from a cerebrovascular accident who appears depressed. It may be appropriate for you to refer the client to a professional who treats depression. Other clients may need the services of a speech-language pathologist who specializes in treating a particular disorder that you cannot treat effectively. For example, a client who has had a laryngectomy may come to see you to learn esophageal speech. If you or your supervisor is not skilled in this area, you should refer the client to a colleague who is. Still other clients may be difficult to schedule because of your caseload. Instead of asking them to postpone treatment, you might suggest an equally competent speech-language pathologist. Finally, there may be clients who cannot afford to continue your services. You may know of other speech-language pathology services that are available for free or at a reduced cost. All such clients should be referred to other professionals who can provide more effective or economical services than you can. It is customary to provide several names of qualified professionals when making a referral. You should not refer clients to an individual practicing speech-language pathology or audiology who does not have current ASHA certification. Your practicum site will have a list of qualified professionals for referrals. Your referral list may include other speech-language pathologists, audiologists, psychologists, otolaryngologists, orthodontists, dentists, and physicians.

It is important to refer to individuals who are both qualified and cooperative. If you have had difficulty obtaining necessary information from a professional, you may want to avoid referring to that individual.

As with all other major clinical decisions, you should not make a referral without first discussing the matter with your clinical supervisor. Your clinical supervisor must approve the reason for the referral and to whom the referral will be made.

Discrimination

The code prohibits discrimination. Decisions related to delivery of service must not be based on "race or ethnicity, gender, age, religion, national origin, sexual orientation, or disability." You will provide speech-language pathology services for a wide variety of individuals. Obviously, there will be certain persons you enjoy working with more than others. In fact, as you progress in your training program, you may decide you want to work only with a specific population. For example, you may choose to specialize in treating individuals who stutter. In this case, declining to serve someone with aphasia would not be discrimination. However, discrimination exists if you solely base service delivery decisions on race, ethnicity, gender, age, religion, national origin, sexual orientation, or disability. It is important to remember that clinical judgments and recommendations must be made on your expertise and clinical data and not on unrelated factors. As part of a research project, you may need to select certain participants based on their ethnicity, race, disability, and so on. However, you may not choose or exclude participants who otherwise qualify for the research simply because of their age, gender, ethnicity, disability, sexual orientation, race, or religion.

Informed Consent

The code covers several rules on providing information to clients. Basically, clients must be given enough information so they can understand all relevant aspects of clinical services that affect them. They can then make a rational decision to seek services or not. Such a decision is informed consent. Individuals must be given information related to possible consequences of treatment as well as no treatment.

University clinics do not, as a rule, require individuals refusing treatment to sign written statements verifying such refusal and their understanding of possible consequences of a refusal. Private clinics may ask clients to sign a statement to that effect. However, most clinics require clients to initial or sign a plan of treatment to confirm their knowledge of the proposed services. If clients are not required to submit a written acknowledgment of the treatment plan, you should note in the records when the plan was discussed with the client and the client's apparent understanding of the discussion (Flower, 1984). Each off-campus site will have its guidelines for obtaining client consent that student clinicians should follow.

Clients must be *informed fully regarding the nature and possible effects* of the service. Also, they must be provided prognostic information. Beginning clinicians sometimes do not know how to reply to clients who ask if a specific treatment will cure them or even how a specific procedure will affect their communicative disorder. As you know from reading the Code of Ethics, you are forbidden from guaranteeing treatment results. However, you can make an informed, reasonable, prognostic statement. For example, you should not say, "After 6 weeks of treatment, you will no longer stutter." You may say, "This type of treatment has been successful with many individuals who had problems similar to yours. Based on the diagnostic information I have and what I think is your level of motivation for change, the chances of improvement in your speech fluency are good." Ethically justified prognostic statements are those that are probabilistic statements based on valid and reliable information about the client and the accumulated scientific evidence in the discipline. Therefore, prognostic statements should not be made without first ensuring that all necessary information has been obtained and is accurate. If there is a gap in your information, you should make it clear to the client. If a satisfactory prognostic statement cannot be made, the reasons should be explained to the client. You must discuss your client's prognosis with your clinical supervisor before you report it to the client.

Informed consent also requires that clients be told if the treatment they receive is part of a research program. Your clients must be *informed clearly of the nature of research, the procedure to be used, the benefits of participation, and the possible negative effects.* The clients must be given a free choice to participate in the treatment research or to opt for other kinds of treatment programs. The clients who agree to participate in an experimental treatment program retain their right to withdraw from it at any time and without prejudice. Potential participants should fully realize this. Prior to its use in a research study, the informed consent form should be approved by the Human Subjects Protection Committee (also known as Institutional Review Board) in your department.

Clients also must be fully informed about who is providing the speech-language pathology services and what his or her qualifications are. In the university clinic, as well as at off-campus sites, it is explained clearly to the client that student clinicians provide services under the supervision of a certified professional. You must *never misrepresent your status* to the public. In many settings, you will be asked to wear a name tag or identification badge that will give your name and title.

Before providing services, you should check to ensure that your client has signed all consent forms. Each site will have different forms. Check with your clinical supervisor if you are not sure what forms are used at your site.

Treatment Efficacy

In medical and health care professions, the concept of evidence-based practice is now well established. The concept has been accepted by general and special educators as well. Simply put, the treatment or teaching methods used must have scientific evidence supporting them; treatment or teaching procedures should have been shown to be effective in experimental research (Hegde, 2003). ASHA's Code of Ethics underscores evidence-based practice by stating that clinicians should evaluate the effectiveness of treatment offered to the public and offer only those services that are reasonably expected to be beneficial. This implies that clinicians should not offer treatment whose effects have never been evaluated in appropriate research studies. It also implies that services should not be provided to clients who may not be expected to benefit from treatment. The code also prohibits continuation of unnecessary treatment. Student clinicians and professionals who are knowledgeable in research methods—especially the experimental designs that help establish treatment efficacy (Hegde, 2003)—will be better equipped to judge the appropriateness of various treatment options for given disorders than those who lack such knowledge.

There are issues that often are difficult for student clinicians to resolve. Professionals and agencies sometimes disagree about these issues. For example, a speech-language pathologist may judge that a patient with brain injury could benefit from speech-language services. However, the insurance company, judging that the patient would not benefit from treatment, may not approve payment for the services. In this instance, the clinician, who may feel frustrated because the needed service cannot be provided, has not acted unethically in recommending treatment.

Financial factors may adversely affect the decision making of those clinicians who are unclear about their values and ethical choices. Unfortunately, economic factors are important in maintaining private businesses, and the business that holds little regard for ethical practice may attempt to put a speech-language pathologist in a compromising position. For example, a speech-language pathologist may be instructed to provide services for a specific number of patients per day. If there are not sufficient numbers of appropriate patients, the clinician may be pressured to increase the caseload by enrolling patients for whom the benefit of treatment is questionable. Clinicians who enroll patients in treatment because of such pressures when they are reasonably sure that a patient would not benefit from treatment (e.g., because of the patient's extremely poor health) will have violated the Code of Ethics and will have acted unethically.

With due regard to adhering to the Code of Ethics, professionals may disagree on who benefits from treatment and for how long. For example, two speech-language pathologists may not agree on the appropriate chronological age for treatment of a specific communicative disorder. Also, progress of some individuals (for instance, a person with a severe cognitive impairment) may be extremely slow and efficacy of treatment difficult to assess. Clinicians who maintain objective and accurate records of client behaviors will be better able to judge the client's response to treatment than those who rely on subjective judgment and memory to evaluate client progress.

Is it considered unethical to not record every response of a client? No. However, failure to maintain adequate records is unethical. Adequate records should document changes or lack of changes in the target behaviors over a span of treatment sessions. Continuing the same treatment when repeated measures show no change in client behaviors is certainly unethical. Do you necessarily have to dismiss the client? No. But you certainly should change the treatment procedure.

There is no single formula to determine which individuals can benefit from treatment or when treatment should be discontinued. Social, educational, psychological, and health factors affect your decision. You should evaluate your clients and attempt to make the appropriate determination, but you should never try to enroll or dismiss a client without first discussing the matter with your clinical supervisor.

Confidentiality

Clients' rights to privacy are protected under the Code of Ethics. You are directed to *maintain client confidentiality*, except when you must reveal information to protect your clients' or the community welfare or because you are directed to do so by law. In addition, legal protection of a client's right to privacy is provided by federal and state laws. The **Health Insurance Portability and Accountability Act (HIPAA)** of 1996 is discussed later in this chapter. HIPAA, which many universities and off-campus sites must adhere to, gives specific guidelines regarding the maintenance of client confidentiality.

Client confidentiality is of ongoing concern at university clinics. There are two reasons for this. First, much of the learning at the university level occurs by individuals sharing information and experiences with each other. Second, persons not directly involved with treatment may observe clients receiving services. Early in your academic career, you will be called on to help ensure client confidentiality. You will observe many clinic sessions, you may present information about clients in certain courses, and you will be involved in student and faculty discussions about clients' evaluations, treatments, and counseling sessions. In all these situations, the clients' rights to privacy must be respected.

Because students frequently discuss their clients with each other, client confidentiality may be violated easily. Observers not directly involved with service delivery may discuss clients in such a way as to violate client confidentiality. You need to be aware of your clients' right to confidentiality and monitor both your written and verbal communications to ensure those rights.

Flower (1984) discussed three types of consent related to disclosure of confidential information: *implied consent, written consent,* and *consent inherent in the private interests of the client.* **Implied consent** means that individuals seeking services implicitly approve access to their records by staff or support personnel without the need for written authorization. For example, it is not necessary for the clinic administrative assistant to obtain written authorization before accessing a client's record, because reviewing client records is typically a part of an assistant's duties.

Release of information to individuals or agencies outside of a facility requires a written authorization, or written consent. The clinic administrative assistant at your university clinic or at an off-campus practicum site can give you information on the consent form required and the procedures for completing it.

Inherent consent that is in the private interests of the client is assumed when release of information is in the best interest of the client. This form of consent generally occurs between the professional and members of the client's family. For example, your client may discuss with you a desire to commit suicide. Of course, you will want to share this information with the client's spouse or other family member. In another instance, you may suspect your client is a victim of child abuse. In this case, you will follow your site's procedures for reporting your concern to the proper authorities. Again, without first discussing a specific situation with a clinical supervisor, you should treat all client information as confidential. This precaution will allow you to avoid the need to justify disclosure of confidential information.

The nature of university training programs requires that everyone is aware of and respects client confidentiality. Students constantly observe assessment and treatment sessions. Consequently, the clinical services offered to individuals through the university training programs are less confidential than those that are offered in private clinics. This is acceptable as long as the client has given informed consent for being observed.

Guidelines to Help Ensure Client Confidentiality

1. *Do not discuss your client by name,* except with your clinical supervisor, clinic staff, or as necessary during clinical meetings. On campus, you will be involved in meetings with your supervisor and clinic staff. Off campus, you may have hospital rounds, student study team meetings, and meetings with your on-site and university supervisors. Obviously in private clinic meetings with your supervisor or affiliated staff, it is perfectly acceptable to identify your clients by name. In fact, you would probably be thought somewhat odd or obtuse if you never mentioned your clients' names.

2. *Do not discuss your client in public areas.* Avoid discussing information about your clients in hallways or waiting areas. If you need to talk about your clients or with your clients, move to a private room. Your discussion will also probably be more profitable if you take the time to find an area where people are not freely moving about and distractions are minimized.

3. *Do not mention your client's name in class presentations or discussions.* As part of class assignments, you may be required to present case histories on various clients you have observed or worked with. You can easily refer to your client as "the client" or give each client an alias.

4. *Do not leave client reports, lesson plans, or other written information unattended.* Promptly file documents in your clients' folders. If you are submitting reports or lesson plans to your supervisor, be sure they are not left on a table or desk that is accessible to the public.

5. *Follow all office rules regarding checking out and returning client folders and reports.* As a general rule, client files are not to be taken from the clinic area. If files are taken to be used during a clinic session, staffing, or meeting, checkout procedures should be followed, so the clinic administrative assistant can retrieve the files, if necessary.

6. *Do not take client folders home and do not remove information from them.* If you need information from your clients' files, allow time to take the necessary notes. Keep all such notes confidential; do not have client names in your notes. Information must remain in your clients' files to document service delivery.

7. *Do not discuss your client with others.* Unless your client or your supervisor has approved the communication, do not discuss your client with other professionals or persons in other agencies.

8. *Remind your observers that they should respect client confidentiality.* When you are working as a student clinician, other students may want to discuss their observations of your clinic session with you. Help them remember the rules of client confidentiality by modeling appropriate behavior and, if necessary, asking them not to discuss your clients in front of other people.

9. *Obtain written consent to make videotapes or take photographs of clients.* A separate consent should be obtained for any photographs or videotapes used for public viewing, such as at a health fair or community education program. Your clinic administrative assistant should have the necessary forms.

10. *Comply with all clinic rules regarding release of information.* Your clinic will probably have a specific form that must be completed and signed by the client before information is released to another agency. Check with your clinic supervisor or the clinic administrative assistant for additional information. When giving information over the telephone, you also must respect client confidentiality. For example, if you have clients who also are receiving speech-language services in the public schools, their school clinicians may phone you. Be sure you do not

(continues)

reveal confidential information without prior approval from the client. If in doubt as to when you may give information over the telephone, discuss it with your clinic supervisor.

11. *Honor client confidentiality during communications on the Internet.* There are several Internet listservs and chat rooms operating that provide forums for clinical discussions. Students and professionals post questions, concerns, and comments about clients. If you participate in such a listserv or chat room, be careful to respect your clients' rights to privacy. Do not discuss your clients by name or use any information that could identify them. For example, in certain circumstances your client could be identified by such a statement as, "My client is a 3-year-old female whose mother is a local pediatrician and whose father is a high school principal." It is acceptable to discuss clinical issues, but be cautious and use good judgment.

The rules of ethics prohibit individuals from providing clinical services solely by correspondence; however, the rules allow clinical practice through telecommunication where allowed by law. As a student clinician, you probably will not be involved in telepractice, but it is gaining interest and there are increasing numbers of professionals providing services through the Internet. It is important that you understand your limitations when you are unable to meet with a client face to face.

There are several other rules related to the importance of client welfare. Most of these are self-explanatory, such as not charging for services not provided, maintaining adequate records, and not assessing or treating an individual only by correspondence.

Principle of Ethics II

Individuals shall honor their responsibility to achieve and maintain the highest level of professional competence.

Competency is minimally defined as holding ASHA's CCC. Individuals providing independent speech–language pathology services, or supervising the delivery of those services, must hold the CCC in Speech–Language Pathology (CCC-SLP). Supervision of speech–language pathologists completing their SLPCF also must be provided by an individual with a current CCC-SLP. As you know, the CCC is the minimum standard, and additional training in specific areas may be necessary to ensure competent service delivery. Your master's degree offers you a foundation on which to build your knowledge. After you graduate, you will be ready to learn and integrate much of the skills that you peripherally touched on in college. As a professional, make it a part of your job to routinely participate in appropriate continuing education activities, read professional journals, and network with other speech-language pathologists.

Scope of Competence

The field of speech-language pathology is growing rapidly. Service delivery encompasses more and more aspects of client care. Speech-language pathologists work with clients of all ages. Some work with infants, providing early intervention services, sometimes while the infants are still in the hospital. Other clinicians primarily work with school-age children, adults, or geriatric clients. Still others specialize in serving clients with specific problems, for example, clients who stutter, clients with head injuries, or clients needing augmentative communication devices. Obviously, the needs of an infant in the *neonatal intensive care unit* (NICU) will differ from the 8-year-old child with a language delay, and the needs of a client who recently has had a laryngectomy will differ from the needs of an adult who stutters. Therefore, every certified speech-language pathologist may not be competent to provide services for every client. The Code of Ethics mandates that speech-language pathologists only work in their areas of competence based on their education, training, and experience. Some of ASHA's SIDs have or are in the process of developing certificate options as a method by which speech-language pathologists can show that they have obtained certain skill levels in specialized areas. The certification is optional and not typically required to engage in clinical practice.

As noted in previous discussions, you may not be expected to know everything needed to serve all your clients, but you should have the basic knowledge and skills to research new information. Your supervisor will always be your resource person, but you should strive constantly to learn on your own and to expand and extend your knowledge.

Continuing Education

As you know, the CCC implies that the minimum educational and clinical qualifications have been met. The Code of Ethics expands on these qualifications by addressing the need for continuing education.

To maintain a high standard of professional competence, speech-language pathologists must continue their education, even after they have earned their CCCs. You may have already discovered that researchers and clinicians rapidly and constantly produce new information about communicative disorders. Some of what you learned in many undergraduate classes may be outdated by the time you start your clinical practicum. You are busy keeping up with coursework, but you must remain current. You can begin the practice of self-study by reading journals and recently published books in speech-language pathology. You also can attend many conferences and workshops to gain current scientific and professional information.

To maintain ASHA certification once you have completed your SLPCF, you must accumulate three CEUs within a 3-year period. Your state may have additional requirements for maintaining your license or your credential. CEUs are obtained through various avenues of professional development. ASHA's policy on continuing education includes the following:

- *Each CEU is equivalent to 10 contact hours.* Therefore, the three CEUs required for maintenance of the CCC equal 30 actual contact hours.

- *CEUs may be earned in several ways.* You may attend conferences or workshops that are sponsored by ASHA-approved CEU providers (this will be written on conference and workshop brochures). You may study independently by participating in certain internships, developing courses, engaging in research, or attending programs offered by non–ASHA-approved CEU providers. Also, you may use self-study to continue your education. Self-study may involve listening to audiotapes or watching videotapes and responding to test questions that are then submitted to the CEU provider. You may also earn CEUs by reading SID newsletters and completing the accompanying quizzes. College or university courses may be used for professional development. Two semester units (or three quarter units) are considered equivalent to 30 contact hours. There may be other activities that you want to use as part of your required professional development. Check with ASHA if you have a question about whether they fall within its parameters for professional development.

- *ASHA randomly verifies CEUs.* It will be important for you to keep a record of your professional development activities. For an annual fee, ASHA offers you the option to have them maintain a record of your continuing education activities in their CEU registry.

Supervision

The Code of Ethics directs individuals to be well prepared for the services they provide and to require individuals under their supervision to be well prepared. The supervisor is responsible for ensuring that support personnel are appropriately supervised and that other professional staff provide services only within their levels of competence. As a professional you may be assigned a speech assistant to help you provide services. ASHA guidelines require speech assistants to be supervised by speech-language pathologists who have their CCCs, at least 2 years of experience, and some education in supervision. As a student clinician, you will not be qualified or expected to supervise a speech assistant; by observing your supervisor, you may gain knowledge regarding various supervisory skills. In training programs, the student uses the supervisor's license and certification to learn the techniques of the profession. If supervisors determine their student clinicians are not qualified or prepared to work with certain clients, they may assign the clients to other individuals. Also, your supervisor may not allow you to engage in research activities if you are not prepared to do so. You must be well prepared to work with your clients in your clinical and research assignments. As part of your preparation, you must acquire and organize information about typical and disordered communication, methods of assessment and treatment, various diagnostic and therapeutic materials, and all clinical procedures, including the Code of Ethics.

Equipment

Being well prepared includes using correct equipment that is in good working order. In your academic and clinical training you will learn to perform various activities to ensure your research or clinical equipment is working properly. When using such equipment as augmentative communication devices, audiometers, or auditory feedback devices, it is important that you perform any preparatory activities before your session with your clients.

Principle of Ethics III

> Individuals shall honor their responsibility to the public by promoting public understanding of the professions, by supporting the development of services designed to fulfill the unmet needs of the public, and by providing accurate information in all communications involving any aspect of the professions, including dissemination of research findings and scholarly activities.

Accurately represent your services, products, and profession. Principle III instructs that speech-language pathologists must not inaccurately portray their ability, education, credentials, or experience. Also, the clinicians should not portray research evidence inaccurately. Statements regarding services or products must be accurate. Misrepresentation of services or products is clearly unethical. All information provided to the public should be clear and accurate. Advertising is appropriate but only when it is not misleading and complies with contemporary professional standards.

Directly related to accurate representation at the university training program is the need for clients to fully understand that students in the program provide services. This information is given to clients who contact the speech and hearing clinic to inquire about available services. The clients also are told about the clinic schedule and fees. Individuals who want to find other services are referred to qualified speech-language pathologists in the locality.

Adhering to the rules of Principle III is fairly simple. Be truthful.

Principle of Ethics IV

> Individuals shall honor their responsibilities to the professions and their relationships with colleagues, students, and members of allied professions. Individuals shall uphold the dignity and autonomy of the professions, maintain harmonious interprofessional and intraprofessional relationships, and accept the professions' self-imposed standards.

Effective professional relationships are important. As a speech-language pathologist you represent the entire profession. In providing optimal client service, you may interact with various professionals. These professionals may be other speech-language pathologists or individuals in allied professions. ASHA recognizes the importance of effective professional relationships by addressing them in the Code of Ethics. In certain instances you will be expected to model appropriate professional behavior; in other instances you may be required to regulate others' professional behavior.

Supervisor Responsibility

The Code of Ethics holds supervisors responsible for individuals working under their direction. In the university training program, your supervisors are responsible for ensuring your behavior is professionally appropriate. As you now know, there are many aspects to professionally appropriate behavior, including adequately preparing for clinical sessions, protecting client confidentiality, maintaining effective working relationships with other professionals, and so on. In your clinical assignments your supervisors will be evaluating your professionalism as well as your technical and academic skills.

Assigning Credit

The Code of Ethics directs that credit (or recognition) be proportionally given to individuals who have contributed to a written work, including research and clinical reports. Your reports submitted for academic or clinical coursework must contain references and credit other individuals involved in the work. You should learn to paraphrase research literature in your own words and, when quoting an author, you should know how to give credit—avoid plagiarism. If you and another student collaborate in evaluating a client and writing the assessment report, both of you should sign the report. (Your supervisor must also sign the report.) If you are reporting information described in a different clinical report, the name of that clinician and the date of the report should be noted.

Professional Judgment

Regardless of who your supervisor, employer, or referral source is, you must always use your own professional judgment in making clinical decisions. For example, as a student clinician and, later, as a professional, you routinely will determine which clients need and could benefit from speech-language pathology services. Even though there may be economic issues to consider, your decision on service delivery must be based on clinical data. Do not let other individuals' priorities cloud your professional judgment. As you begin your clinical practicum, clearly evaluate not only what your clinical service plan is but also what the rationale behind the plan is. This will help you begin to develop your own problem-solving skills.

Maintaining Professional Demeanor

The code prohibits any behavior that adversely reflects on the profession. As you know, many of these behaviors are specified in the various Rules of Ethics. Expressly prohibited are dishonesty, deceit, fraud, and sexual harassment. In addition, the code prohibits sexual activities between clinician and client or supervisor and student. Be conscious of what words you use and how you use them. Also, be aware of your actions and how others may interpret them. Remember that others may misinterpret certain words or actions innocently made, and you do not want to be accused of behaving inappropriately.

Upholding the Standards of the Profession

Individuals must comply freely with the standards of the professions, in this case, the standards ASHA suggests in its Code of Ethics and other guidelines. In addition to individually upholding the code, clinicians who believe that another ASHA member has violated the Code of Ethics must report the violation to the *Board of Ethics*. However, the student clinician reports such incidents to the clinical supervisor. The clinical supervisor, the clinic director, and the department chair will decide on what action might be taken.

So far, we have highlighted the major sections of the Code of Ethics with which student clinicians may commonly be involved. The code also contains additional rules. Read the Code of Ethics in Appendix D. Then determine which of the following situations would involve a violation of the Code of Ethics.

What Would Be an Ethical Way to Handle Each Situation?

1. You were busy studying for midterm exams and "just didn't have enough time" to completely prepare for your clinical session. What would you do?

2. You are beginning your second year of graduate school. A speech-language pathologist in private practice telephones and asks you to work as an aide. How would you reply? Are there any specific requirements you would need to comply with to be employed as a speech aide? Could you earn clinical clock hours? Could you perform other clinical services?

3. The mother of one of your clients contacts you and asks if you would be available to tutor her child. How would you respond?

4. A clinical supervisor allows students who were continually ill-prepared for their clinical assignments to continue in clinical practicum. Is the supervisor acting unethically?

5. You are working with a client who also is receiving speech-language services at another facility. You do not agree with the type of treatment being provided by the other speech-language pathologist. What would you do?

(continues)

6. Your supervisor suggested that you use certain treatment procedures with one of your clients. You were unsure of how to implement the procedures but could not get to school during your supervisor's office hours to discuss the procedures. You decided to work with your client anyway, because if you do something wrong, your supervisor will see it and come to help you. Is this an ethical violation or a commonsense solution?

7. A man you have been working with for 2 months tells you that he just tested positive for human immunodeficiency virus (HIV) infection. He wants to continue treatment but does not want anyone to know about his medical history except you. Do you need to add this information into your report or do you need to maintain the client's right to privacy?

8. You have the opportunity to participate in a research project related to adult dysarthria. You have not yet had coursework in this area but have observed various clinic sessions for clients with dysarthria. What factors would determine if you could work with clients as part of this research project?

9. You feel overwhelmed by your coursework and it is almost time for you to take your comprehensive exams. You have 4 more weeks at your medical internship but feel that you have pretty much learned everything you need to know to work in that setting. At the last minute you call in sick. Later you ask your supervisor if you can miss a few days so you can catch up on your studying. Is this unethical behavior or just a reflection of the stress of being a graduate student?

10. You are completing your school internship. Your supervisor seems to have much confidence in your skills and tells you to "just go and work with the students." The supervisor is always available to answer questions but no longer observes you or the students with whom you work. What, if anything, would you do?

Other Codes and Regulations

Health Insurance Portability and Accountability Act (HIPAA)

Client confidentiality, privacy, and welfare are extensively discussed in ASHA's Code of Ethics as well as other ASHA documents. In addition, the federal government's Department of Health and Human Services (HHS) developed standards intended to protect client privacy and to improve the efficiency and effectiveness of the health care system. These standards were adopted under the HIPAA. HIPAA required that all health care providers, including speech–language pathologists and audiologists, who engage in electronic transactions involving health information be in compliance with the standards. In your medical internship, you will hear much about HIPAA, and your information reporting will be guided by its standards. Even in such nonmedical settings as the public schools, your practice will be influenced by HIPPA standards. For example, you may have to request a hospital report that was done for one of your students. To obtain this information, the hospital will require you to adhere to their HIPAA standards for disclosure of patient information. Therefore, it is important that you have a general understanding of certain HIPAA regulations.

Basically, compliance with HIPAA standards for patient and client privacy is commonsense. Similar to the guidance provided by ASHA, you want to do everything you can to protect patient privacy. However, under HIPAA, if you carelessly or purposely violate the regulations, there could be a criminal penalty.

> **Protected health information (PHI)** is a term used to describe any health information that is created or received by the health care provider; relates to the past, present, or future physical or mental health diagnosis, treatment, or payment; and can or does identify the individual. As the term implies, *Individually Identifiable Health Information* (IIHI) simply defines PHI. Both of these terms refer to such communications as e-mail, telephone conversations, exchange of insurance information, and other written and oral communications.

Except in cases of protecting the public interest (including abuse, neglect, or domestic violence), before you can disclose any PHI for treatment, payment, or health care operations, your patient must give his or her consent. In addition, patients have the right to see their medical records and make corrections to the records. Patients have the right to receive advance notice of disclosure policies and to obtain a history of who, if anyone, has had access to their records.

To maintain patient privacy, comply with the rules outlined earlier in this chapter. Also, adhere to specific rules at your internship site. Your site will provide specific guidelines regarding any required patient notice and consent forms, accessing and storing patient charts, and disposal of any confidential information.

HIPAA also provided guidelines regarding **Electronic Data Interchange (EDI).** EDI refers to any electronic transaction that happens between a provider and an agency such as a hospital or third-party payer. HIPAA requires that providers, hospitals, and third-party payers use the same terminology with EDI. Your internship site will provide you with any needed information related to EDI and various codes.

Scope of Practice

ASHA has outlined service delivery for professionals in communicative disorders through its scope of practice statement (American Speech-Language-Hearing Association, 2007a) and its preferred practice patterns statement (American

Speech-Language-Hearing Association, 2008. The scope of practice statement describes professional activities and defines which professionals may perform those activities. For example, speech-language pathologists may not perform audiological evaluations; however, they may perform pure-tone air conduction hearing screenings and tympanometry screenings as part of a complete evaluation of a client's communicative performance and to determine if the client should be referred for additional audiological evaluation and treatment. Remember that you must adhere to the scope of practice defined under your state's license or credentialing law. If an activity is approved (or not explicitly prohibited) in ASHA's scope of practice statement, but prohibited under your state law, you cannot legally perform that activity in your state. Refer to ASHA's Web site (www.asha.org) for a copy of the Scope of Practice in Speech-Language Pathology.

Preferred Practice Patterns

In addition to identifying what types of services specific professionals may provide, ASHA's preferred practice patterns statement also outlines clinical processes, clinical indicators, equipment specifications, expected outcomes, safety and health precautions, documentation, and related references. As with the Code of Ethics, one of the guiding principles of the preferred practice patterns is the importance of client welfare. Refer to the preferred practice patterns as an introduction to your research when gathering new information about each of your clients.

Reporting Suspected Child Abuse

Although students should first assume that all client information is confidential, there are specific state laws governing disclosure of information to protect the well-being of a client or of the public. A clear example is a clinician's responsibility to report suspected child abuse. Child abuse can include physical, emotional, or sexual abuse. Neglect and child endangerment can also be included in the category of child abuse.

Based on federal laws and regulations, states have established laws regulating the reporting of suspected child abuse. The reporting requirements differ across states. The definition of child abuse, the age range of victims, and the agency to whom the suspected abuse is reported vary also from state to state. Nevertheless, suspected child abuse must be reported. In most states, the individual suspecting the abuse must report it. The individual cannot leave the reporting to the agency he or she works for. Child abuse is not always visible or easily identified. Most children are very active and consequently suffer various accidental scrapes, bruises, and broken bones. You must not jump to conclusions, but you must not disregard signs of possible child abuse. If a child arrives with a bump, bruise, bite, burn, or broken bone, you may want to ask how it happened. If you have a child who repeatedly arrives with various injuries, report it to your clinical supervisor. Again, this may not be a case of child abuse, but your supervisor can investigate further or take other necessary action.

Signs of Possible Child Abuse

1. Burns, broken bones, bruises, bites, and cigarette burns. These are indicators of physical abuse.

2. Scratches or bruises on areas of the body other than elbows, knees, or shins. These may be indicators of child abuse, rather than those of an active child.

3. Bilateral injuries.

4. Inadequate or inappropriate clothing. Examples may include the child who wears sandals in the winter or a warm jacket during hot summer months. Be aware of different cultural influences in evaluating this category. In some cultures, certain items of clothing such as sandals (without socks) are worn throughout the year regardless of the outside temperature.

5. Unexplained injuries.

6. Frequent school absences when there is no record of a serious illness.

7. Behavioral difficulties. These may include lack of trust, depression, hostility, compulsive behavior, lethargy, or withdrawal.

8. Overly sophisticated sexual knowledge.

9. Seductive behaviors with peers and adults.

10. Dirty or malnourished. These are indicators of neglect and may be accompanied by unmet dental and medical needs. (Burke, 1990)

When you suspect child abuse, inform your supervisor immediately. Each clinical site will have its reporting procedure. You should know these procedures and follow them when necessary.

Dress Code

When people first meet you, they judge you by your appearance and demeanor. With clients, you must quickly establish a degree of trust through your professional demeanor, attire, and general appearance. A neat appearance and appropriate clothing will positively influence your clients' first impressions of you.

There is no universal dress code that you must follow in all practicum sites. However, all clinics have guidelines for what they consider appropriate professional attire. Contrary to some beliefs, you are not expected to go out and purchase an entirely new wardrobe. Typically, shorts, jeans, sandals, and strapless dresses are not considered appropriate for professional clothing.

If you have a question as to whether something is appropriate to wear, do not wear it.

At off-campus practicum sites, dress may be more or less formal than at the university clinic. If no information is offered, ask your off-campus supervisor about the dress code or guidelines at the site. Occasionally, a supervisor will say that "Anything is okay to wear," while the supervisor and the rest of the staff dress very formally. In this case, it is best to dress as similarly to the staff as possible. In all cases, dressing with a view to appearing professional is desirable.

Being a student during certain times of the day to being a clinician at other times of the day can be a difficult mental transition. Donning professional dress helps you make that transition. It also prompts the client to regard you more as a professional person and less as a student.

Professional Liability

Although you are a student in training, you still provide direct client services when you engage in clinical practicum. You will be expected to provide a certain standard of care and you will be held responsible for your actions. You may be liable for any inappropriate or negligent service that results in damage or harm to a client. ASHA has published a technical report on professional liability and risk management (American Speech-Language-Hearing Association, 1994a). Read this report early in your clinical practicum.

All student clinicians should have liability insurance before beginning their clinical practicum. You can obtain information from your clinic office regarding the procedures for obtaining liability insurance. In some locations, students pay for insurance directly to the university. In other locations, students are required to independently purchase insurance and then provide the proof of coverage.

Insurance typically is purchased on an annual basis. A low-cost group insurance is available for students and professional practitioners. Information can be obtained at your clinic or by contacting ASHA.

To avoid any suspicion of negligence or malpractice, you must closely follow the ASHA Code of Ethics, comply with all clinic procedures, and maintain appropriate communications with your supervisor. You also should be knowledgeable in current standards of care for the disorders you treat. As you know, periodically ASHA publishes position statements and guidelines. These documents specify ASHA's official position on controversial clinical or scientific issues, recommend appropriate courses of professional actions, and summarize state-of-the-art information on selected issues. Keep yourself current on these position statements and guidelines.

Health and Safety Precautions

Because you will be working closely with people, you must follow certain health and safety precautions. These precautions help provide protection for you and your clients from various communicable diseases or injuries.

Because you work with many different individuals, you are at a greater risk for exposure to a communicable disease than, for instance, a computer programmer might be. Also, you will work with certain clients who are very susceptible to infection, such as patients in the NICU, elderly patients, and critically ill patients. Many sites follow universal health care precautions. Under universal precautions everyone (patients and professionals) is considered a risk for infection (Kemp, Roeser, Pearson, & Ballachanda, 1995). Materials that require universal precautions include blood, semen, vaginal secretions, cerebrospinal fluid, synovial fluid, pleural fluid, any body fluid with visible blood, any unidentifiable body fluid, and saliva from dental fluid.

Each practicum site may have different health and safety regulations. You must follow the regulations of your clinical assignment.

General Health Procedures

1. *Get a rubella vaccination.* All individuals should have a rubella vaccination. It is required only one time. Rubella, also known as German measles, is a viral disease often accompanied by a fever and a rash. Although children who contract rubella rarely have any complications, the virus active in a pregnant woman can be a teratogen to a developing fetus, with the possibility of causing intrauterine death, spontaneous abortion, or many types of congenital defects (Heymann, 2004).

2. *Get a mumps vaccination.* Mumps is a viral disease. It is accompanied by fever and tenderness and swelling of one or more of the salivary glands. There is no clear evidence linking mumps during pregnancy with congenital malformations. However, because of the incidence of testicular mumps in the male population, male health care providers often are advised or required to have a mumps vaccination. The frequency of mumps has decreased since common early childhood immunization has become available; however, an increase in mumps was reported in the United States in both 1986 and 1987 (Heymann, 2004).

3. *Get a hepatitis B vaccination.* Like the mumps vaccination, this vaccination is not always required but is recommended. Hepatitis B is a form of viral hepatitis and can be transmitted through contaminated blood, needles, or instruments. Onset is rapid and infection can cause severe liver damage.

4. *Have a tuberculin skin test (purified protein derivative [PPD]).* Tuberculosis is an infectious mycobacterial disease. Generally, it has decreased in occurrence in developed countries but has stabilized or increased in frequency in the population of persons testing positive for HIV infection. Tuberculosis most often involves the lungs and, if left untreated, can result in death or other serious complications. The initial infection to tuberculosis

(continues)

often is not recognized. This is one of the reasons students, who are in close contact with a variety of individuals in their clinical experiences, are required to have a tuberculin skin test on a regular basis. Clinics may require a skin test annually. Public schools often require the skin test less frequently, because the incidence of tuberculosis is less in children and increases in the aging population (Heymann, 2004).

5. *Protect any wounds or skin lesions.* Use a waterproof dressing or gloves, or both, to protect any wounds, sores, or skin abrasions you may have.

6. *Use gloves.* Wear latex gloves when performing oral exams, during any invasive procedure of the oral cavity (such as dysphagia assessment or treatment), or during any contact with blood or bodily fluids with visible blood (American Speech-Language-Hearing Association Committee on Quality Assurance, 1990). To protect the client against infection, do not touch your pencil, furniture, or other unsanitized objects when wearing gloves.

7. *Wash your hands after removing latex gloves.* Your hands may become contaminated as you remove your gloves. Therefore, be sure to wash your hands after removing gloves.

8. *Wash your hands before and after working with a client.* Hand washing is considered one of the best ways to prevent the spread of disease. In addition, avoid touching your hands to your mouth, eyes, or nose when working with your clients.

9. *If necessary, wear eye and mouth protection.* If you are working with a client and blood, saliva, or other bodily fluid splashing is possible, you may need to wear eye goggles and a mouth mask (Golper, 1998).

10. *Disinfect or sterilize equipment.* Follow your practicum site's procedures regarding sterilization and disinfection of equipment. Disinfection can be performed using 1:100 solution of household bleach (sodium hypochlorite) to water (American Speech-Language-Hearing Association, 1989a). Commercial disinfectant also is available. McMillan and Willette (1988) advise that environmental surfaces such as tables, tape recorders, and audiometers be disinfected prior to and following each client contact. However, more recent information suggests that "equipment not contaminated by blood or bodily fluids containing visible signs of blood need not be cleaned after each use" (American Speech-Language-Hearing Association, 1989a).

11. *Use disposable materials.* Whenever possible use disposable materials. After using these materials, follow your clinical practicum site's guidelines regarding disposal of used items.

12. *Stay home if you are ill.* If you are ill, cancel your clinical appointments. You probably will not be very effective as a clinician anyway and may transmit your illness to your client.

13. *Treat the blood of all patients as potentially contagious.* Although it is important to be aware and assess the risk of exposure with each of your patients, you cannot determine the need for infection control based on a patient's case history. Remember that the use of universal health care precautions protect you and your patient.

14. *Be informed about communicable diseases.* There are many diseases you could be exposed to. However, knowledge about the transmission and prevention of the disease is one of the first steps in defense against the disease. For obvious reasons, the spread of AIDS/HIV infection currently is a major health concern (American Speech-Language-Hearing Association, 1989a; McMillan & Willette, 1988). Acquired immune deficiency syndrome (AIDS) is considered the last clinical stage of HIV infection. Present information indicates that transmission is by sexual exposure and exposure to blood or tissue. Although progress is being reported in the drug treatment for HIV infection, there is no known cure for AIDS (Heymann, 2004).

Depending on the work environment, there are other diseases of which the speech-language pathologist should be aware. However, this chapter cannot outline all possible diseases to which one may be exposed. It is hoped that students will seriously consider the potential for exposure to communicable diseases and the potential for exposing others to infections—both the inconvenient types as well as the life-threatening ones—and closely follow all disease control procedures established at clinical practicum sites.

In addition to following health care precautions, you will help decrease the chance of injury to the client by following some basic safety rules.

Safety Fundamentals

1. *Make sure the clinic area is clean and orderly.* This will help avoid such accidents as tripping over small items left on the floor.

2. *Do not leave children unattended in the clinic.* Children who are left without supervision may cause mischief or injury to themselves and others. They may swallow small objects, play with electrical outlets, pull furniture over, or fall.

(continues)

3. *Do not let children stand on tables or chairs.* If, for some reason, you want a child to stand on a table or chair, hold him or her with at least one hand.

4. *Check with the parent before giving food.* Occasionally, you may want to use food in your treatment program. Before doing so make sure you have the parent's approval and that the child does not have any food allergies, is not on a restricted diet, or does not have swallowing difficulties. If you are working with an adult who is under the care of a spouse or caregiver, check with that person before giving your client food.

5. *Make sure clients who are in wheelchairs lock their brakes.* If they do not do so automatically, advise them to lock their brakes. If they cannot do so independently, lock their brakes for them.

6. *Before pushing clients who are in wheelchairs, make sure their feet are in the footrests or lifted off the ground.* Sometimes clients use their feet to propel their wheelchair and end up resting their feet on the ground. You need to be aware of where your client's feet are so that they do not inadvertently get caught under the wheelchair as it is moved forward.

7. *Do not allow smoking in the clinic area.* Typically, clinic areas are non-smoking areas. If you see a client or a client's family member smoking in a nonsmoking area, politely tell them of the nonsmoking policy at your clinic.

8. *Know where the fire extinguisher is.* In addition, it is important to know how the fire extinguisher works. If there is an emergency, you will not have time to read the instructions on the canister.

9. *Locate the nearest emergency telephone.* Most sites will have a telephone or intercom available for emergency communications.

10. *Adhere to safety procedures at your site.* As you know, each practicum site may have different safety precautions. Do not second guess these. Know and follow all rules established at your practicum setting.

Client Bill of Rights

By now it is obvious that there are many rules governing your behavior for the protection of the profession and your clients. Under these rules, you have certain obligations to your clients, and your clients have certain implied rights. However, ASHA thought that implied client rights were not sufficient. ASHA's Task Force on Protection of Clients' Rights (ASHA, 1994b) published a technical report in which the Model Bill of Rights for People Receiving Audiology or Speech-Language Pathology Services was outlined and discussed. This is a generic document encompassing both children and adults across all service delivery settings. It applies to both speech-language pathology and audiology services and was designed to be easily understandable to the consumer. Many of the principles advocated in the Bill of Rights reflect the rules in the Code of Ethics. For example, one of the rights is "that services be provided without regard to race or ethnicity, gender, age, religion, national origin, sexual orientation, or disability" (p. 61). Before working as a student clinician, read this Bill of Rights.

In abiding by the Code of Ethics and state and federal laws, you may occasionally encounter guidelines that could be interpreted in different ways. In all such cases, you must consider the well-being of your clients as the most important basis on which to make decisions. Your supervisor or clinic director will be there to help you make appropriate and ethical decisions. ASHA, your state speech-language-hearing association, and your state licensure agency also are important institutions that help resolve professional questions.

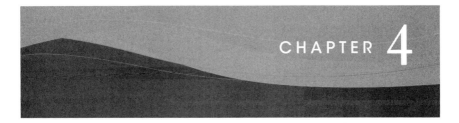

CHAPTER 4

The Clinical Supervisor and the Student Clinician

Chapter Outline

· ·

- The Role of the Clinical Supervisor
- Off-Campus Clinical Supervision
- Responsibilities of the Student Clinician

An essential component to the success of your clinical practicum as a beneficial learning experience is the interaction between you and your supervisor. As you may expect, your clinical practicum in speech-language pathology is a three-way process involving you, your supervisor, and your client. Your supervisor is your clinical mentor. In many ways, your supervisor helps you acquire the knowledge and skills necessary to become an independent and competent clinician who can provide quality service for clients. The effectiveness of your practicum experience depends, partly, on the relationship developed between you and your supervisor. Each of you has different roles and responsibilities in the development of your clinical skills.

The Role of the Clinical Supervisor

· ·

Training student clinicians while ensuring quality clinical service to clients is the primary role of the clinical supervisor. In a sense, the student clinicians are the supervisor's clients. It is a supervisor's responsibility to maximize students' learning opportunities.

95

Also, the supervisor must fulfill other managerial or academic obligations. Many university clinics have a staff of full-time supervisors who do little or no classroom teaching. Many other university clinics have academic faculty members supervising clinical practicum. Supervisors also may be assigned a variety of administrative duties.

It is important that a student clinician understand the scope of a supervisor's main responsibilities and some of the limitations to avoid misunderstandings or incorrect expectations. It is equally important that a clinical supervisor be aware of a student clinician's prior experience and clearly defines practicum guidelines and expectations.

What to Expect From Your Clinical Supervisor

The supervisor is your clinical mentor. He or she facilitates your practicum experience. This facilitation includes direct teaching of clinical methods, self-evaluation, clinical analysis, and problem-solving skills. ASHA has developed various regulations and guidelines on supervision (American Speech-Language-Hearing Association 2008b, 2008c, 2008d). ASHA's Special Interest Division II focuses specifically on administration and supervision, and several books have been written on clinical supervision. ASHA's Ad Hoc Committee on Supervision in Speech-Language Pathology developed a *Knowledge and Skills* report to reflect the importance of effective supervision and to outline the information, understanding, and abilities needed to provide supervision in speech-language pathology (American Speech-Language-Hearing Association, 2008d). The supervisor's required knowledge and skills were defined under 11 core elements:

1. Preparation for the supervisory experience

2. Interpersonal communication and the supervisor-supervisee relationship

3. Development of the supervisee's critical-thinking and problem-solving skills

4. Development of the supervisee's clinical competence in assessment

5. Development of the supervisee's clinical competence in intervention

6. Supervisory conferences or meetings of clinical teaching teams

7. Evaluating the growth of the supervisee both as a clinician and as a professional

8. Diversity (ability, race, ethnicity, gender, age, culture, language, class, experience, and education)

9. Development and maintenance of clinical and supervisory documentation

10. Ethical, regulatory, and legal requirements

11. Principles of mentoring

Much of this information has been integrated into the following sections, providing an overview of what student clinicians can expect from their supervisors.

Tasks of Supervision

Although updated and expanded models of supervisory competencies and the role of supervisors across settings have been developed, the thirteen tasks of the clinical supervisor identified by ASHA in 1985 (American Speech-Language-Hearing Association, 1985a) continue to be central duties of the clinical practicum supervisor.

1. Establishing and maintaining an effective working relationship with the supervisee

2. Assisting the supervisee in developing clinical goals and objectives

3. Assisting the supervisee in developing and refining assessment skills

4. Assisting the supervisee in developing and refining clinical management skills

5. Demonstrating for and participating with the supervisee in the clinical process

6. Assisting the supervisee in observing and analyzing assessment and treatment sessions

7. Assisting the supervisee in the development and maintenance of clinical and supervisory records

8. Interacting with the supervisee in planning, executing, and analyzing supervisory conferences

9. Assisting the supervisee in evaluation of clinical performance

10. Assisting the supervisee in developing skills of verbal reporting, writing, and editing

11. Sharing information regarding ethical, legal, regulatory and reimbursement aspects of the profession

12. Modeling and facilitating professional conduct

13. Demonstrating research skills in the clinical or supervisory process.

Develop and Maintain Effective Communication

In preparation for the supervisory experience, it is important that you and your clinical supervisor *establish a cooperative working relationship* to enhance your clinical practicum experience and ensure the delivery of quality services. *Supervisors know the importance of the supervisor-supervisee relationship and of effective communication.* Some clinical supervisors are available before, during, and after clinic sessions to discuss issues and questions with you. Other clinical supervisors assign specific conference times. It is the responsibility of the clinical supervisor to provide a forum for appropriate and effective communication between supervisor and student clinician. However, you share in this responsibility. In truth, you may be initially intimidated by your first clinical supervisor. To complicate matters, because of other obligations, the clinical supervisor may not always be readily available to you. Therefore, it is important to remember that (1) your supervisor is available to answer questions; (2) your supervisor is not a mind reader; and (3) that there may be times when you need to be assertive in seeking advice. Your supervisor will try *to match his or her style of supervision to your knowledge and skill level.* If you are a beginning student clinician, your supervisor may provide more direct instruction; as a more advanced clinician, your supervisor may demand that you do more independent research and *self-reflection* to advance your skills. Regardless of the level of supervision provided, your supervisor will do the following:

- Help you understand the supervisory process and your responsibilities within that role

- Understand your level of experience with the types of clients that you are assigned and provide an appropriate supervisory style based on these variables

- Objectively collect and analyze data to assist you with your acquisition of clinical knowledge and skills

Provide Guidelines of Practicum Requirements

Initially, your clinical supervisor will discuss the *organization of your clinical practicum* with you. He or she will outline expectations for your performance and requirements of your practicum assignment. For example, your supervisor will explain how and when you will be evaluated and on what basis. In addition to requirements of clinical performance, your supervisor will discuss scheduling, attendance, submission of written reports, and mandatory clinical meetings. *Legal and ethical guidelines* related to each practicum experience will be provided.

Your supervisor should encourage you to discuss any questions or concerns you may have at the beginning of your clinical assignment or as your practicum progresses. As you continue your practicum, issues related to future practicum assignments or requirements may arise. If your clinical supervisor is unavailable or unable to answer your questions (possibly because the supervisor is a part-time member of the university staff), your clinic director or advisor should be able to assist you.

Provide Consistent Feedback

Your clinical supervisor will provide consistent feedback on your clinical performance; of course, different supervisors have different supervisory styles. One supervisor may give written feedback at the end of each session. Another supervisor may provide verbal feedback or modeling during a session and written feedback after the session. A different supervisor might never interrupt a session unless the well-being of the client is jeopardized. At the beginning of your practicum assignment, your supervisor will discuss the type of feedback he or she will provide.

To maximize learning, your supervisor may arrange client staffing, role playing, or other forms of clinical teaching sessions. These sessions may be held on a regular or intermittent basis and before, during, or after clinical practicum sessions. Your supervisor arranges these added learning experiences for your benefit. It is important that you take them seriously by being prepared and an active participant.

Informative feedback may take the form of identifying a behavior that you need to change. Just as it is not advised to always simply give your clients such general verbal reinforcement as "good job," it is not useful for you to simply hear from your supervisor, "good session." Therefore, your supervisor will provide you with *objective feedback* that includes specific behaviors that you demonstrated (or did not demonstrate) during the session. For example, beginning clinicians tend to use questions instead of statements: "Can you say /r/?" versus "Say /r/." To give objective feedback, the inappropriate use of questions may be charted by the supervisor. Then your supervisor would share these data with you and ask you to eliminate or decrease the use of such questions by a certain amount. Following up on this communication, your supervisor would again observe a clinical session and chart your use of the question, "Can you say /r/?"

If you think that you are not receiving sufficient feedback or that the feedback is unclear, discuss this with your clinical supervisor. Your supervisor may believe that you understand the feedback that has been given, and if you do not make appropriate changes, your supervisor may think you are disregarding his or her recommendations. Remember, feedback does not necessarily imply negative criticism. It is a teaching method that you will frequently use with your clients.

Assist in Planning Clinical Objectives

Typically, your supervisor will direct you to review your clients' charts or case histories and *develop an assessment or treatment plan* for your first session with your clients. Before your initial meeting with your clients, your supervisor will review these plans with you. The less clinical experience you have had, the more assistance your clinical supervisor will expect you to need.

Your supervisor will help you learn to *critically evaluate* your clients' speech and language behaviors and learn to *develop measurable clinical objectives*. Each practicum site will have different ways of writing appropriate objectives. For example, in the school setting, you will write objectives related to your students' educational performance. In the hospital setting, you may write objectives related to your patients' ability to successfully complete such daily living activities as stating when they want something to eat. Your supervisor also will help you establish priorities for treatment objectives. Chapter 7 describes some general guidelines for selecting target behaviors. Note, however, that your clinical supervisor must approve all major clinical decisions, including what to teach your clients and how.

Your supervisor also may identify or help you *identify personal objectives* for you to achieve. You may be asked to describe areas of professional growth and how you plan to achieve it. For example, your supervisor may suggest that you need more information related to the nonverbal child, or you may identify your own weakness in that area when assigned such a child as a client. To supplement your knowledge in this area, your supervisor might direct you to specific resources or advise you to research the subject area and report your findings to him or her.

Assist in Developing Diagnostic Skills and Assessment Strategies

Two of your supervisor's key duties are to assist you in *developing clinical competence in assessment and intervention*. Your supervisor will guide you in understanding and using *best practices based on current research* for assessment and intervention with your clients; in addition, he or she instructs you on various *interpersonal and counseling skills*.

Your clinical supervisor will observe a sufficient amount of your clinical sessions to assist you with your assessments. You will get feedback on your *selection, administration, and interpretation* of tests. Your supervisor may suggest certain tests or test administration sequences. It is your responsibility to learn each test before you attempt to administer it to a client. To ensure the test is appropriate for your client, you should carefully read the test manual. If possible, practice using the test by administering it to friends. After you have familiarized yourself with a test and practiced administering it, your supervisor will give you additional help if needed. For example, your supervisor may model both general and specific test administration procedures. Your supervisor also will advise you regarding *informal observation procedures* and client-specific assessment procedures, and assist you in integrating results of standardized tests and nonstandardized observations.

Demonstrate a Variety of Clinical Skills

Beginning student clinicians sometimes are unsure of how to implement the myriad of treatment techniques and principles about which they have read and observed. For example, if you exhibit difficulty with effectively reinforcing a desired behavior, your *supervisor will demonstrate* the appropriate strategy. Some clinical supervisors prefer to actually demonstrate with a specific client during treatment sessions. Other supervisors do not interrupt sessions, but may demonstrate a technique after a session and expect you to implement it the following session. Often, supervisors will inform you in advance if they intend to demonstrate a specific technique during a clinical session. You should request demonstration of certain procedures when you do not clearly understand your supervisor's instructions.

Facilitate Development of Client Management Skills

After you develop your treatment goals, you must determine a progression of treatment. Your supervisor will assist you in *evaluating the needs of your client*, including such variables as determining the initial level of treatment, developing intervention strategies, establishing the performance criteria for each level, and accurately charting treatment results. Your supervisor will encourage you to evaluate the effectiveness of your clinic sessions and determine what, if any, changes should be made in your treatment goals or strategies.

In evaluating each of your sessions, it is necessary for you and your supervisor to have accurate information on your clients' performance. You will discover that a set method of charting responses will not be appropriate across all clients and that you may need to experiment with different methods. Your supervisor will suggest different ways to maintain accurate records.

In addition to analyzing client performance, you may expect your supervisor to *require you to analyze your own behaviors* and how they affect client responses. One way your supervisor may assist you in evaluating your performance is by videotaping clinical sessions. You may be required to watch the video independently or jointly with your supervisor. Your supervisor also may chart some of your clinical behaviors (such as your use of positive feedback or method of evoking responses) to show you what you do.

Describe Record-Keeping Requirements

As you know, accountability and documentation are important components of clinical service delivery. Certain record-keeping requirements are common across settings and other requirements may be unique to individual sites. Regardless of the documentation method, closely adhere to the requirements. Whether your client is able to continue treatment or whether your site receives payment for services provided are only two reasons why appropriate record keeping is essential. Your supervisor will *describe the documentation and record-keeping requirements* specific to your setting. The methods utilized to ensure confidentiality of clinical records also will be outlined and monitored by your clinical supervisor.

Encourage Independent Problem Solving and Self-Analysis

The importance of the clinical supervisor in providing direct guidance and assistance to student clinicians should not be minimized. Nonetheless, an important role of clinical supervisors is to *teach clinicians independent problem-solving skills and critical self-analysis*. Regardless of the number of practicum hours completed, you still will encounter clients exhibiting communicative disorders with which you have had little or no experience. Also, although clients with the same diagnoses may exhibit similar communicative performance, each client will have unique problems and behaviors. However, if you have developed the ability to critically analyze both your clients' behaviors as well as your own clinical behaviors, you will be able to make appropriate clinical decisions in a variety of clinical situations. This is not to suggest that each clinician is, or even should be, highly qualified to work with every type of speech and language disorder. Clinicians who specialize can better serve specific clients. However, the clinical decision-making process includes knowing when it is necessary to seek additional information or to refer clients to other speech-language pathologists or different professionals.

Your supervisor will provide guidance based on your level of clinical experience. At each level of your practicum experience, your supervisor will involve you in the problem-solving and analysis process. The supervisor will make suggestions but will expect you to expand on those suggestions and to generalize ideas across clients and settings. Your supervisor also will expect you to seek information, rather than just waiting to receive instruction or direction. As you progress in your practicum, your supervisor, although continuing to monitor your performance, will provide less and less assistance with decision making and allow you to perform with increasing independence.

Help Develop Verbal and Written Skills

Your supervisor will facilitate the development of your verbal and written reporting skills by providing you with opportunities for practicing both types of activities (Hegde, 2010). Content requirements and formats of clinical reports vary across supervisors and settings; therefore, your supervisor should provide you with an *outline of professional writing requirements* of your assignment. Also, to help guide you, your supervisor may provide you with samples of reports.

Although reporting styles may vary, the need to write clear, concise, and logical reports does not (Hegde, 2010). Your supervisor will *edit your clinical reports* or suggest specific changes. Do not be surprised if you must revise a report more than once. When your supervisor first edits your report, the most obvious problems may be noted. However, after these errors are corrected, more subtle problems may be observed, requiring you to revise your reports further.

Verbal reporting skills will be required at each of your practicum sites. For example, at the university clinic, you will need to share information with your clients and their family members. In the medical setting, you may be required to share information with clients' family members and various health professionals. In the educational setting, you will be required to share information with such people as clients' family members, teachers, family physicians, and psychologists. Therefore, your supervisor may require you to *practice your verbal reporting skills* during client staffing, consultation with other professionals, and sharing information with clients and their families. If you have little previous experience with verbal reporting, you might find it beneficial to write out the information you want to cover and practice presenting it aloud. It is also helpful to try to anticipate questions that might arise and prepare answers in advance.

Provide Current Resources

Information is changing rapidly in the field of communicative disorders. Experts continue to suggest new assessment and treatment methods. New instruments and technological devices also are developed frequently. Your supervisor will expect you to use current information, instruments, procedures, and technology and will assist you in locating them. The supervisor will *help you research current information* and use many campus resources, including the library, computer laboratories, writing clinics, and so forth. Much information is available on the Internet. For example, ASHA has made many of its position papers, guidelines, and other resources available through its Web site. *Before using material that you find on the Internet, be sure the information is accurate.* Only use information that you obtain from a reliable site that offers research-based scientific and scholarly information (such as PubMed,

ScienceDirect, ERIC, or asha.org) or find a second source that validates information you obtain from the Internet. Be critical of information offered in blogs and wiki entries that are often opinions of individuals; many are not written by experts. Before you begin clinical practicum, you will have begun to develop a library of various texts and journal articles. Although these texts and articles may be only 1 or 2 years old, by the time you begin clinical practicum, they may already be outdated. It is essential to routinely read your journals and maintain current information on a variety of subjects. ASHA encourages its members to update their clinical information through its continuing education program. Also, some state licensure laws and credential regulations require continuing education units.

Model and Demand Professional Behavior

Your supervisor will model the behavior expected of you. For example, your supervisor will be punctual, dress appropriately, protect client confidentiality by not talking about clients in public areas, and so on. Your supervisor will treat you as a professional and will expect to be treated as one. Regardless of your clinical practicum site, your supervisor will expect you to know and comply with ASHA's Code of Ethics. Your supervisor will outline the requirements of your clinical site, including the dress code, health regulations, and clinical practicum schedule. If you have any questions about the parameters of professional behavior for your site, ask your supervisor for clarification.

Evaluate Your Clinical Work

Your clinical supervisor also is an instructor who must evaluate your clinical work and assure that you are developing appropriate *knowledge and skills* to advance in your academic program and meet ASHA's requirements for certification. Every supervisor must strive to *make objective and constructive evaluation* of your clinical work. Although there may be times set aside for formal evaluations, every time you receive feedback from your supervisor, you will have received some level of evaluation as well. In conjunction with your clinical practicum, you may receive a letter grade or grade of credit/no credit. Your supervisor will follow your university's guidelines for *evaluation of student clinicians*, but most evaluations include areas such as knowledge of disorders, competence in administering tests and interpreting results, proficiency in developing and implementing treatment plans, readiness to implement and expand on supervisory suggestions, and so on. Many universities are using rating scales that help supervisors assess students' abilities and assist them in improving their clinical skills. Your performance may be compared in terms of accuracy, consistency, and need for supervisory guidance to an optimum clinical behavior called a *clinical competency*. If you have questions about your clinical practicum evaluation, discuss them with your clinical supervisor.

Help, Guide, and Support You

In addition to ensuring quality patient care, a primary responsibility of the clinical supervisor is to *provide appropriate training for the student clinician*. During training, sometimes it may be necessary for your supervisor to give you feedback that seems negative. However, your clinical supervisor's aim is for you to learn, so try not to feel that your supervisor is picking on you. As a conscientious student clinician, you can expect your supervisor to be there to help, guide, and support you. The supervisor will expect you to have confidence and trust in him or her. Your supervisor is not only your mentor, but also your advocate.

Off-Campus Clinical Supervision

Often the off-campus clinical supervisor is a professional employee of your practicum site. Off-campus clinical supervisors have their CCCs in speech-language pathology. Your university training director will have discussed ASHA's requirements for supervision and may have provided a general background of your experience level. However, off-campus clinical supervisors may or may not be fully familiar with your university's training program. Consequently, they may not act or hold the same expectations as the supervisors at the university clinic. As the following list shows, your off-campus supervisor will perform many of the same activities identified in the previous section.

What to Expect From Your Off-Campus Supervisor

- Develop and maintain effective communication
- Provide guidelines of the practicum requirements
- Provide ongoing feedback
- Assist in planning clinical goals
- Assist in developing diagnostic skills
- Demonstrate clinical methods
- Assist in developing client management skills
- Describe record-keeping requirements
- Encourage independent problem solving
- Facilitate development of reporting skills
- Provide current resources
- Model and demand professional behavior
- Evaluate your clinical work
- Help you and support you

However, you should not expect off-campus clinical supervisors to be exactly the same as the university clinical supervisors in performing all these and other duties.

Frequency of Supervision

At your off-campus site, the frequency of supervision may be different from what you are used to at on-campus clinical sites. The amount of supervision offered at off-campus sites may be more or less. Minimally, the *off-campus supervisors will meet ASHA's guidelines* for the type and frequency of supervision. However, at an off-campus site, you are expected to be able to work relatively independently, but you may be supervised more closely than when you were less experienced. This increased amount of supervision does not mean that the supervisor does not have much confidence in you. The off-campus supervisors may only have one student clinician to supervise; university clinic supervisors may supervise up to four clinicians at one time. In addition, in certain cases, you may be working with critically ill patients or providing a therapy that, if done incorrectly, could compromise the client's health. The off-campus site also may have additional supervisory requirements for compliance with insurance requirements.

Unique Aspects of Practicum Sites

Each of your practicum sites will offer you unique learning experiences and have requirements specific to that site. Your off-campus supervisor will let you know about the special components of clinical work in his or her setting. In the beginning, your off-campus supervisor may have to spend extra time in getting you familiarized with the special clinical populations served at the site and the unique clinical and administrative procedures to be followed. Your clinical supervisor may model certain techniques and give you samples of different documentation procedures.

Progress Toward Independence

Expect your supervisor to demand fairly independent performance from you. This sounds like a contradiction, based on the probability that you will receive greater one-to-one supervision than at the university clinic; however, it is not. Inherent in an internship placement is the assumption that you are fairly advanced and able to make independent judgments. Because of this, your clinical supervisor certainly will expect you to act relatively independently in planning assessment and treatment sessions, problem solving, researching additional information, and asking necessary questions.

Supervisor Expectations

Your off-campus clinical supervisors may have a general understanding of your clinical experience and academic coursework, but they probably will not know your specific academic background in detail. They may know what courses you have had but may not know the scope and orientation of those courses. Consequently, their expectations may be different from those of your supervisors at the university clinic who probably know the curriculum content and orientation of courses you have had and the level of your clinical experience. But the off-campus supervisors may not be familiar with the full details of the university's training program. The supervisors' expectations of you may be based on their general experiences with students of your background. Some supervisors may base expectations on their own educational experiences and the requirements they faced. This is not necessarily a disadvantage but something of which you should be aware.

Responsibilities of the Student Clinician

Student clinicians must fulfill numerous responsibilities to ensure a successful practicum experience for themselves and to provide effective services to their clients. In essence, though, student clinicians should (a) learn to assess, treat, counsel, and professionally work with their clients and their families and (b) show systematic progress in their learning of those professional skills.

Throughout your clinical practicum experiences, many of these responsibilities will remain unchanged as you progress in your practicum. However, the expectations of the clinical supervisor change. As you advance and gain experience, you will be expected to fulfill your clinical responsibilities with less guidance from your clinical supervisor. Although individual university departments may have additional requirements, the following sections provide a general overview of the student clinician's responsibilities.

Adhere to ASHA's Code of Ethics

As you know from Chapter 3, ASHA's Code of Ethics describes various acceptable professional behaviors. In all clinical practicum settings, abide by ASHA's Code of Ethics. It is your responsibility to be aware of the intent of the Code of Ethics and its various principles and rules. You do not want to jeopardize your career as a speech-language pathologist because you have violated the Code of Ethics.

Know ASHA Preferred Practice Patterns

The ASHA Task Force on Clinical Standards developed an extensive list of speech-language pathology and audiology procedures (American Speech-Language-Hearing Association, 2004b). The preferred practice patterns paper was written in generic terms and provides a framework under which service may be provided across various work settings. Intended to be flexible in nature, the preferred practice patterns are designed to outline current practices and to be updated as the profession changes. Paramount to the preferred practice patterns is the welfare of the client, although many professional issues are covered. The fundamental components of the preferred practice patterns include identification of professionals who perform a procedure, expected outcomes, clinical indications, clinical process, setting and equipment specifications, safety and health precautions, and documentation. In most cases, ASHA policy and related references are also given. Each of these areas is discussed in greater detail in Chapter 3. As you might imagine, knowledge of these preferred practice patterns is important to the student clinician. Referring to the different procedures will provide you with a general guide to a variety of procedures such as speech screening, language screening, augmentative and alternative communication assessment, fluency assessment, and speech-language pathology treatment.

Understand ASHA's Scope of Practice Guidelines

American Speech-Language-Hearing Association's (2007a) Scope of Practice guidelines define the role of the speech-language pathologist. To gain a good understanding of the range of professional practice, you will have a variety of clinical practicum experiences and work with a number of allied professionals. Because of the diversity of clinical experiences, it is important that you know what kinds of services are provided in which clinical setting. Your state's licensure laws will also influence your scope of practice. As you know, ASHA guidelines are not legal mandates, but licensure laws are.

Understand and Follow Clinic Policies and Procedures

The many clinic policies and procedures student clinicians must follow may appear unwarranted to the new clinician. Yet, these policies and procedures enable a clinic to operate effectively and efficiently. Each clinical site will have different policies and procedures you must follow. Typically, the clinic administrative assistant or your clinical supervisor will let you know the policies. Many practicum sites will make procedural handbooks available to you.

The following subjects commonly are addressed at the university clinic and any off-campus practicum sites: enrolling in clinical practicum, scheduling clients, ensuring client confidentiality, reserving and checking out materials and equipment, maintaining and working with clients' folders, utilizing the clinic telephone, maintaining clinic records, fulfilling insurance and health requirements, quality improvement, health precautions, and complying with the site's dress code. If you are unsure of a specific procedure or policy at your clinical site, you must get the information from your clinical supervisor.

Maintain Client Confidentiality

Because of its importance, the necessity of ensuring client confidentiality has been addressed in several places in this book. Remember that all information regarding a client is confidential. Do not discuss a client or a client's family by name in public areas. Public areas include reception areas, workrooms, waiting rooms, and other places outside the clinic. Do not leave clients' records unattended at desks or in workrooms. As a general rule, never remove permanent records from the clinic area. Follow established procedures regarding release of client information to other agencies.

Respect Clients' Personal and Cultural Beliefs

You will work with many clients who have varied cultural and ethnic backgrounds. You are not expected to share each client's values and beliefs, or even to know every culture's traditions; however, your willingness to accept your clients' diversity will maximize the effectiveness of your service delivery. You should be aware of assessment, treatment, and counseling considerations in serving a diverse clinical population. Chapter 6 contains specific information about serving multicultural populations.

Prepare for All Clinic Sessions

Know the administration and evaluation of diagnostic assessment procedures. Review them before every diagnostic session. Inspect the tests you plan to administer before meeting with your client to make sure the tests are complete, that they contain all required materials, and that the necessary test response forms are available. Although it may be another person's job to stock the treatment rooms, it is your responsibility to have all the necessary materials. In the middle of an oral-peripheral examination, you cannot blame someone for not providing the needed supplies. To avoid wasting assessment or treatment time, prepare and organize all materials and forms in advance of each session.

Check any equipment that you plan to use in your clinical sessions to ensure it is working properly. Make sure you know how to operate equipment you plan to use. Some distressing problems can occur with common tape recorders. They may be broken or the batteries may be dead. Not infrequently, student clinicians have recorded an entire clinical session only to find that the pause button was depressed instead of the record button.

Carefully review data obtained in previous sessions to determine appropriate beginning levels and possible sequences of treatment for the sessions for which you are preparing. Make sure the materials you have selected are the most appropriate for the target behaviors you plan to teach. The best organized and most creative materials are ineffective if the target behaviors are inappropriate or unrealistic. If you are working with a new client or in a medical setting where others place information in your client's chart, review the chart before beginning each treatment session.

Choose Appropriate Diagnostic Instruments

Select and use evaluation procedures and instruments that are appropriate to the client. Select procedures and instruments that are valid, reliable, nonbiased, and comprehensive. The evaluation procedures must sample behaviors adequately. Report with caution the results of tests administered to clients outside the standardization population. Use an assessment approach that integrates the traditional procedures (excluding standardized tests; see Chapter 6 for details) with alternative approaches that are more suitable to individuals of diverse ethnocultural background (Hegde & Pomaville, 2008). Use informal or naturalistic observation of a client's communicative skills as a part of each evaluation. This type of assessment is used to provide a more comprehensive analysis of a client's spontaneous speech and to provide a basis for evaluation when standardized instruments are not appropriate. Standardized tests can supplement information obtained from analysis of a client's conversational speech.

Write Measurable Treatment Objectives

Write measurable treatment objectives based on diagnostic results or reassessment of a client's current communicative skills. You may continue to work on objectives established the previous semester, if they still are appropriate for the client. Do not believe erroneously that you are always required to develop "original" objectives—even though the previous semester's objectives may still be applicable.

Submit Written Assignments Promptly

Your clinical supervisor will notify you of time lines and due dates for written assignments. Each practicum site will have different writing requirements. University clinics typically require an initial written summary, daily lesson plans or a semester treatment plan, and a final summary or progress report. Submit written assignments on time; this is important for many reasons. First, completing assignments on time suggests that you are dependable and that your practicum assignment is a high priority to you. Second, your written work reflects your knowledge of your clients, their communicative disorders, and of assessment and treatment procedures you plan to implement. A promptly submitted report will help the supervisor give you timely feedback. Third, your reports may suggest to the supervisor the level of supervision you need to work effectively with your client. To understand the formats and to practice writing various kinds of professional reports before or during your clinical practicum assignment, see Hegde (2010).

Write Effective Treatment Plans

An effective treatment program may fail if it is poorly sequenced for an individual client. For example, if the initial target behavior is defined as the correct production of a phoneme in sentences, you may never get started at all. Therefore, plan and sequence treatment using the initial and continuous assessment data. Plan realistically for the time available within each session. Design maintenance procedures early in the treatment sequence. Include the family in the treatment process. Use clinical procedures based on replicated research and technology. Finally, include the client as an active participant in the intervention process. Read the second part of this textbook and other books for details on treatment procedures (Hegde, 1998a, 2008c).

Maintain Accurate Clinical Records

Maintain an accurate and comprehensive record of your clients' clinical histories and related information in their permanent files. Maintain clinic files in the order established by the clinical site.

Continuous measurement of target responses throughout the treatment sessions and charting them in the form of line or bar graphs will make it easier to see client progress or lack of it. Such graphic and other quantitative measures enable you to find out quickly if treatment is appropriate or if modifications are needed.

Graphs also allow you to provide the client (or parent) with a visual representation of progress. Therefore, record and analyze your clients' responses during all assessment and treatment sessions. Learn efficient and accurate charting skills to record client responses.

Maintain an accurate and complete chronological log of clinical activity. This log is a necessary part of the documentation and analysis process. A review of a client's file should show his or her progress. Record-keeping requirements are discussed in more detail in Chapter 5.

Apply Information Learned in Academic Courses

In planning for evaluation and treatment sessions, draw from the information you learned in your academic courses. This seems like a fundamental assumption that should go without mentioning, but occasionally there are students who differentiate between material learned in academic courses and material learned in practicum assignments. Some students fail to see the relevance of what they have learned in the classroom to clinical work. The more you integrate academic and clinical assignments, the greater is the value of both. You also will find that information learned in one class that focused on a particular disorder can be expanded and generalized to other communicative disorders. The information you acquire in your academic studies is the foundation on which you build your independent professional skills and clinical experience.

Seek Research Information

Research information will be needed to fulfill your clinical assignments. Your clinical supervisor may provide you with resources or you may independently locate materials. Know the library resources, including current and past periodicals, latest books, and computerized data search programs that are available for finding research information. If you are unsuccessful at resolving a particular clinical question independently, request assistance from your clinical supervisor.

Ask Questions

Although expected to work increasingly independently, you must learn to seek assistance when you have questions. You should not continue an aspect of your practicum when you are not sure of something. If you are unclear about clinic policies and procedures, if you are not certain about implementing a specific treatment plan, if you are not sure about directions given by your supervisor, or if you just forget something that was said, ask for clarification.

Your clinical supervisor does not always immediately know when you need help. If you think you are not getting enough assistance from your supervisor, evaluate your own behavior before assuming that your supervisor "doesn't have time" or "doesn't care." Some clinical supervisors will be structured in scheduling times for questions, meetings, and staffing. Others will be less structured and expect student clinicians to approach them with questions as they arise.

Self-Evaluate Your Clinical Performance

Do not expect your clinical supervisor to evaluate all your sessions. To make independent clinical judgments and to modify assessment or treatment procedures, learn to self-evaluate your clinical work. You will learn to analyze your clients' behavior and your behavior objectively. This self-analysis is an essential part of clinical practicum. The skill will enable you to improve your initial assessment and treatment plans. Eventually, it is your good self-evaluation skills that will make you an independent and effective clinician. You will then continue to build on your past clinical experience and integrate new research information into professional practice.

There is an ever-increasing number of assessment instruments in communicative disorders. To further confuse students, there are many contradictory theories and treatment strategies. If you can objectively evaluate your clinical behaviors and those of your clients, you can establish the most effective treatment for your clients. Also, you will be better able to find out what academic areas or clinical skills you should target for personal improvement.

You are not expected to know automatically how to evaluate your clinical sessions. Your supervisor is responsible for helping you acquire this skill. In helping you acquire self-evaluation skills, your supervisor may respond to your questions with additional questions. Your supervisor may suggest areas of research rather than giving you a specific manual or reference. Also, when you are having trouble working with a client, your supervisor may not immediately step in but allow you time to analyze and resolve whatever problem you are having.

Maintain Regular Attendance

Attend all scheduled clinical sessions promptly. If you are ill or have a personal emergency, *notify your clinical supervisor* and, if part of your clinic's protocol, your clients. Studying for examinations, leaving for a vacation, or simply being unprepared are not acceptable reasons for canceling a clinical appointment. Also, begin and end your clinical sessions on time.

Act Professionally

Sometimes it is difficult to be a student on the one hand and a professional on the other. But even though you are in training, you are a professional helping people with communicative disorders.

Know how to make others view you as a professional. Model your supervisor's behaviors. Observe the behavior of senior clinicians. Do some of your fellow students generate more of an aura of professionalism than others? If you look at their behaviors, you probably will find individuals who have spent much time becoming knowledgeable about their clients' communicative disorders. They will have prepared thoroughly and organized their clinical sessions. They also will have given thought to how they speak, dress, and interact with clients and their families.

Student clinicians who present themselves as professionals also treat their clients, supervisors, clinical staff, and other professionals with respect. In turn, the student clinicians are treated as professionals.

Maintain a Clinical Clock Hour Log

You are responsible for maintaining a log of the clinical clock hours you have earned. Maintain both a daily and a semester log. University speech and hearing clinics and ASHA have formats for recording clock hours. Carefully follow the documentation requirements of your training program, because you may not get credit for incorrectly recorded clock hours. Appendix C contains a sample of ASHA's KASA form that helps document your clinical and academic progress.

Maintain an Effective Clinical Supervisor Relationship

You will work with many supervisors. Each may have a different supervisory style. Regardless of your practicum site or the supervisor you have, it is important to maintain contact with your supervisor. If you have any questions or concerns about your assignment, contact your supervisor. If you had a great experience in the clinic, let your supervisor know. Do not expect your supervisor to know everything that happens in each of your sessions. Also, do not expect your supervisor to always know when you need help. Work cooperatively with your supervisor and assume some of the responsibility for maintaining effective communication with him or her.

The interaction between the clinical supervisor and student clinician is the basis for learning in the practicum setting. To ensure optimal training for the student clinician and quality service for the client, the supervisor and the student clinician should diligently fulfill their respective responsibilities.

Enjoy Practicum Experience

All this work and all this responsibility and now you have to enjoy yourself? Yes! As you gain knowledge and clinical independence you should at least feel some personal fulfillment. Often, your clients will know if you dislike what you are doing. More importantly, if you never find joy or satisfaction in your clinical practicum, you should reevaluate your professional objectives, because you may have chosen to pursue the wrong career. But if you enjoy your work with people with communicative disorders, and if their success gives you personal satisfaction, you know you have chosen the right path to a fulfilling career.

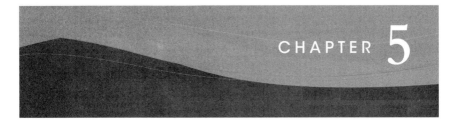

CHAPTER 5

Working with Clients

Chapter Outline
....

- Scheduling Clients
- Assessment of Clients
- Reassessment of Clients
- Establishing a Working Relationship with Client and Family
- Report Writing
- Record-Keeping Procedures
- Working with Other Professionals
- Establishing Collaborative Relationships with Other Professionals

In your academic coursework, you were responsible for learning, assimilating, and evaluating new information. As a student clinician your major task is to learn professional skills in working with clients who have communicative disorders or swallowing disorders, or both. These skills include scheduling clients, evaluating their communicative and swallowing performance, developing and implementing intervention plans, writing a variety of reports, maintaining adequate records, working with families, and coordinating services with other professionals.

Scheduling Clients

Scheduling clients is an initial step in beginning clinical work. Depending on your clinic's policy, either you or the clinic's administrative assistant may schedule your clients. It is your responsibility to confirm appointments with the administrative assistant, regardless of who is responsible for the initial scheduling. Several factors influence the scheduling of clients.

Factors That Influence Scheduling of Clients

1. *The student clinician's schedule.* Your clients will need to be scheduled around your class schedule, your work, and other obligations. Remember that your clinical practicum is viewed as a professional responsibility and your outside employment may not take precedence over it. You may be asked to change your employment schedule, if scheduling around your job cannot be accomplished.

2. *The supervisor's schedule.* Supervisors may have obligations, such as teaching academic courses, advising, or serving on university committees, that will influence their availability. Also, part-time supervisors may be hired. In these cases, the supervisors may only be available after their full-time job is over. For example, one of your supervisors may work full-time in the public school setting and part-time at the university.

3. *The student clinician's clinical experience and level in the academic program.* As a rule, student clinicians are not assigned clients with disorders in which the students have had no academic training. Therefore, if you have not had any courses on stuttering, you will not be assigned a client who stutters. Client family issues, behavioral issues, or complexity of a disorder will also influence scheduling. Beginning student clinicians will be assigned clients with less complex needs as much as possible.

4. *The type, frequency, and duration of service needed.* The needs of each client will influence the type, frequency, and duration of service provided. Many variables are involved. For example, certain clients may need individual intervention, with other clients benefiting from interaction in a group setting. In other instances, clients with more severe disorders may be seen more frequently (e.g., 4 to 5 times per week), whereas clients who are close to being dismissed may be seen as few as 1 or 2 times per month. The severity of the disorder, as well as client health and ability to attend to task, influence the duration of appointments. Sometimes clients with more severe disorders need to be seen frequently, but for shorter periods of time. Certain clients fatigue easily because of health problems. Other clients' optimal attention to tasks may be 20 to 30 minutes.

5. *The population served.* For the convenience of working adults, the clinic hours may include many evening appointments. Your clinic may have both day and evening hours to accommodate a variety of schedules.

6. *The clients' cultures.* Cultural and religious factors also can affect scheduling. Religious holidays must be considered. While it is rare for services to be provided on a Sunday, certain individuals may not be available for service on a Friday or Saturday. Also, clients with certain cultural backgrounds may prefer not to be grouped with members of the opposite gender. Other cultural and religious factors must be considered.

7. *The clinical site.* Each clinical site has different priorities regarding client scheduling. At a university clinic, clients must often be scheduled around the needs of the students and supervising faculty. At a hospital, however, the clients' health care and the schedules of allied professionals must be considered. In private practice, the convenience to the client is paramount.

8. *Financial resources.* The policy for payment of services will vary at each clinical site. In some cases, the client's ability to pay for services will determine the length and duration of the intervention. For example, a client may have insurance that pays for 10 hours of speech-language pathology services and he or she can afford to pay for 5 more hours. Unless the site is willing (and able) to waive any remaining fees, the client's intervention would be restricted to 15 hours.

University Clinic Schedules

University clinics schedule clinical sessions based on the availability of clinical supervision, convenience for clients, the schedule of student clinicians, and the operating times of the clinic. Because of the number of variables involved, university clinic schedules may change from semester to semester.

Most university clinics usually operate during regular business hours, Monday through Friday, with some evening sessions available for clients who cannot attend during the day. Clients typically are scheduled for 2 to 3 sessions per week, ranging from 30 to 60 minutes. Diagnostic sessions may be scheduled for 1 to 2 hours. Clients are scheduled for individual or group treatment sessions.

Initial Client Contact

You will receive your clinical assignment at the beginning of the term. You will be given your clinic schedule and your supervisor or clinic director will assign you appropriate clients. Beginning clinicians are assigned one or two clients, with the more advanced clinicians possibly working with three to four clients.

At many schools, student clinicians are responsible for telephoning their clients to schedule them. If one of your clients cannot attend at the proposed time, notify your supervisor and the clinic's administrative assistant. You will be assigned another client to contact.

The initial contact with your clients is an important step. You should plan what you want to tell the clients or their families. Use the following general guidelines to make your initial telephone contact with your client.

1. *Introduce yourself, your credentials, and the purpose of your call.* For example, "Hello, this is Jennifer Jones, a graduate student clinician at the University Speech and Hearing Clinic. I'm calling to schedule speech services for your daughter, Lisa." If the client has not been seen previously at your clinic, be prepared to answer questions about the clinic's policies and procedures. New clients will have questions about fees, clinic schedules, parking, the type of supervision provided, the frequency of supervision, qualifications of the supervisors, length of the semester, qualifications of the student clinicians providing services, and related services available (e.g., audiology).

2. *Discuss the client's schedule.* Tell the client when his or her appointment is. Some clinics also may send written appointment cards to clients. If you contact your clients more than 5 or 6 days in advance, telephone them again the day before their first appointment to remind them of the date and time. This will help reduce the number of missed appointments.

3. *Clarify ambiguous information and request additional information.* For instance, parents sometimes complete a line incorrectly on the case history; they may write the current date on the line requesting their child's date of birth. In addition, you may want to review information that seems too brief. Also, request that clients or parents bring all reports from other speech-language pathologists or related specialists they have seen. As appropriate, verify the primary language of the parents and the client. Discuss the need for an interpreter.

4. *Give information about parking permits and clinic fees.* Tell clients where they can park. If a free parking permit is possible, tell them how they can acquire one. If clients state they are unable to afford the clinic fee, ask them to see your clinic director (or follow the policy already established at your clinic). You do not have the authority to make decisions about fee reduction or to set up a payment schedule.

5. *Give directions to the clinic.* New clients may not know where the university clinic is. You are familiar with the campus and may not think in terms of how to get to the clinic from other areas of the community. Therefore, have a map of the campus and city available when you first contact your clients. With the help of the map, give accurate directions. Redundant information is usually helpful to an individual unfamiliar with the campus.

6. *Give directions to the clinic waiting room.* Tell your clients that you will meet them in the waiting room after they have completed any business at the clinic office. Each clinic has its procedures for the first meeting with clients. Follow the procedures at your university.

7. *Ensure that the client has the correct appointment date and time before ending the phone call.* After answering the client's questions and giving directions, tell him or her the appointed date, time, and place, for example, "Okay, I'll see you on Monday, September 2nd, at 9 a.m. at the clinic waiting room."

Hospital Schedules

Your hospital schedule will coincide with the typical business day, usually from 8 a.m. to 5 p.m. Because many hospitals provide speech-language pathology services 6 days a week, you may be asked to schedule practicum on some weekends. There will be many variables to consider in your hospital schedule, and one of the keys to success is flexibility. Do the following to schedule patients in the hospital setting:

1. *Determine the frequency and duration ordered for speech-language pathology services.* In medical settings, inpatients often are scheduled for speech services 5 to 6 days a week.

2. *Determine the optimum schedule for your patient.* Attempts are made to schedule services at times that are most beneficial to patients. Patients may be seen one or two times a day. One factor influencing their intervention schedule is the length of time they are able to effectively participate in evaluation or treatment. For example, clients may have been prescribed speech-language services five times per week for 60 minutes each day. However, if they are unable to attend for a full 60 minutes, they may be seen for 30 minutes during the morning and again for 30 minutes during the afternoon. Another factor influencing the schedule is the type of treatment provided. For example, if you are working with a client who has dysphagia, you may coordinate his or her intervention with the meal schedules. Sometimes, you may go in early to work with the patient before or during breakfast or you stay late to work with the patient at dinnertime.

3. *Coordinate your schedule with the nursing staff.* Though your hospital assignment may require you to begin at 8 a.m., you may not immediately begin direct patient contact. Much of the nursing patient care occurs early in the morning. This care may include such activities as administering medications, providing breakfast, toileting, and bathing. Therefore, you must coordinate your schedule with the nursing staff.

4. *Coordinate your schedule with other patient rehabilitation services.* Besides speech services, a patient may be receiving other rehabilitative services, such as physical and occupational therapies. To determine your schedule, you will need to check with other professionals providing services to your patients.

5. *Allow time for meetings and conferences.* In the hospital setting, conferences are scheduled to discuss patient care and progress. These conferences are called rounds and are attended by the physician and other members of the medical team. The rounds may be specific to patient rehabilitation, in which case members of the rehabilitation team attend. Rounds are often scheduled early in the morning.

6. *Adjust your schedule around a regular family visit.* Often, you need to train certain family members to work with your patient in the hospital and at home after discharge from the hospital. In such cases, find out when it is

most convenient for the family member to attend the intervention sessions. Although you want to involve the family in your patient's intervention, there also should be times when the family can be with the patient to just visit. There is the occasional family member who can be at the hospital only at a certain time because of transportation, work, or school obligations. Schedule your sessions so your patients will have some private moments with their families.

7. *Adhere to your schedule.* After you have consulted with other staff and determined a schedule of therapy for a medical patient, remain with the same schedule as much as possible. As patients are discharged and new patients enrolled, some schedule changes will be necessary.

8. *Be punctual.* Your patients' schedules may be full. Many specialists may have scheduled services. The doctors, nurses, physical therapists, occupational therapists, and family members all want to have time with your patients. To ensure your patients receive the total amount of intervention they are entitled to, begin and end your sessions on time.

9. *Schedule time for indirect services.* Schedule time for report writing, consultation with other professionals, and family consultation. Because, generally, patients stay in the hospital for a short period of time, educating families about the patient's disability and intervention is imperative. Allow sufficient time for transition and discharge planning. Also, schedule time for your own breaks and lunches.

10. *Verify your appointments with the administrative assistant.* If you are working in an outpatient setting, the receptionist or administrative assistant may schedule your clients. Clients are scheduled for a regular time during their entire enrollment as much as possible. For example, one of your clients may be scheduled for speech-language pathology services every Monday, Wednesday, and Friday from 10:00 to 10:45 a.m. Your schedule will change as clients are discharged and new clients are added.

School Schedules

In the educational setting, caseloads may be large and several service delivery models may be used. (Refer to Chapter 2 for additional information on different service delivery models.) Because of this, scheduling may seem overwhelming to the beginning clinician. When scheduling students in the school setting, consider the following:

1. *Determine the type of schedule.* The two common types of schedules are block (intensive cycle) and intermittent. In **block scheduling,** specific students (or schools) receive services 4 to 5 days a week for a certain number of weeks (for example, 6 weeks). After the predetermined length of time, service is rotated to the next group of students (or schools). In **intermittent**

scheduling, all students and schools are served each week. For example, the speech-language pathologist assigned to serve two schools might provide services on Mondays and Wednesdays at one school, and Tuesdays, Thursdays, and Fridays at the other school.

2. *Determine what types of service delivery models you will use.* Your schedule will be influenced by the service delivery model used. Many school clinicians provide a combination of the traditional pull-out model, consultation model, and classroom-collaboration model. Each model requires different amounts of time and considerable coordination with the other professionals involved. For more information on these models, refer to Chapter 2.

3. *Determine how often each student on your caseload will receive service.* Certain students may require more intensive service than others. Generally, students who are close to attaining their objectives and being dismissed are seen less frequently than students who are just beginning to learn new behaviors. Students with more severe disorders may be seen more frequently than students with less severe disorders. You must provide services for the amount of time specified in the student's IEP.

4. *Determine if students will receive intervention individually or in a group.* Certain students require individual intervention and other students may benefit from intervention in a group setting. Although students receiving individual speech-language pathology service receive more of your individual attention, group intervention also has advantages. The group setting may better reflect students' school environment than does a student's interaction with only the speech-language pathologist. To aid generalization and maintenance in a private practice, you can ask family members and the client's friends to attend and participate in the intervention. However, in the public school setting this is rarely possible. So, effective use of the classroom setting or group setting can aid in generalization and maintenance by better reflecting the students' school environment by enlisting other students to assist with your clients' intervention. In addition to becoming discriminative stimuli (see Chapter 9) for the target behaviors trained, other children can act as models for the target behaviors.

5. *Consider school and class schedules.* You must find out the times of recess, lunch, class dismissal, school assemblies, and so on. Several of your students may be receiving services from other professionals, including the school psychologist, resource specialist, adaptive physical education specialist, or physical therapist. There also will be certain periods of the class that the teacher does not want the student to miss on a regular basis.

6. *Allow time for consulting with teachers, testing, writing reports, and meeting with parents.* Consultation and collaboration with classroom teachers is essential to your effectiveness in the school setting. Be careful to allow sufficient time to work with them. Generally, this time will have to be scheduled before or after school or during the teachers' breaks. Even if you are working directly

with students in their classrooms, you should not interrupt your treatment or the teachers' work to discuss the needs of the students or the program. Also, testing students, writing reports, and meeting with parents are important components to your school service delivery. To avoid canceling sessions, schedule blocks of time for these activities in advance.

There are many factors to consider in developing your schedule for service delivery in the schools. The preceding items provide a brief overview of issues faced in school scheduling. Appropriate implementation of any type of schedule requires effective communication with the classroom teachers and other specialists serving the students on your caseload. When you participate in your school internship, your supervisory clinician or the university supervisor will provide you with practice in scheduling and decision making regarding scheduling options.

Scheduling Guidelines Summary

Because of the number of factors involved, scheduling a client (or patient, or student) can become an art form of its own. Although frequency of service and procedures for scheduling clients will differ across settings, there are some general issues to consider at any site.

Common Factors to Consider in Scheduling Clients at Any Practicum Site

1. *Schedule sessions to optimize the effectiveness of intervention.* Make decisions about time of day, length of session, frequency of intervention, group or individual intervention, and direct or indirect (e.g., consultative) service delivery. In making your decisions, follow clinic and site guidelines.

2. *Coordinate speech-language pathology service with other services.* Avoid conflicts with other professionals by developing effective communication with them. Make sure you know what other professionals your client is receiving services from, when the services are provided, and what the intervention objectives are.

3. *Follow your schedule.* Be punctual in beginning and ending sessions. Alter your schedule as little as possible and communicate any changes in your schedule to all individuals affected by the change.

4. *Allow time for indirect services.* Schedule time for paperwork, evaluations, conferences, and breaks.

Assessment of Clients

Before enrolling for treatment of communicative or swallowing disorders, individuals must have a complete speech-language assessment or speech-language and swallowing assessment. The assessment allows you to determine if disorders of communication, speech, language, literacy, or feeding/swallowing exist. If one or any combination of these disorders exist, you should then determine the nature and extent of that single or multiple disorder. In addition, the evaluation allows you to gather enough information for recommendations on possible treatment objectives, treatment procedures, and time lines for treatment.

Many university training programs have a "diagnostic clinic" designed for the sole purpose of evaluation. Other clinical settings may have clinicians who only perform assessments and are not involved in treatment. However, most speech-language pathologists are involved in both assessment and intervention.

It is not the purpose of this section to provide a comprehensive assessment guide, but to give an overview of the components of evaluation, with emphasis on the university clinic setting. Read one of the many books on evaluation and diagnosis (Emerick & Pindzola, 2007; Hegde, 2008b; Tomblin, Morris, & Spriestersbach, 1999) and read Chapter 6 for information on *alternative and integrated assessments*. Also, refer to specific texts on assessment of swallowing disorders (Crary & Groher, 2003; Leonard & Kendall, 2007; Logemann, 1998).

University Clinic Assessment

At the university clinic, the initial assessment procedure begins after an individual has contacted the clinic regarding a communication problem. Under your clinical supervisor's direction, you will assess individuals with a variety of communicative disorders. Typically, you will not assess swallowing disorders as part of your university clinic assignment; however, you may assess certain feeding problems (e.g., difficulty with certain food textures, specific food aversions, inability to manipulate utensils, etc.). Assessment procedures vary, depending on disorders, clients, and clinicians. However, the following procedures are common to all assessments.

1. *Discuss your assessment plans with your clinical supervisor before meeting with your clients.* Also, notify your supervisor of the time of the scheduled evaluation.

2. *Obtain a case history.* A completed case history form is required before scheduling an individual for an evaluation. Occasionally, the clinician and client may complete the case history during the initial interview. The case history can be extensive and often includes prenatal, birth, and developmental information; medical, social, educational, and occupational history; and previous related evaluation and intervention results. When you assess individuals after they have experienced a traumatic event (e.g., stroke, head injury, accident, etc.) you will also include questions about the client's **premorbid** abilities

(knowledge, skill, and performance levels before the incident resulting in communicative or swallowing disorders). An evaluation is scheduled following receipt of the necessary information in the clinic office.

3. *Interview the client (or parent)*. The interview allows you to clarify information reported on the case history and obtain additional information either omitted or inferred from it. Information obtained during the interview suggests the types of testing that you will need to perform. Also, the interview is an information-giving process in which you explain the assessment procedures and results to the client or parents, or both.

In some cases, *the interview can be the beginning of intervention*. For example, you might ask the parents of a child with a fluency disorder what they are doing to intervene during the child's dysfluent moments. The question, "How's that working for you?" following the parents' response can assist in initiating a new intervention strategy. Discuss the positive aspects of the client as well. This will help you later in determining individual and family strengths that will assist with your intervention. Pay attention to the amount of speaking that you do versus the amount of talking of the client or client's caregiver. If you are speaking more than the person who you are interviewing, then you may not be obtaining all of the information that the interviewee has to share.

Each interview will vary depending on the type of disorder, related problems, and so on. Some interviews will be relatively short and others may be lengthy. Typically, the more complicated the medical history, the longer the interview. You also may be involved in a lengthy interview with clients who have received intervention from other agencies. When an interpreter is required, the interview time must be extended. Interviews also may have different formats. To assess the communication skills of a child, you will interview the parent. You may or may not include the child in the interview. For example, you may want to include the child with a fluency disorder in the interview, but a child with a language disorder may not be able to participate because of limited expressive vocabulary. In addition, you will want to discuss everyday routines and activities in which the child interacts; later you can incorporate naturally occurring activities into your intervention.

Avoid Common Problems during Interviews

1. *Difficulty establishing rapport*. A common problem beginning student clinicians experience—difficulty establishing rapport—stems from an extremely formal and stiff disposition inexperienced clinicians may exhibit. The use of the case history form as an interview guide creates

an unnecessarily cold format. Instead, use a more warm, conversational style to gather information.

2. *Asking too many "yes" or "no" questions.* Ask open-ended questions and create conversational interactions. For instance, instead of asking, "Does he play well with other children?" say, "Tell me about how he interacts with other children."

3. *Asking redundant questions.* Do not ask questions the family has adequately answered on the case history form. For example, do not ask, "Has Josh had ear infections? Has he had any seizures? Has Josh had mumps?" and so on if such questions have been answered on the form. Generally, it is more effective to summarize information on the case history and request verification. For example, "You wrote on the case history that Josh was sick for several weeks as an infant. Tell me a little bit more about that." Ask redundant questions or rephrase your questions only when the informant fails to give information clearly or to clarify information.

4. *Ignoring, or bypassing, important information.* Some clinicians simply ask a set of questions when they rely on an interview "script." Instead, listen to what the informant says and ask follow-up questions. Pay attention to anecdotes reported by the client or the family; these often contain behaviors that will give you more in-depth information about the client and about the family dynamics. Simply sticking to a set of prepared questions will make it difficult to get additional information from the informants. It is important to direct the interview, but it is equally important to listen and respond to all that is said in the interview. Appendix E contains a sample of an interview.

5. *Entertaining preconceived ideas about the clients and their families.* Avoid stereotypic notions about people, their presumed levels of cooperation, openness, and what they will or will not say. Approach the interview with an open disposition to interact naturally and professionally to get the information you need.

To get detailed and accurate information from the informants during interviews, consider the following strategies:

- *Paraphrase* what clients or their family members have said. Listen to clients and, to check for understanding, rephrase, in your own words, what you heard. Clients will correct you if you misunderstood the intent of their comments or confirm the information if you correctly understood their remarks.

- *Repeat* clients' or family members' words back to them. Be careful not to overuse this technique.

- *Check* your beliefs by verbalizing them. For example, a man with aphasia may be discussing the emotional effects the disability has had on his family. Additional information may help you direct treatment, and you might use such a phrase as, "It sounds like you are very frustrated by the difficulty you have communicating at family dinners."

4. *Perform an oral-peripheral examination.* An oral-peripheral examination is performed to investigate the structural and functional integrity of the speech mechanism. There are several published oral-peripheral examination instruments you can purchase that will provide you with a standard format to follow.

Integrate the following procedures in your oral-peripheral examination:

- *Systematically evaluate* the oral-peripheral mechanism during each examination to avoid overlooking any areas; that is, always evaluate structures in a certain sequence. For example, some clinicians begin with general facial features, then progress to examination of lips, teeth, tongue, hard palate, and so on. Other clinicians begin by examining the oral cavity first and then the peripheral areas.

- *Verbally describe* your observations while audiotaping. It is helpful to orally record the evaluation. This step will allow you to continue the examination without having to stop and write notes.

- *Observe* the speech mechanism during activities such as laughing, speaking, and eating, if the client refuses to allow invasive procedures during the oral examination. Perform the examination later in the evaluation session or in a treatment session, if the client is enrolled for speech services.

5. *Screen the client's hearing.* ASHA guidelines require audiometric screening as part of a speech and language assessment. University clinics routinely screen the hearing of clients as part of a speech and language assessment. In other practicum settings, an audiometer may not be available to the speech-language pathologist. Therefore, the clients are referred to an audiologist. In the public school setting, the school nurse, licensed as an audiometrist, often performs hearing screenings. Before evaluating individuals wearing hearing aids, it is important to find out when the person last had an audiological evaluation. Also, perform a hearing aid check to determine if it is functioning.

6. *Obtain speech-language samples.* The speech sample is sometimes referred to as an "informal" assessment procedure, which seems to diminish the importance of its analysis. However, the conversational speech sample is one of the most important assessment instruments available to you. It allows you to evaluate your client's communicative abilities in a natural context. It is essential to the assessment of a client's actual speech and language performance.

When obtaining and analyzing a speech and language sample:

- Obtain more than one sample to ensure the reliability of the speech sample.

- Direct conversation to provide clients with opportunities to produce a variety of language structures (e.g., declaratives, interrogatives, different verb tenses, and so forth).

- Sample conversation in a variety of environments. With adults, use the interview to obtain at least a portion of the conversational sample. In addition, sample clients' speech while they are speaking on the telephone, speaking with the clinic receptionist, or speaking with a bookstore salesperson. With children, obtain speech samples during play and during other interactions (e.g., asking for snacks, requesting information). Avoid asking questions that are answered with "yes," "no," or one word. Instead, imitate their actions and verbalizations. If children are reluctant to engage in play, choose some interesting items and begin playing with them. As they begin to show interest, verbally invite them to join you, or place a toy close to them. Play-based assessment (Linder, 2008) can provide you with excellent information.

- Assess more than just the client's mean length of utterance. In your analysis of the speech sample, include information about the client's semantic, morphologic, syntactic, and pragmatic productions.

- Use the speech samples to examine articulation skills.

- Compute overall speech intelligibility.

- Analyze production of phonemes. Note specific erred phonemes, types of errors (e.g., omissions, substitutions, distortions), frequency of errors, and percentage of occurrence. You also may describe specific phonologic error patterns, known as phonological processes (e.g., syllable reduction, cluster reduction, fronting).

- Observe voice characteristics: quality, pitch, and intensity. Note such behaviors as the number of pitch breaks in a 5-minute speech sample or the absence of adequate breath support.

- Measure the types and frequency of dysfluencies in the sample and calculate the dysfluency rate. Refer to Appendix F for a discussion on types of dysfluencies and how to calculate them.

- Use effective and appropriate stimuli to create conversational speech. To evoke speech from children, clinicians often use pictures, toys, and books. The recurring problem with pictures is that they often evoke single-word responses. The problem with toys is that children just play with them, without talking with the clinician. Books, too, may only evoke a looking response from children. Storybooks with sequenced pictures may be better, however. Children may be prompted to tell the story that unfolds in sequenced pictures. Conversation is probably the best, if that can be evoked. Before bringing out pictures and books to describe, try to engage children in conversation. If a child is school aged, ask about most and least favorite school activities, favorite teachers, what happens to students who get in trouble in the cafeteria, best friends, the school bully, recent vacations, cartoon shows, other favorite TV shows, birthday parties, and so on. Sometimes, you can tell the child something about yourself first to stimulate speech. For example, "I have a puppy that is so silly. Yesterday he ran through the sprinklers and then came and jumped all over me! I bet you have a silly puppy, too. Tell me about your puppy." While a prudent use of play can be effective, you should avoid the trap of letting the child spend too much time playing independently. You, or the parent, must engage the child to obtain a representative sample of his or her communication skills.

If you have a difficult time obtaining a valid sample or if you need a second sample, use one of the following methods.

- Record a short conversational sample between a parent and the child. The two should be alone in the room. Use audio or video recording. Tell parents why and what you are doing. Ask them to talk (or play and talk) with their children as they normally would.

- Ask parents to maintain a daily log of their child's speech for 1 week. Help parents take this request seriously and organize their note taking by providing a small notebook with their child's name written on it. You even may want to attach a pen or pencil to the notebook. This is one way to get a more complete view of the language of a young child who is reluctant to participate in activities in the clinic. Although the information may not be fully accurate, it will give you a better idea of the child's language performance as well as the parent's perception of the child's communication skills. A parent may report that his or her child produces only single words. However, while recording the child's speech for a week, the parent may find that the child produces some two-word phrases. Another parent might report that his or her child has a large vocabulary. The record of verbal productions may confirm or contradict this report.

Refer to Appendix G for information on obtaining and analyzing speech samples.

7. *Administer standardized tests.* There are many standardized tests designed to evaluate communicative disorders. They should adequately sample behaviors. Review tests before administering them; you must know the administration and scoring procedures. If you have to concentrate on remembering administration or scoring procedures to the exclusion of observing your client, you may miss important behaviors exhibited by the client. For example, if you are unfamiliar with the *Peabody Picture Vocabulary Test*, you may be busy figuring out basals and ceilings and miss the child's perseverative responses or uncooperative behaviors. It is important to remember that the information obtained from a standardized test is only as good as the examiner. Standardized tests can be used to substantiate your clinical observations but should not be used to replace those observations.

8. *Use reliable, valid, and culturally nonbiased tests.* Test selection must be appropriate for the client. Read and evaluate the information provided in the test manual. Determine if the test meets reliability and validity standards. Review the normative demographics to ensure your client's ethnicity is adequately represented in the sample. Look at the test stimuli to determine if there are pictures or vocabulary that are culturally biased. In California public schools, certain tests have been prohibited for use with African American students because of potentially biased results. Be sure you follow the guidelines for test use at your site.

9. *Use other evaluation instruments.* Technology is providing speech-language pathologists with an array of computerized equipment to quantify data that were previously evaluated subjectively. Take the time to learn and use any such equipment available at your university clinic or practicum setting.

10. *Conduct disorder-specific evaluation.* Other types of testing and sampling may be performed depending on the type of disorder you evaluate. Most of these will be disorder specific. For example, you will assess stimulability of misarticulated sounds in evaluation of articulation disorders. You may analyze reading samples in your assessments of fluency and literacy disorders. In many cases you may also incorporate useful elements of such alternative assessment strategies as dynamic, authentic, or portfolio assessments into your assessment plan (see Chapter 6 for additional information).

11. *Observe a variety of skills.* Because communication does not occur in a vacuum, you will need to observe more than your client's speech and language skills. For example, with young children you will observe the type of play in which they engage. You can obtain some clues about children's development levels by comparing their language and play skills. This is especially critical when evaluating children who are nonverbal or who have limited or unusual verbal language. You will also want to note your client's fine and gross motor skills. Although you cannot diagnose motor developmental disorders, typically you can determine if your client should be referred to other professionals for additional evaluation.

12. *Discuss impressions and recommendations.* At the end of the assessment, discuss your initial impressions of the child or the client with the family or client. Let them know that a more detailed analysis and a written report will be given soon. Communicate everything in simple and direct language. After discussion with your supervisor, give your recommendation.

13. *Analyze the results and write the report.* Find out the meaning of the combined test scores, oral-peripheral examination, and speech sample results. It is not sufficient to report only test scores without also making both objective and subjective clinical observations. Based on your analysis of the client's speech and language skills, make recommendations for or against intervention. If intervention is recommended, report client-specific objectives, prognosis for obtaining the objectives, and possible duration of intervention.

If intervention is not recommended, state clearly the rationale for not recommending it. Discuss your assessment plans with your clinical supervisor before meeting with your clients. Also, notify your supervisor of the time of the scheduled evaluation.

Multidisciplinary versus Transdisciplinary Assessment

In many settings you will be a member of a team of specialists that evaluates clients. Generally, team assessments fall within the categories of multidisciplinary and transdisciplinary assessments.

As a member of a *multidisciplinary assessment team*, you will assess the communication or swallowing performance of your client and report your findings. Other team members will perform their assessments relative to their specialty and report their findings. Typically, each member evaluates the client individually and then the reports are gathered together, information is reviewed, and recommendations are made.

The *transdisciplinary team* may obtain similar information as the multidisciplinary team but does so in a different fashion. Members of the transdisciplinary team often have prescribed roles in the assessment process but observe and assess the client together. Individuals on the team may also observe cross-identified "professional boundaries" as part of their assessment activities. For example, you may engage your client in conversational speech to determine word-finding skills during spontaneous productions. At the same time, you may notice limited hand mobility. You may ask the client to write or perform other skills that require various hand movements. Although you may make a gross identification of a mobility problem, the occupational therapist will be observing the same skills and make more specific recommendations to improve mobility. In addition, the occupational therapist may begin to more actively guide that part of the assessment process.

Reassessment of Clients

Clients returning to the university clinic for a new term of treatment should be reassessed before continuing treatment. A reassessment of all areas of speech and language typically is unnecessary. For example, it is not necessary to readminister a battery of language tests to a client diagnosed with a fluency disorder who had no previous indications of a language problem. Important reassessment data needed for the continuing client may be the results of a speech sample, hearing screening, oral examination, course of the disorder in the absence of treatment, and baselines of target behaviors. See Chapter 8 for procedures for establishing baselines.

Reassessment is important to establish the progress or improvement in the client's communicative behaviors. In addition to reassessing communicative behavior following a break in service delivery, you will be involved in ongoing assessment (or reassessment) of your client's skills. Ongoing assessment is obviously essential when working with clients with swallowing disorders, but it is also important when working with clients with speech and language disorders. In certain cases, your clients' abilities will change rapidly, and to effectively provide treatment, you will always need to know at which level your client is. This will include such activities as accurate, ongoing record keeping, probes, and self-evaluations. To complete reassessment or ongoing assessment, specific tests may be administered at the clinician's (or supervisor's) discretion.

Additional procedures and time lines for assessment and reassessment of clients are mandated by insurance companies and the public schools. Find out about these procedures and time lines from your supervisor.

Establishing a Working Relationship with Client and Family

To treat clients effectively, you should establish a good working relationship with them and their families. Individuals with communicative disorders and their families initially may feel uncomfortable with the treatment process. They may not know much about the treatment, its duration, and its effects. Clients and their families may not begin treatment with the same level of knowledge or enthusiasm that student clinicians do. Therefore, you should educate clients and their families about their responsibilities, the intervention procedures, and their effects. To this end, you must establish good communication between yourself, your client, and your client's family. Because you are learning to do this, you also should maintain constant communication with your clinical supervisor. When working with clients and their families, consider the following guidelines.

1. *Obtain your supervisor's approval before you discuss important issues with your clients.* Also, when you do not know the answer to your clients' or their families' questions, tell them that you will find out from your supervisor. Then discuss the questions with your supervisor and find out how to answer them. On occasion, because of the complexity of the information to be presented, your supervisor may decide that he or she needs to talk with the family. In such cases, the supervisor will probably include you in the discussion so you will learn how to handle such issues.

2. *Give an overview of the planned services at the beginning.* Briefly describe to the clients or families the assessment results, the planned intervention, expected results, and what the family members should do at home, along with follow-up and booster intervention procedures. In talking with clients and their parents, use simple, direct language. Do not give obscure answers that are couched in incomprehensible speech-language jargon. When you need to use technical terms, describe them, define them, and give everyday examples. However, do not talk down to people. For example, when the father of a child with a language delay is a professor of English, do not try to explain prepositions that you want to teach the child. Similarly, if the mother of a child is a physician, it is not necessary to try to describe the velopharyngeal mechanism in everyday language (Hegde, 1998a).

3. *Repeat important information.* Your clients may be hearing a lot of new information at one time. Do not be afraid to repeat important information several times. For example, you may explain something at the beginning of a discussion and ask if they understand your description. Later, using different words or putting it in a different context, you may give the same information. At the next meeting, you may repeat the information again. It is not unusual for clients to report that they "were never told that." It's not because they are trying to be difficult, but because they were hearing so much new information at once that they did not assimilate (or learn) all of what you said.

4. *Always give accurate information.* Do not bluff. Often-asked questions include, What caused the speech or language problem? Why does my son stutter? Why can't my youngest child talk, while two older children are doing fine? The parents assume that research will have provided answers. But the research information may not provide a clear-cut answer that satisfies clients or their families. If there is a well-researched answer to your clients' questions, then provide that information in terms they can understand. If there is not an evidence-based answer to your clients' questions, then let them know that.

5. *Tell parents and clients that it is often difficult to point out the cause of a disorder in a given individual.* Our knowledge of disorders and their potential causes are applied to groups of persons, not to specific individuals. For example, you can say that we know many potential causes of stuttering, including hereditary predisposition, faulty learning, environmental stress, instability in the nervous system, and many others. But clinicians cannot say why a given child or adult stutters, because several factors may come together to produce a problem and most of the factors may be obscure. The etiology of a specific disorder may be apparent for such clients as those who have suffered a CVA or TBI that has resulted in swallowing, speech, or language disorders. In these cases, with medical test results and a well-documented premorbid history of your clients' communicative skills or swallowing, or both, you will be able to relate the disorders to certain specific factors.

6. *Discuss the sequence of treatment with your clients.* Explain that treatment will begin at a simple level and progress gradually to more complex levels. For example, "I will begin training the /s/ sound in single words. First, I will teach the sound at the beginning of words. After Jason masters the sounds in words, he will learn to use them in phrases and sentences. Finally, Jason will learn to produce the sounds correctly in conversation—here at the clinic and at home and school." Explain too that, although a target behavior may be established quickly in the clinical setting, it takes additional work to establish that behavior in everyday communicative situations.

7. *Allow sufficient time for clients and their families to ask questions.* Any time you give technical information, make sure the clients and their families understand by inviting questions and comments.

8. *Answer questions on treatment outcome in probabilistic terms.* You may tell the parents that they may see some improvements in their child's fluency after 3 months of treatment, but you may not say that "John will be speaking fluently in 6 months." Point out to parents that the effect of treatment will depend on many factors, including the motivation of the client, the amount of family support, duration of treatment, and so forth. Recall that ASHA Code of Ethics specifies that you not guarantee treatment outcome.

9. *Ask family members to observe treatment sessions.* This helps the family to understand the treatment process and the abilities of the client. Schedule time to discuss what they see with you. Answer questions they may have and give information to begin integrating the family into the therapeutic process. Be sure to tell the client and family that their questions and input are always welcome.

10. *Empower family members to be active participants in the client's treatment.* Let family members know the importance of their involvement in the treatment process. Early on, give family members responsibility for working with the client during therapy sessions and when at home. To help formalize the family's involvement, provide charting forms or other written material. Routinely ask for feedback regarding the family's and the client's progress when working at home. Give positive feedback and supportive instructions. Make any necessary changes in the client's and family's homework. When a client is reluctant to comply with family members' instructions, give the home assignment and explain that it is you, not the family member, who is expecting it to be completed.

11. *Review the treatment progress with your client and his or her family regularly.* Give periodic progress reports to the parents of child clients. Invite parents into the treatment room. Allow sufficient time for you to share information and answer questions. You may obtain valuable information related to your clients' treatment if you periodically schedule 10- to 15-minute sessions with parents. Discuss their child's progress only in the treatment room. Avoid discussions in the hallway, waiting room, and such other places, because they compromise client confidentiality. Also, such discussions usually are hurried and noncommunicative. Again, repeat important information; use redundancy to help clients and their families remember.

The ultimate goal of treatment is to integrate the behaviors trained in the clinical setting into a client's everyday communicative environment. To accomplish this, it is necessary for you to work closely with the client's family so that they support the newly established communicative behaviors at home and in other nonclinical settings. Therefore, families are an integral part of the treatment process. Family members can provide important information regarding not only your clients' disorders but also the family dynamics. Family members can be invaluable in assisting with generalization and maintenance of target behaviors. In medical settings, other health care providers can also be used to assist with generalization and maintenance of target behaviors. In school settings, teachers are invaluable members of the intervention team and can provide help with generalization and maintenance. Maintenance strategies are described in Chapter 10.

The Internet's Role

The use of technology has expanded rapidly. Twenty years ago, only a few people envisioned the future of the personal computer. Students understand better than many people the opportunities technology and the Internet present. Because of electronic mail (e-mail), students can readily communicate with professors and other students. They can discuss theoretical and clinical issues with experts and other students thousands of miles from their home. The Internet also offers easy access to libraries, papers, electronic journals, and support groups. However, students are only a handful of the individuals using the Internet for communication and research.

Before parents or family members bring clients in for an evaluation, it is not unusual for them to have made inquiries related to their concern about the client. For example, prior to the inexpensive availability of the Internet, if parents suspected their child had autism, they may have discussed their concern with their pediatrician and their child's preschool teacher. Also, they may have read an article or two in a popular magazine. Now parents and family members who have Internet access often have spent numerous hours researching their concerns. They may have accessed journals published by different professional associations, support groups composed of parents with similar concerns, professional discussion groups, specialized associations and organizations, articles from popular magazines, and advertisements for materials, intervention techniques, speakers, and other people and materials that offer all the answers and "cures."

Parents, family members, and clients who have taken the time to do Internet research before meeting with a speech-language pathologist may be quite knowledgeable about a disorder. Some people may be motivated and willing to apply their knowledge to assist with intervention. Occasionally, their understanding of a particular disorder may be helpful in completing the evaluation and may decrease the amount of intervention time needed. Unfortunately, other people may be misinformed. As you know, there is much misinformation published on the Internet. Also, it is easy to take information out of context or without understanding the background or related information. You can reeducate many people by explaining what is known and what has been proven to be effective in working with specific disorders. In addition, you will encounter people who resist learning the facts. They may insist that you provide a certain therapy that they read about on the Internet. If the therapy the client or the caretakers insist on using is judged inappropriate, your supervisor may decline to offer the questionable therapy to the client.

Regardless of the type of client or family member you encounter, it is important that you be well informed. Know as much as you can about the disorders your clients have. In addition, know what information and misinformation is published on the Internet. Know the latest fads and be able to explain why certain interventions are or are not appropriate; include information on the research that supports your comments.

Report Writing

Speech-language pathologists write different types of reports on clients they serve. **Diagnostic reports** provide comprehensive information on a client's pretreatment status. **Treatment plans** describe short- and long-term goals and the procedures used to obtain those goals. **Lesson plans** (in the school and some clinic settings) describe treatment planned for one or a few sessions. Client performance is described in different formats, including progress reports, final summaries, and **discharge reports**. See Hegde (2010) for a variety of clinical reports and opportunities to practice them.

In addition to generic reports, public agencies have specific reporting requirements. IEPs are required in the public schools for individuals with disabilities, 3 through 21 years of age. The **Individualized Family Service Plan (IFSP)** is required for individuals with disabilities, birth through 2 years of age, and their families.

In medical and rehabilitation settings, assessment of functional skills is often the focus. Occasionally, a checklist may be used in lieu of a written report.

The general format and content of a variety of reports are discussed in the following sections. Written report requirements will vary from one practicum site to another. You should find out what specific reporting procedures must be followed at each practicum site.

General Guidelines on Report Writing

Written reports satisfy many needs, and there are several reasons why clear, comprehensive reports are essential. Written reports *document the status of a client* and thus provide a basis for future comparisons. They also *provide an efficient form of communication* with other individuals. In clinical training programs, supervisors judge a student's knowledge and writing skills by his or her written reports. Insurance companies and other third-party agencies also use reports as a *basis from which to determine if payment will be made* for speech-language pathology services. Besides, many different individuals, including allied health professionals, educators, clients, and the clients' family members, also read the reports. Each person who reads a clinical report is likely to make certain assumptions regarding the clinician's training and professional skills. Sometimes families judge if the clinician represents their family member's abilities fairly and concludes if the clinician "likes" the client.

Although content is the most important element of your report, clear, concise presentation, neatness, and accurate use of vocabulary, grammar, spelling, and punctuation also are important. In fact, the first impression formed of your report is probably based on how the report looks, which may or may not have anything to do with your clinical abilities.

How to Write Good Reports

- Use the practicum site's format.
- Write in complete sentences.
- Spell all words correctly.
- Use correct punctuation.
- Present information in a logical sequence.
- Do not use nebulous or ambiguous statements.
- Provide as much detail as necessary to clearly describe the client's skills.
- Avoid making inferential judgments without substantiating data or qualifying statements.
- Avoid the use of jargon.
- Avoid the use of such qualifiers as "like," "very," "rather," and so on.
- Do not use sexist or culturally biased statements or make assumptions based on stereotypes.
- Use correct margins and line spacing. Follow the format requested by your supervisor.
- Use the required type of paper. Most clinics require you to use nonerasable white bond paper.
- Proofread and sign your reports before submitting them.
- Submit only high-quality computer printouts.
- Do not submit anything without page numbers.
- Always keep a copy of your report.

Some beginning student clinicians may not know where or how to begin their first reports. Find out if your university provides report-writing guidelines or samples of reports as references. If neither of these are available, refer to past reports for a writing format. The university clinic often requires more detailed reports than are typically required (or necessary) at other practicum sites. The rationale behind the overly detailed reports is that if information is not included in the report, then, possibly, you did not observe or consider it. Also, if you know how to write a detailed report well, you can always write brief reports equally well. See Hegde (2010) for multiple exemplars on general, technical, and professional writing.

The following sections offer guidelines for writing different kinds of reports. Follow the requirements on the format, style, and content of reports specified at each of your practicum sites.

Treatment Plans

After the assessment has been completed, write treatment plans that describe short- and long-term objectives and the procedures for achieving those objectives. A well-written treatment plan and accurate progress notes will allow another clinician to review the client's records and begin treatment based on the supplied information. Written treatment plans are reviewed and changed as the client's needs change. Paul-Brown (1994) recommends that the discussion of the treatment plan with the client and the client's family be noted on the treatment record. ASHA (1994c) states that the following information should be in a treatment plan:

- Dates the plan was established and discussed with the client or family as well as the dates of any interdisciplinary conferences and the date the plan is scheduled to be reviewed;

- Prognostic statements;

- Written long- and short-term objectives based on conclusions and recommendations of an evaluation;

- Statements regarding type, frequency, and duration of treatment;

- Follow-up activities; and

- Signature and title of the qualified professional responsible for the treatment plan. Both you and your supervisor will sign your reports.

In addition to this information, treatment plans include descriptions of target behaviors, stimuli to evoke responses, topographical aspects of responses, performance criteria, response consequences, probes to measure generalization, maintenance training, dismissal criteria, and follow-up treatment (Hegde, 1998a, 2010). This information is discussed in detail in the following section.

The preparation and writing of treatment plans will vary from setting to setting. Public schools, clinics, and insurance companies have their own formats. In the following section, common components of treatment plans are presented, along with examples specific to certain clinical settings. You are likely to receive additional instructions at individual practicum sites.

Writing a Treatment Plan

The comprehensive treatment plan describes the beginning of treatment to the maintenance of trained behaviors in natural environments. It details the client's and the clinician's performances as well as the interaction between the two. The treatment plan does not have to be lengthy, but it should be comprehensive (Hegde, 1998a, 2010). When you write a treatment plan, you should do the following:

1. *Briefly summarize identification data.* Describe background information, current performance levels, and purpose of treatment.

2. *Describe target behaviors.* Include both long- and short-term objectives in your description. Write objectives that are client specific (i.e., appropriate

and useful to the client), valid, and measurable. Ideally, you will have established baselines of target behaviors before preparing a treatment plan. Chapter 7 provides information on the selection of target behaviors.

3. *Describe stimuli to evoke responses.* You must determine if pictures, objects, conversation, or orthographic symbols will be used to obtain a specific response. You also must decide if visual, auditory, or tactile stimulation will be used. You must identify the setting in which treatment will be offered (e.g., in the clinical setting, in the client's home, and so on). It is not uncommon for treatment to begin at a single-word level with the presentation of pictures in the clinical setting and advance to the spontaneous speech level with conversational interaction in extraclinical environments.

4. *Describe topographical aspects of responses.* Response topography identifies the level at which treatment is initiated (e.g., at the syllable level) and the levels of progression. Response topography is not disorder specific but is used in treatment across all communication disorders. For example, a client with a voice disorder initially may sustain an appropriate pitch only during single-word productions. A client with an articulation disorder may only produce or imitate the target phoneme accurately at the single-word level.

5. *Specify performance criteria.* Describe the rate of accuracy that will be accepted as the criterion for moving through the treatment hierarchy. Distinguish between modeled and evoked responses.

6. *Describe response consequences.* Describe how you increase desirable behaviors and decrease undesirable behaviors. Specify any treatment modifications in the progress report or final summary. Response consequences that increase or decrease behaviors are discussed in Chapters 8 and 9, respectively.

7. *Describe probes for generalization.* Probes measure generalized production of the behaviors taught. However, they frequently are absent from treatment plans, perhaps because some clinicians think they are implied within the treatment sequence. To ensure that probes are not omitted, describe their use in the treatment plan. Answer the following questions in describing probes: When will probes be administered? What type of probe will be utilized? What is the criterion? What happens if the criterion is or is not met? See Chapter 8 for details on probe procedures. Appendix H has a sample probe procedure and recording sheet. A reproducible form also is provided for your use.

8. *Describe the maintenance program.* Describe how you program maintenance of target behaviors. Include in the description how you plan to teach other individuals in the client's environment.

9. *Describe the dismissal criterion.* This criterion typically reflects production of the target behaviors in conversational speech in both clinical and extraclinical settings. Written dismissal criterion helps ensure accountability. See Chapter 7 for the recommended criterion.

10. *Describe follow-up or booster treatment.* After clients have met a certain performance criteria, they are dismissed from frequently scheduled intervention sessions. However, many clients require follow-up sessions to maintain a certain proficiency level. For example, a fluency client who has established 98% fluent speech in clinical and extraclinical settings may be dismissed from twice-a-week intervention sessions. However, he or she should be scheduled for periodic follow-up sessions to assist in maintenance of fluency skills. You should specify the intervals for follow-up sessions in your initial treatment plan. Refer to Appendix I for a sample treatment plan.

Lesson Plans

Writing Lesson Plans

Although you have written a comprehensive treatment plan, you also may be required to write lesson plans, which are a description of session-by-session or weekly activities planned for the client so the supervisor knows what you are doing in a given session. As part of your planning and preparation for clinical sessions, you will write lesson plans for each of your clients. At the university clinic, lesson plans commonly are developed on a weekly basis and submitted to the clinical supervisor in advance for approval. The lesson plan typically contains the following information:

- *Treatment objectives.* Write the treatment objectives for your client. For example: The production of /s/ in word initial positions at the evoked level, with 90% accuracy.

- *Procedures and materials for obtaining the objectives.* Describe how you will implement the treatment objectives; include materials and treatment procedures. For example: The /s/ picture cards and /s/ objects will be presented to the client. The client will be required to name each picture. All correct /s/ productions will be verbally reinforced. All incorrect /s/ productions will be interrupted by a verbal "No" or "Stop."

Information contained in the lesson plan may be similar to items identified in the treatment plan (e.g., response typography, criterion levels, management of consequences). However, the lesson plan does not always allow for a complete view of the client's treatment. The lesson plan describes what is done in a session or two, whereas the treatment plan describes the total sequence of treatment for a given period. Refer to Appendix J for a sample lesson plan and Hegde (2010) for additional examples.

Individualized Education Programs

Writing Individualized Education Programs

Public Law 94-142 (and its many amendments) mandates a free, appropriate public education and related services for all children and youth who have a disability. Speech-language pathology is a part of **designated instructional services (DIS)** under special education services. A written IEP is required for each child, ages 3 through 21 years, who receives special education services.

IEPs originally were formulated to provide for management, communication, and accountability in special education services. More than a treatment plan, the IEP is a management plan that links the child's needs, individual services, and educational outcomes. It is also a contract between the school and the family. The IEP describes what will be trained but not the specific training procedures. Specific rules regulate the development, writing, and implementation of IEPs. There are many legal requirements regarding the time lines for services, identification, referral, assessment, enrollment and dismissal of students, the rights of parents, and due process. The following section gives you guidelines on writing the speech-language IEP.

Content of the IEP

A speech-language pathologist writes an IEP for each student he or she serves. The parents are important members of the IEP team and provide input regarding the delivery of special education services for their children. An IEP must be developed before a student can receive services. An annual meeting to review the IEP is required, although meetings may be held more frequently. IDEA 2004 authorizes the development of three-year IEPs for students age 18 and older. Emphasis is placed on the collaboration and coordination between public schools and adult programs. In addition to annual review of students' progress, periodic progress reports are required. Many IEP forms are used, but the basic content is the same. To provide a comprehensive management plan, the following information must be included on an IEP (Moore-Brown & Montgomery, 2005; California State Department of Education, 1989; Dublinske & Healey, 1978).

1. *Give the identifying information.* Write the child's name, address, phone number, birth date, and parent's name(s) on the IEP. Also write the student identification or folder number on the IEP, and note the child's grade, native language, and English language proficiency. The influence of limited English on academic performance must be considered when developing the IEP.

2. *Describe the child's present level of performance.* State current communicative performance, including both receptive and expressive speech and language skills, behavioral problems noted or reported, related educational strengths or weaknesses, and contributing history or current developmental or health information. Also report learning styles. Present levels of performance must be based on at least two assessment procedures. Report test scores as standard scores or percentiles. Both standardized tests and speech samples typically are used to describe communicative skills. Sometimes you may refer the reader to a separate diagnostic report rather than repeating the information; for example, you might write "For additional information, see diagnostic report 4–10–08." Report sufficient information to develop appropriate objectives. Information about the student's strengths should be noted. Include relevant information obtained from interviews with parents and teachers.

3. *Describe how the disability affects the student's educational performance.* Indicate how the disability affects the student's involvement, progress, and participation in the typical curriculum. You must report the child's present levels of performance as compared to educational performance. For instance, report how the 6-year-old child's speech intelligibility of 50% affects his or her educational performance. For example, *Sandy's speech in the classroom is 50% intelligible and does not allow her to successfully participate in oral presentations. Also, her teacher is not able to understand many of the questions and responses Sandy produces in class.*

4. *Describe objectives.* When required, write goals to describe the child's expected performance for an entire school year. Objectives (or short-term goals) reflect steps necessary to obtain the long-term goal. In some cases these objectives are referred to as **benchmarks.** Write measurable objectives (or benchmarks) that have a completion date and performance criteria. For example:

Goal: Increased sentence length in classroom conversation and oral presentations to a minimum mean length of utterance of 4.0 words by _____ (specify a date).

Objective: By _____ (specify a date), following picture presentation, Jennie is expected to produce 10 sentences, containing a minimum of 4 words, with 90% accuracy at the evoked level over three sessions. Progress will be measured by response charting.

Base the long-term goals and the objectives on information reported in the present levels of performance. The goals and objectives should help meet the student's needs that were reflected in the description of the present levels of performance. Develop objectives that demonstrate incremental steps toward the goal. As much as possible develop goals that relate to educational benchmarks (or goals). Other IEP team members, especially the parents, provide input regarding the development of the student's IEP goals and objectives. The speech-language pathologist will guide the selection of treatment goals that are appropriate to the student's current abilities. At the annual review meeting, note the status of the goals and objectives. Some of these may have been met; others may not. Work on some goals or objectives may not have begun yet. There is no required number of goals or objectives.

5. *Describe special education services required.* Specify the type of service that will be provided, the frequency of the service, the duration of each session, and the location of the service on the IEP. For example, speech services may be provided as follows:

Group therapy/2x per week/40 minutes each session in the speech-language pathologist's office.

or

Teacher consult/1x per month/30 minutes each session in student's classroom.

6. *Describe the amount of time the child will spend in the regular educational program.* Note the child's participation in regular education on the IEP. For the speech IEP, you may abbreviate the amount of time the child will spend in regular education as a percentage (e.g., 95% per week).

7. *Describe when the services will begin and end.* Write the beginning and ending dates of service on the IEP. Services should begin with minimal delay. Initiation of service often begins the next school day or week after the IEP meeting. If an IEP meeting is held at the end of the school year, services begin as soon as school resumes. Because an annual review is required of each student enrolled in special education services, you must write the duration of service for 1 year or less. Note this in month/day/year format (e.g., 06/01/2009).

8. *Describe how progress will be reported.* In addition to the annual review of the IEP, you must report the child's progress to parents regularly. On the IEP, note if you will periodically report progress by sending a report card, progress report, or other type of communication.

9. *Specify the rationale for special education services.* The rationale or justification for service is based on an established criterion for enrollment. In an IEP, indicate if the child is to be enrolled in, continued in, or dismissed from special education services.

   The criteria for speech–language pathology services are based on legal requirements and are not always consistent with the common practices in the professional community. As noted before, a 5-year-old child with a frontal lisp may receive speech–language pathology services through a private agency but may not be eligible for speech services in the school until he or she is 8 years old. Your school district will provide you with a summary of its eligibility criteria for speech–language pathology services.

   The justification for service can be brief or lengthy:

   Language needs cannot be met in the regular education setting. Standardized test scores reflected performance 1.5 standard deviations below the mean in all language areas. Analysis of a conversation sample revealed errors in syntax and morphology and limited semantic abilities, which hamper progress in the general education class.

   Conversational speech is 15% dysfluent and student cannot make effective oral presentations that are required in general education class. Speech needs cannot be met in the regular education classroom.

10. *Describe all professionals providing services.* The child receiving speech–language pathology services also may be receiving other special education services. Include related services that are educationally necessarily. Give the names of all services and all service providers on the IEP.

Some common services and the individuals responsible for providing them include the following:

- Counseling: School psychologist

- Medication follow-up: School nurse

- Speech services: School speech–language pathologist

- Special reading lessons: Reading specialist

- Hearing services: Educational audiologist

11. *Get the signature of all individuals attending the IEP meeting.* The names, positions, signatures, and dates of participation of all the individuals attending the IEP meeting must appear on the IEP. Regular education teachers have a place to sign, as does the special education teacher. Other specialists such as the school psychologist and the school nurse may sign the IEP. Get the parents' signatures on the IEP, indicating consent with the IEP for their child's placement in special education. Parents dissenting with the recommended IEP may be provided a separate line to sign or box to check, but a signature may still be required to indicate attendance at the meeting. The child also may attend and be a member of the IEP team. If appropriate, have the child sign the IEP form. If an interpreter is used at the IEP meeting, get the interpreter's signature and write his or her title on the IEP.

12. *Note additional IEP information.* Write (or check) the following information on the IEP:

- Date of annual review;

- Date of 3-year evaluation;

- Eligibility for extended school year; and

- Recommendations for specific materials, methods, or equipment needed to accomplish the goals.

To reduce paperwork, many school districts use computerized forms or checklists for their IEPs. Computer-generated and checklist formats should be diverse enough to allow the development of an individualized program. This is not a problem with most programs. If none of the already written objectives are appropriate, there usually is a space for other objectives to be written. Your school site will supply you with IEP forms.

Individual Family Service Plan (IFSP)

As an amendment to P.L. 94-142, P. L. 99-457 Part H established an early intervention program for infants and toddlers and their families. This program requires that an IFSP be written for children with disabilities, ages birth through 2 years. The IFSP must be developed by a multidisciplinary team of professionals and the child's parent(s).

The Contents of IFSPs

- Present levels of performance (physical, cognitive, communicative, and self-help)

- Family needs and strengths related to assisting the child

- Intervention goals and the ways progress will be measured

- Types of services the child will receive

- Initiation and duration of services

- The name of the case manager

The IEP and IFSP are similar in that they both describe clinical and educational objectives, types of services to be provided, and the beginning and ending dates of services. The IFSP differs from the IEP because of its emphasis on family involvement. The IFSP targets not only the needs of the child but also the strengths and weaknesses of the family and how these influence the child's development. Emphasized in the 1997 and 2004 revisions of IDEA is the location of services. Services should be provided in the **natural environment.** For young children, this often translates to providing services in their homes, at a playground, in an activity center, or in any other location where nondisabled children could typically be found. The IFSP incorporates public school services and the services of other public agencies (e.g., families may need respite care services or social welfare services, as well as educational and rehabilitation services). The case manager is selected based on the needs of the child and the family. Basically, the case manager is responsible for identifying, coordinating, and monitoring services. The case manager may be a speech-language pathologist, audiologist, special education teacher, psychologist, social worker, or other professional. A review of the IFSP is required every 6 months, compared with the IEP's annual review.

Diagnostic Reports

Diagnostic reports are written following the evaluation of a client. A diagnostic report is a summary of case history, assessment data, clinical impressions, conclusions, and recommendations. It provides a clear, written statement of the client's communicative abilities at the time of the evaluation. It also provides a forum for communicating with other professionals. At times the diagnostic report may be used to help obtain payment from an insurance company for the services provided. At other times it may be used for research; therefore, it is important to clearly document information and differentiate between subjective statements and objective data.

Each client's file must contain a diagnostic evaluation. A copy of an evaluation performed at another facility may be included in a case file. When you are assigned a client who has been evaluated by another clinician, in accordance with the guidelines at your site obtain a copy of the diagnostic report for the client's file.

There are several formats for writing diagnostic reports (Emerick & Pindzola, 2007; Hegde, 2010; Knepflar & May, 1989). In addition, reporting requirements vary at each practicum site. To write a diagnostic report, use the following outline, or modify it for different practicum settings.

1. *Give identification information.* Give this information at the beginning of the report. Include the following: the client's name, file number, address, phone number, date of birth, age, diagnosis, date of evaluation, name of the evaluator, and the name of the individual who referred the client. If applicable, also note the client's occupation or school level and parents' names.

2. *Write a statement of the problem.* Describe briefly the client's presenting complaint. To be explicit, write the client's comments verbatim and identify them as such in the text. For example: *(1) Mrs. Applegate stated her voice was "scratchy and old sounding." (2) Mr. Thomas reported that he stuttered. He said that his "blocked speech" occurred most frequently when he spoke on the telephone.* Note the client's words by using quotation marks. If someone other than the client was the informant, indicate it: *Mr. John Jones, who accompanied Johnny to the clinic, was the informant during the interview.*

3. *Write the diagnostic report in the past tense.* You are writing about performance that you observed during the assessment. For example, write: *Joan omitted final consonants in her spontaneous speech.* Your observation of the client is limited to a specific time and your statements must be limited to those observations.

4. *Give background information.* Describe the client's background. Obtain this information from the client's case history, client interview, and reports by other professionals. Detail relevant information in this section. Do not report unrelated provided information. Include the client's developmental history, medical history, social and family history, and educational history in this section. For some clients, it will be necessary to report only certain areas; for other clients, all areas will need to be documented. For example, for a child with language problems, educational background must be described in some detail; but for an adult man with a hoarse voice, detailed educational history may not be necessary. If the reported medical history was unremarkable for speech and language development, just say that: *The reported medical history was unremarkable.* However, if a number of illnesses were reported, or if many medications were prescribed or were continued to be prescribed, then carefully document this in the report. Note in this section any previous speech-language pathology services the client has received. Report previous diagnoses. If you summarize information from another professional's report (another speech-language pathologist, a physician, a teacher), always give the professional's name, credentials, and date of report.

5. *Summarize assessment information.* Describe results of the pure-tone audiometric screening, oral peripheral examination, and speech and language assessments.

6. *Include statements regarding the client's general behavior.* Include in your behavioral observations such information as the client's attending behavior and cooperativeness. For example: "The client was cooperative and attended to all tasks with minimal verbal prompting throughout the 1-hour evaluation session. Results were considered representative of the client's abilities."

7. *Perform an audiometric screening.* This is a part of all speech-language evaluations. If it is impossible to perform the screening, note this in the diagnostic report and refer the client for an audiological examination. If a client is wearing hearing aids, perform a hearing aid check before the speech and language assessment to ensure that the hearing aids are functioning.

8. *Perform an oral peripheral examination.* This is a standard part of diagnostic evaluation. The amount of information that must be written in the report will depend on the results of this examination. If no abnormalities were observed, then briefly describe the results. Write in detail any structural or motorical deviations observed.

9. *Describe in detail the speech and language assessment.* Include information about the client's articulation, voice, fluency, receptive language, and expressive language. You should report results of standardized testing, language sampling, and informal clinical observations of communicative abilities. Do not just list test scores; instead, say what they mean. For example, the statement that "The client obtained a raw score of 9 on the auditory comprehension subtest of the Preschool Language Scale 4" means little to your readers, unless they have memorized the test or have the test administration booklet in front of them.

10. *Quantify results of your client's speech sample.* Report the total number of words in the sample. When reporting certain behaviors (e.g., correct use of plural /s/), give the percentage of occurrence or the specific number of times its production was evoked. For example: *The client produced the plural /s/ correctly 75% of 27 obligatory contexts in which it was evoked.* This statement is more meaningful than *The client three times produced the plural /s/ correctly.* If the client omitted specific speech or language structures, give the total number of opportunities (or obligatory contexts) he or she had to produce them. For example: *The client did not produce the plural /s/ in 10 phrases that should have contained the plural /s/.*

11. *Present the information in a logical and organized sequence.* Describe observations relevant to speech, language, voice, fluency, and other aspects in separate paragraphs. Do not confuse the reader by writing about articulation performance in sections describing fluency and voice.

12. *Write a statement about each parameter of speech.* This will document that all aspects of the client's speech and language were evaluated, even if no disorder or deviation was exhibited in some areas. For example, if you made no mention of fluency in your report on a child with an articulation disorder because you found no problem with it, the reader cannot be sure of this.

Therefore, it is necessary to write such a statement as: *Analysis of a 200-utterance speech sample revealed 97% fluent speech.*

13. *Do not cross professional boundaries.* When you present assessment information, limit yourself to speech-language functions. A common problem occurs when guessing at cognitive levels. The speech-language pathologist cannot report IQ scores. Neither can you diagnose psychological disorders (depression, mental retardation, etc.). However, you can report behavior that you have observed. For example, you might write: "The boy appeared withdrawn throughout the evaluation. That is, he sat with his arms crossed through most of the evaluation and was never observed to make eye contact with the examiner."

14. *Summarize your impressions.* This section is a summary and interpretation of all the information gathered in your assessment. Report the type and severity of any communicative disorder in this section. Also report if no communicative disorder was exhibited. If a cause for a found disorder is known, you may report it in this section. You may make a statement about the prognosis here or report it in the recommendations section.

15. *Write recommendations.* In this section include the type and amount of service needed, further assessment required, and/or referral to other professionals. Although specific areas of need should be identified, do not report exact objectives. As you know, additional evaluation, including baselines, may need to be performed before starting intervention. You must confer with your clinical supervisor before making specific recommendations.

16. *Sign the report.* Conclude the report with your name, title, and signature. Your clinical supervisor also must sign the report; therefore, type his or her name and title. Refer to Appendix K for a sample diagnostic report and to Hegde (2010) for a variety of examples.

Progress Reports

Progress reports provide information about intervention procedures, a client's performance, and further recommendations. There are several types of progress reports. Two types of commonly used progress reports are described in this section. The first type of progress report is written daily or for every session to document the client's performance. Because they are brief, daily progress reports often are called progress notes. The second type of report is written periodically to summarize a client's progress for a specific treatment period. At the university clinic, the periodic report may be called a *final summary* or *progress report* written at the end of a semester or quarter. Both types of reporting document necessary clinical information.

Daily Progress Notes

You should chart your client's performance in each session. Your practicum site may provide you with a recording form or you may develop your own. This recording form will include spaces for the client's name, the date of the session, the objective(s), stimuli, client responses, response consequences, and remarks. If you are using unique materials or equipment, you may want to note that on the recording form. A sample treatment recording form is illustrated in Appendix L.

Record the results of each clinical session on a chronological log as soon as possible after the session. This enables you and your supervisor to review the treatment session and make necessary modifications. It also provides a means of communication among professionals. It gives enough information for another clinician to serve your client if you are unable to do so.

One form of charting and reporting client progress is referred to as *SOAP notes* (Flower, 1984; Golper, 1998). "SOAP" stands for "subjective," "objective," "assessment," "plan."

Guidelines on Writing SOAP Notes

1. Describe your impressions of the client in the subjective section. For example: The client appeared very alert and cooperative. He stated, "I'm ready to work hard today."

2. Write measurable information in the objective section. For instance: The client produced four-syllable phrases with 80% accuracy in 40 out of 50 trials (40/50).

3. Describe your analysis of the session in the assessment section. You also may compare the client's performance across sessions in this section. For example: (a) Production of /r/ increased from 65% accuracy during the last session to 90% accuracy during today's session; (b) Withdrawal of visual models resulted in a decrease in accurate production of single syllable words from 90% to 65%.

4. Outline the course of treatment in the plan section. You might simply state: (a) Continue current treatment activities; (b) Continue training production of functional CVC words at the imitative level.

SOAP notes are more commonly used in the medical setting but also may be used at other practicum sites. If a lesson plan has been prepared in advance of each session, you may sometimes write the results of the session directly on the lesson plan. Because the lesson plan has already detailed the activities, you may just specify a percentage after an activity. For example: *Initial /s/: 90% at the word level. Medial /l/: 30% at the phrase level.*

Regardless of the form of recording, the data should be accurate and recorded during each session. At the end of the sessions, you may write additional notes. You may make subjective statements, but do not confuse them for observed facts. Also, support your statements with observable data.

Guidelines on Writing Progress Reports

- Write legibly.

- Date entries.

- Use a pen (some agencies require you to use a specific pen color).

- Initial or sign your name on all progress notes. At certain clinical practicum sites your supervisor will cosign your progress notes.

- Be accurate.

- Report objective data.

- Avoid qualifiers such as "seems to" or "appeared," unless you report specific behaviors to support your assumptions.

- Record progress notes immediately following your clinic session.

- Use only those abbreviations or jargon that others will understand. These usages may change depending on the site.

Several abbreviations are used in writing progress notes. Refer to Appendix B for some of the commonly used abbreviations. Appendix M contains a sample of progress notes.

Periodic Progress Reports

In medical and private clinics, periodic progress reports are written to summarize a client's treatment and its results. Procedures and their effects on the client's communicative behaviors are described. Again, depending on your practicum assignment, there will be different requirements for writing progress reports. In writing progress reports:

1. *Give client identification information.* List the client's name, age, address, phone number, occupation or school status, and birth date. If applicable, give the name of the parent or spouse.

2. *Describe the period covered by the report.* Note the dates that the treatment period began and ended. Also note when treatment was originally initiated, if different from the beginning period of the report.

3. *List the number of sessions the client attended.* You will want to carefully document how many sessions your client actually attended. You may be reporting on a treatment period covering 3 months in which your client only attended six sessions.

4. *List the length of the treatment sessions.* You will see clients for differing lengths of time. Some clients may attend 60-minute sessions and others

only 30-minute sessions. Include the length of time you spend with your client in each progress report.

5. *Briefly summarize the client's status at the beginning of the treatment period.* State the client's status before the reporting period. Also, do not write as detailed a description of the client's status at the beginning of the treatment period as you did in your diagnostic report. Give only a brief overview of his or her communicative abilities at the beginning of the treatment period. For example, you might state: *An analysis of conversational speech in the clinic setting revealed 85% fluency. Analysis of an audiotaped sample of the client's conversational speech at home revealed 82% fluency.*

6. *Summarize the treatment plan.* Describe the treatment objectives and procedures. Include enough information for the reader to know what your progression of intervention was and what stimuli and response consequences were used. If the procedure described in the treatment plan was modified, describe the changes and justify them.

7. *Describe the client's performance.* Describe how the client's target behaviors changed during the course of the intervention. Make such objective statements as *At the beginning of treatment, Tom's voice was judged hoarse on 90% of his utterances. At the end of the semester, he was judged hoarse on 10% of his utterances.* Include tables and graphs that summarize quantitative data and show changes over the course of treatment.

8. *Summarize your conclusions and recommendations.* Include in this section your overall impressions of treatment effectiveness. Make a prognostic statement and recommendations based on that prognosis. Did your client make progress? Do you expect your client to continue to make progress? What type of intervention will enable the client to continue to progress? For example: *John demonstrated progress throughout this treatment period. Based on his performance over the past 3 months, prognosis for continued progress is good. It is recommended that John continue to receive treatment for his voice disorder. To be most effective, treatment should be given two times per week for a minimum of 30 minutes each session.*

9. *End your report with your name, title, and signature.* Also include your supervisor's name, title, and signature. Refer to Appendix N for a sample progress report and to Hegde (2010) for multiple exemplars.

Final Summaries

At the end of each semester, you must prepare a report for each of the clients you served at the university clinic. This is a report of the client's treatment. The final summary is sometimes interchangeable with a progress report. It contains information similar to a progress report but often provides more detailed information. As in a progress report, include the following in a final summary:

- The client identification information

- The period covered by the report

- The number of sessions attended by the client and the length of the sessions
- Summary of the client's status at the beginning of the treatment period
- Summary of the treatment plan
- Description of the client's performance and improvement
- Your conclusions and recommendations
- Names and signatures (yours and your supervisor's)

See Appendix O for a sample final summary and Hegde (2010) for multiple exemplars.

Discharge Reports

A discharge report is written at the time clients are dismissed from treatment. Clients are dismissed because they no longer need intervention or do not benefit from it. Others may be dismissed because they do not attend intervention sessions regularly or have stopped coming to the sessions. Some clients may be dismissed or may dismiss themselves from treatment because they cannot afford treatment.

The discharge report follows a format similar to that of the final summary. It covers the treatment period from the beginning of treatment to the discharge date. Regardless of the title of the report, a final report is always prepared when a client leaves treatment at any facility. In this case, the discharge report and final summary may be the same.

Record-Keeping Procedures

Besides writing various kinds of reports, student clinicians are responsible for maintaining client files and an accurate log of their clinical practicum hours. Therefore, you should know the general procedures of maintaining client records and your practicum records.

Client Files

Because they are confidential, clinic files are kept in a secured area such as a locked room or in a locked file cabinet. As noted previously, you should never leave clinic files unattended, release copies of reports to other professionals or agencies without prior written approval from the client, or take clients' files home.

You are responsible for maintaining your clients' files in a complete and orderly fashion. Follow the procedure established at your clinic for filing documents, recording phone calls, and so on.

To ensure that all necessary information is in their files and is current, review your clients' files periodically. Ask your clients if the phone numbers and addresses in their files are correct. Note all changes in the clients' folders and report them to your clinic secretary. To maintain adequate records, follow the general guidelines (Paul-Brown, 1994) and the specific requirements of the clinic.

Information to Be Included in Client Records

- Client identification information: telephone number, address, file number, and so forth

- The name of the individual or agency that referred the client

- Client history including any related information from other agencies, such as copies of medical reports, IEPs, psychological evaluations, and so on

- The name of the speech-language pathologist (and student clinician) responsible for service delivery to the client

- A diagnostic report (may have been performed at another facility)

- A current treatment plan, including specific objectives and prognosis

- Indication of when the treatment plan was discussed with the client or the responsible member of the client's family

- Notations regarding conferences held with other professionals

- Treatment reports, progress reports, and final summaries

- A chronological log of all services provided for the client

- Daily progress notes reflecting current status of treatment objectives

- A signed and dated consent for release of information

At the university clinic, client files should also contain a signed and dated consent to be observed. All records must be signed by an individual holding current ASHA certification.

Practicum Hours

Student clinicians are responsible for maintaining a log of their clock hours earned in clinical practicum. Your university probably will provide you with a form for reporting these hours. Such a form may be a part of your academic file and will include ASHA's *KASA*. Because you will not always be seeing clients for an entire hour, you may need to report fractions of hours. Use a consistent system for recording clock hours earned. For example, do not report a 30-minute session one time as 1/2 hour, another time as 30 minutes, and still another time as .5 hr. At the end of the term, totaling your hours will be much easier if your reporting is consistent and systematic. Use the following guidelines for reporting clock hours and fractions of hours.

60 minutes = 1.0 hour	30 minutes = .5
55 minutes = .9	25 minutes = .4

50 minutes = .8	20 minutes = .3
45 minutes = .75	15 minutes = .25
40 minutes = .7	10 minutes = .2
35 minutes = .6	5 minutes = .1

All clock hours must be verified by a signature of the supervising speech-language pathologist. Chapter 1 describes the activities that may be counted as practicum hours.

Working with Other Professionals

To provide effective services to their clients, speech-language pathologists frequently must work with other specialists. You often will see clients who receive services from such professionals as a physician, physical therapist, psychologist, or special education teacher. You may need to coordinate your services with the services delivered by these professionals. You also must refer clients to other specialists for services. For example, you probably will refer an individual who comes to see you about a voice problem to an otolaryngologist for a laryngeal evaluation. You will refer the individual who does not pass his or her hearing screening to an audiologist for an audiological examination. (Refer to Appendix P for a sample referral letter.) You will consult with professionals in allied health and education professions. To enhance services to clients, speech-language pathologists must develop a working relationship with these professionals.

To work effectively with other professionals, you should know about their services. Following is a summary of the services provided by different specialists with whom you may work.

Health and Allied Health Professionals

To work effectively with other professionals, you must know something about their roles. Following is a summary of the services provided by different specialists.

1. **Audiologist.** *The audiologist is a specialist in the identification, measurement, and rehabilitation of hearing impairments.* Whether you work in a medical setting, private practice, or educational setting, you will work closely with audiologists in many instances. For example, you will refer clients who do not pass their hearing screenings to audiologists. Also, you may find that some of your clients have hearing aids that are not functioning correctly. The audiologist may recommend repair, modification, or replacement of the hearing aids. You may work closely with the audiologist in developing a rehabilitation program for a child with a hearing impairment or in developing a program for community access to assistive listening devices. Audiologists and speech-language pathologists collaborate in treating an individual who has had a cochlear implant. Also, the audiologist is trained to screen for the presence of a speech or language disorder and may refer individuals to you for speech or language services.

2. **Board Certified Behavior Analyst.** *The Board Certified Behavior Analyst (commonly referred to as BCBA) is an individual who conducts behavioral assessments and designs and supervises interventions based on the principles of applied behavioral analysis (ABA).* The BCBA has a master's degree, has completed a specified number of practicum hours, and has passed an examination. In some areas, the BCBA has become the professional of choice to develop and oversee intervention programs for children with autism. If you work with young children with autism, it is likely that you will encounter BCBAs and often work in collaboration with them. Communication between you and the BCBA professional will not be difficult for you since you have had similar coursework and also focus on observable behaviors rather than theoretical frameworks.

3. **Cardiologist.** *The cardiologist is a physician with specialized training in cardiovascular diseases (heart and circulatory disease).* Because of the nature of their specialty, cardiologists most frequently work with adults, but there are children who also require their services. You may not work frequently with cardiologists, but occasionally you will work with children or adults who have some form of cardiovascular disorder. For example, some of your clients may have a genetic syndrome. Many such syndromes are associated with a high incidence of cardiovascular disorders. Some of the prematurely born infants and children you work with also may have cardiovascular problems. The cardiologist may refer individuals to you who have voice problems because of their reduced lung capacity. You need to find out from the cardiologist what physical abilities you reasonably can expect from your clients. You also need to know if medications your clients are taking may affect speech or behavior (e.g., lethargy, attention span, memory).

4. **Dietitian.** *A dietitian is a professional with training in nutrition and diet. The dietitian is responsible for planning and managing the food service in health care settings.* In certain settings, you may work closely with the dietitian in treating patients with swallowing disorders. You will need the dietitian's assistance in providing appropriate foods for your patient's treatment and meals.

5. **Neurologist.** *The neurologist is a physician with specialized training in function and disorders of the nervous system.* Within neurology, there are subspecialties such as pediatric neurology. It is not unusual for the neurologist to work with individuals who also have speech or language disorders. The neurologist may work with individuals recovering from a CVA, head trauma, or a variety of other neurological disorders.

   The neurologist may request a speech and language assessment of a client recovering from a CVA or head trauma. You must provide detailed information, including prognosis for speech and language rehabilitation and treatment recommendations.

   Your clients with aphasia, Parkinson's disease, or Alzheimer's disease may be seeing a neurologist or may already have seen one. The neurologist can provide information about the extent and location of brain involvement, effect of current medications, and prognosis.

Neurologists also work with individuals with behavior disorders. For example, you may be working with a child who begins receiving medication for aggressive behavior. You may need to document any change in speech or language performance after the child takes the medication.

If you work with a client with a seizure disorder, he or she likely will be receiving services from a neurologist. If you suspect a client of having undiagnosed seizures, you may refer the client to a neurologist. You will want to know from all your clients if they are taking medication that may affect their speech, attention span, or alertness.

6. **Occupational Therapist.** *The registered occupational therapist (OT or OTR) provides evaluation and treatment of daily living skills for individuals with disabilities.* This includes assessing and retraining such skills as dressing, cooking, and bathing. The OT also may be involved in training clients in the use of adaptive living devices. Adaptive living devices help individuals live more independently. They include such equipment as modified eating utensils, modified cooking equipment, adaptive equipment for self-dressing, and so forth. More and more OTs work with children with autism providing "sensory integration (SI)" therapy, which is based on little empirical evidence but has been supported anecdotally by some parents and professionals. In SI therapy the OT works with the individual to either decrease or increase the effects of various environmental factors (e.g., noise, touch, odors, and so on). In some settings, the OT provides "cognitive therapy." Basically, cognitive therapy involves the same activities you provide in language therapy that involve comprehension, memory, judgment, and reasoning. Your most common interaction with the OT will be in working with patients with dysphagia. Depending on the setting, either the OT or the speech-language pathologist heads the dysphagia team. There has been much discussion between speech-language pathology associations and occupational therapy associations regarding which profession should be responsible for treating dysphagia and providing cognitive therapy. Follow the guidelines provided at your clinical site.

Because of the overlap in services, it is essential that you regularly communicate with the OT. You want to provide maximum clinical service without duplicating efforts. To provide effective clinical service, the OT will need to know your role in treatment of dysphagia and communication. Also, the OT will need to know the patients' communicative abilities. You will provide the OT with information on the patients' receptive and expressive language and give suggestions on how he or she can help enhance the patients' communicative skills.

7. **Orthodontist.** *The orthodontist is a specialist in dental occlusion.* You will work closely with the orthodontist providing services for a client with cleft palate, other craniofacial anomaly, or myofunctional disorder. The orthodontist may request a detailed speech evaluation from you. In some instances, your reports will be critical in helping the orthodontist determine

the course of treatment for the client. As always you should provide accurate, detailed information.

8. **Otolaryngologist.** *The otolaryngologist (commonly called an ENT) is a physician specializing in evaluation and treatment of disorders of the ear, nose, and throat.* The speech–language pathologist often has a close working relationship with the ENT. You and the otolaryngologist may share clients with voice disorders, chronic otitis media, hearing loss, or laryngeal cancer. A few instances in which you might work with an otolaryngologist are described in the following paragraphs.

If you are working with a child who has a history of chronic otitis media, you should find out what types of medical treatment the child is receiving from the otolaryngologist. You should closely monitor the child's hearing and refer to the physician if there is a decrease in hearing abilities.

If you have a client who has been diagnosed with vocal nodules, the otolaryngologist may consult with you regarding treatment. The otolaryngologist may suggest a trial period of voice treatment before recommending surgical intervention. Carefully document progress in voice treatment and refer your client back to the otolaryngologist.

You may work with the otolaryngologist in educating the individual facing a laryngectomy. After you receive a referral from the otolaryngologist, you will educate the client about communication options following laryngectomy. The laryngologist will inform you of the surgery schedule, and you will meet with the client soon after the surgery to provide an immediate method of communication. You also may arrange for a person who already has had a laryngectomy to meet with your client before and after surgery.

9. **Pediatrician.** *The pediatrician is a physician specializing in the medical care of children.* You may refer children to their pediatricians because of suspected hearing or vision problems, chronic health problems (allergies, colds, and so on), or unusual behaviors such as poor attention span.

You will encounter some pediatricians who are knowledgeable about communicative disorders and many who are not. Unfortunately, a few pediatricians continue to erroneously advise parents that their children will outgrow a communication problem. One of your responsibilities is to educate pediatricians about early intervention for speech and language disorders. One way to do this is to provide regular progress reports regarding any of their patients for whom you may be providing services.

10. **Physiatrist.** *The physiatrist is a physician with specialized training in rehabilitative medicine.* The physiatrist directs the rehabilitation of a patient who is disabled. Although there are many reasons for the disabilities experienced by the physiatrist's patients, often the disability is caused by CVA or head trauma.

In the medical setting, you may work closely with the physiatrist who may refer patients to you. He or she may request that you give a detailed report on patients' communicative skills, speech and language prognoses, and recommendations. You also may offer suggestions to assist in patients' reentry into their school, work, or home.

11. **Physical Therapist.** *The registered physical therapist (RPT or PT) provides assessment and treatment for disorders related to physical and musculoskeletal injuries.* In the hospital and rehabilitation setting, the speech-language pathologist and physical therapist often provide services for many of the same patients.

    The physical therapist provides you with information about patients' motor abilities and optimum positioning and posture. This information can be essential in developing an appropriate eating program or successful implementation of an augmentative communication device.

    You will provide the PT with information about patients' communication skills. The PT may want to know what types of instructions (e.g., single-word commands) a patient can understand.

12. **Prosthodontist.** *The prosthodontist is a dentist with specialized training in the development and use of prosthetic appliances.* The speech-language pathologist and prosthodontist may consult regarding a client with insufficient velopharyngeal closure. You may refer a client with velopharyngeal incompetence (VPI) to a prosthodontist. A prosthodontist may ask you to help assess velopharyngeal adequacy in a patient before and after a prosthetic appliance is used. You also may be asked for suggestions regarding choice of appliances.

13. **Radiologist.** *The radiologist is a physician specializing in the evaluation and treatment of disease with radioactive substances (X-ray).* The radiologist may perform brain imaging for patients with aphasia. You and the radiologist also may share patients with laryngeal cancer and swallowing disorders.

    Your most frequent contact with the radiologist may involve patients with swallowing disorders. The radiologist may perform videofluoroscopy for patients with dysphagia. You may give suggestions regarding positioning of the patient and textures and types of foods to use during the evaluation. You will work closely with the radiologist in evaluating results of the videofluoroscopic examination.

14. **Registered Nurse.** *The registered nurse (RN) is responsible for most medical care prescribed by the physician for the patient.* Because registered nurses work closely with patients, it is important for the speech-language pathologist and nurse to develop effective communication. The RN can provide information on a patient's daily communicative skills. Another part of patient care is provided by the licensed vocational nurse (LVN) or licensed professional nurse (LPN). The LVN is frequently identified as a nurse's aide, has less medical training than the RN, and delivers such care as bathing and feeding patients and taking vital signs.

    The nursing staff will request information from you on the patient's receptive and expressive abilities. The staff may give you information about patients' communicative attempts. They also may help identify patients needing your services. Because the nursing staff typically has the most contact with the patients and their families, it is critical for you to develop a good working relationship with them.

15. **Social Worker.** *The social worker is often a member of the hospital's rehabilitation team working closely with the patient's family.* You can obtain information about community services that your clients may need from the social worker. You also may ask the social worker to intercede with your patients' families who are having difficulty. For example, if you are serving an elderly patient in his or her home, you may observe that neither the spouse nor the patient is able to prepare meals adequately. The social worker may be able to obtain part-time help for the couple or arrange for delivery of meals through social service agencies that provide such services as prepared meals delivered to the home.

Educational Specialists

1. **Adaptive Physical Education Specialist.** *The adaptive physical education specialist has specialized training in physical education.* These specialists have been trained to work with individuals with disabilities, such as providing physical education programs. For certain students, they may also provide gross and fine motor activities. You probably will not work closely with the adaptive physical education specialist; however, they often are members of the IEP team.

2. **Educational Audiologist.** *The educational audiologist specializes in working with children in the public schools.* The educational audiologist provides assessment and management of hearing disorders for children in the public schools. As a school-based speech–language pathologist, you may frequently interact with the educational audiologist. You may have children on your caseload who are deaf or have limited hearing. Also, you may have children whom you suspect may have hearing problems or you may be working with a child who has had a cochlear implant. In all these cases you will want to consult with the educational audiologist to ensure optimal service delivery.

3. **Principal.** *The school principal is responsible for the day-to-day operations of the school, including the education and well-being of all students.* The principal can influence a school staff's behaviors and dispositions toward the speech–language pathology program. It is important for you to discuss your program's goals with the principal. Keep him or her informed about such matters as the caseload size and types of disorders. Help principals realize the importance of your role in the educational community by regularly communicating with them, maintaining highly visible and effective service delivery, documenting and communicating results of service delivery, and participating in certain school committees.

4. **School Nurse.** *The school nurse is a registered nurse with additional training in laws related to public schools.* The school nurse often is responsible for screening students' hearing and vision. He or she maintains a health history for each student and often acts as a liaison between the educational staff and other health professionals. Often, the school nurse is knowledgeable about your students' family history and may provide important background information.

   You will consult regularly with the school nurse about students with hearing loss, voice disorders, and chronic health problems. You may refer students to the school nurse who have poor dentition (such as unrepaired dental caries). You also may refer children with suspected hearing or vision problems to the school nurse.

5. **School Psychologist.** *The school psychologist is trained and credentialed to work in the public school setting.* The main duties of the school psychologist include testing students to determine their educational strengths and weaknesses. They also determine appropriate educational placement and recommend intervention techniques. The school psychologist may provide some family and student counseling.

   The school psychologist may request you to perform speech and language assessments with some of the students he or she is also evaluating. He or she will ask your opinion regarding how a child's communicative skills may affect educational performance.

   You may need information from the school psychologist about a student's cognitive abilities. You also may ask for help from the school psychologist on managing a child's behavior problems during your treatment sessions.

   It is important for you to establish an effective relationship with school psychologists because they are often the leaders of the IEP team. They can provide support for your program by making appropriate referrals and abiding by your speech and language recommendations.

6. **Special Education Teacher.** *The special education teacher is a credentialed teacher with additional training in specific disabilities or disorders.* Many students receiving services from a special education teacher also need the services of the speech-language pathologist. Teachers of special education include the following: teacher of the deaf and hard of hearing (DHH); teacher of the learning disabled (LD); teacher of the severely emotionally disturbed (SED); teacher of the orthopedically handicapped (OH); teacher of the severely disabled (SD); teacher of the visually impaired (VI); and resource specialist (RS).

   You may work with many of these educational specialists. You should develop good communication with them so you can coordinate your services with theirs. For example, if the SD teacher is training a child to sit in his or her chair for 5 minutes by using a token reinforcement system, you may follow through with this procedure when you work with the child individually. Conversely, you may be teaching the use of present progressive with a child. You may ask the LD teacher to instruct the child to correctly use the present progressive in the classroom setting and reinforce the correct responses.

7. **Teacher.** *The regular education teacher is one of the most important professionals with whom you will work.* The classroom teacher is responsible for ensuring an appropriate education for each child in his or her class. Regular education teachers are involved in many school activities and work closely with other teachers and parents.

Unless you are assigned such a select caseload as only children with severe disabilities, many of your children will be in typical education classrooms. These children spend the large majority of their day with the classroom teacher and a small fraction of the day with you. In addition, many of your children with severe disabilities may be in regular education. Many schools have adopted a policy of including all children in the regular education class. In inclusive schools, instead of being in a special education program most of the day and sharing only such activities as recess with their peers without disability, children with disabilities are educated in the typical classroom. Special education teachers and other specialists may visit the classroom to support the student and the teacher.

The effectiveness of your intervention may be assisted or hampered by your relationship with the classroom teacher. It is important that you maintain ongoing communication with the regular education teacher. To maximize a child's education and speech therapy, you should understand what and how a teacher is teaching. You may incorporate the curriculum into your treatment. In other cases, you may provide services in the classroom or help the teacher modify his or her method of teaching to increase your student's comprehension and success. Chapter 2 contains additional information about the different types of service delivery models in the schools.

The Speech-Language Pathology Assistant (SLPA)

One or more of your clinical internship assignments may involve working with SLPAs. SLPAs should have completed a training program and may work in any setting in which speech-language pathologists are employed, but their scope of practice differs from that of the SLP. As a student, you will not supervise SLPAs; however, you may work closely with them. For example, you may be asked to determine appropriate activities with which the SLPAs can assist, or you may be asked to train SLPAs to perform a specific task. In other instances, family members or other staff may question you regarding the qualifications of SLPAs. There may be a number of experiences you will gain in working with SLPAs, and it is important that you have an understanding of ASHA's guidelines for the use of SLPAs (American Speech-Language-Hearing Association, 2004a).

What SLPAs May Do Under Supervision

- Implement treatment plans developed by the supervising speech-language pathologist

- Assist with speech-language and hearing screenings, formal and informal assessments, clerical duties, research projects, in-service training, public relations programs, and such departmental operations as scheduling and record keeping

- Document client performance by preparing charts, records, and graphs

- Check and maintain equipment

- Collect and document data for quality improvement

What SLPAs May Not Do

- Perform standardized or nonstandardized testing

- Interpret test results

- Screen or diagnose patients for feeding or swallowing disorders

- Participate in any parent or case conferences without a supervising speech-language pathologist

- Provide counseling

- Develop or modify treatment plans

- Assist with treatment without supervision and without a treatment plan prepared by the speech-language pathologist

- Sign treatment plans, assessment reports, or other formal documents

- Select, refer, or discharge clients

- Disclose confidential information

- Demonstrate swallowing strategies or precautions

The SLPA is held to the same professional standards of other employees at your intern site and, as you can see, can be very helpful in assisting the speech-language pathologist. Read ASHA's various documents on SLPAs to ensure that you understand their role and the role of the speech-language pathologist.

Establishing Collaborative Relationships with Other Professionals

Regardless of your professional setting, you should communicate effectively with other professionals and obtain all needed services for your client. You should show other professionals that the services you provide are valuable and that the client needs your services as much as theirs. The following are some guidelines that can help you accomplish these important goals.

1. *Provide high-quality service.* This will help develop a reputation for excellence. Be well prepared for each clinical session.

2. *Develop good communication with other professionals.* Provide clear, concise, and relevant information. In your reports, describe the effects of your services in direct and measurable terms. Minimize the use of jargon that other professionals may not understand. Provide charts, graphs, and tables when they seem to show the progress of your clients more clearly than just the written narrative.

3. *Be courteous.* Occasionally, you may be angry with another professional or may just be in a bad mood. Regardless of how you are feeling, when you communicate with another person, it is important to be courteous. If you offer an inappropriate or unexpected display of temper, that is how you will be remembered. Also, the other professional may not listen to the content of the message you are trying to convey. As you know, you can disagree and present your viewpoint in a gracious manner.

4. *Understand the services provided by other professionals.* To effectively collaborate with other professionals, it is essential that you understand their roles. Learn not only the definitions of their duties, but also try and understand how their responsibilities to your clients affect their job. For example, teachers who must demonstrate that their class is at a certain academic level may become disheartened when a child with special needs enrolls in their class. It is not because of the child, but because of the other pressures from the administrators or the community, or both. Rather than judging that these teachers do not like children with special needs, work with them to help the student and the class perform optimally.

5. *Respect the services offered by others.* It is important that you understand and demonstrate respect for the role other professionals play in the treatment of your clients. As a student clinician, you are focusing on speech-language pathology. Therefore, you may sometimes feel that your services are the most important. They are important, but others offer equally important services. The amount of training or prestige an individual has does not ensure the importance of his or her contributions. Remember, the assistant who drives your client to the grocery store and the neurosurgeon who removed a tumor from your client's brain both are important in helping your client live successfully.

6. *Respond promptly.* Reply readily and accurately to inquiries from clients and professionals. When you delay responding to clients, parents, or professionals, they may feel that they are not important enough for you to make time for them. They also may have urgent information, concerns, or questions.

7. *Acknowledge referrals.* Send a thank-you letter to all professionals who refer a client to you. He or she may follow up with additional helpful information or provide you with more referrals. Also, acknowledging referrals is a chance to educate others about your services.

8. *Send reports promptly.* With your client's consent, send out assessment and progress reports to those professionals who have referred the client to you. If necessary, talk to the referring professionals during the course of the term to keep them informed of your services.

9. *Educate other professionals about speech-language pathology services.* Any time you discuss a client or your services with other professionals is an opportunity to educate them about speech-language pathology. Offer accurate information about your services and the needs of particular clients. Be a resource person for other professionals.

10. *Respect professional boundaries.* Give information only about speech-language pathology. Do not give information, advice, or treatment that is not within the realm of speech-language pathology. Refer the clients to other professionals for needed services.

11. *Talk to your supervisor before you contact another professional.* Remember that when there is a need to contact another professional, student clinicians must first discuss it with their clinical supervisors to get their advice and approval.

The Internet's Role

The Internet is just one of the many innovations in technology that is affecting speech-language pathologists. Similar to the personal computer, the Internet has been of great assistance to many speech-language pathologists and other professionals. Communication between professionals has increased because of the Internet. For example, on the Internet you will find many *subscriber e-mail lists* and *electronic bulletin boards* that function as communication networking tools for professionals with similar concerns. There is an e-mail list for people involved in the treatment of dysphagia. You may find occupational therapists, physical therapists, radiologists, and neurologists, as well as speech-language pathologists, posting questions, answers, and comments to this forum.

In addition, there are many *journals that can be accessed via the Internet.* You are no longer restricted to the journals offered by ASHA or those that are available through your local library. You can read articles published by other professions. This may give you a more thorough understanding of certain disorders and help you understand the concerns of other professionals.

Telepractice is an application that is beginning to be used in speech-language pathology. You may hear the terms *telemedicine*, *telehealth*, and *telepractice* used interchangeably. *Telemedicine* was one of the original terms used to describe doctors' use of advanced technology for medical applications. The term *telehealth* evolved from telemedicine and has become an overarching term to refer to a variety of health professions using distance technology. *Telepractice* is a broad term to describe distance service delivery. It is becoming more commonly used in areas where there are professional shortages (e.g., a rural area may not have access to a pediatric psychiatrist or a speech-language pathologist with expertise in treating fluency disorders).

Technology may be simple or sophisticated. The telephone may be used for individual or group consultation or conferencing; interactive video or digital broadcasts may be used for "visual" consultations. In addition to "face-to-face" interaction, certain instrumentation (such as an otoscope) may be attached to the recording device. In a telepractice, a patient may be several thousand miles from a specialist providing the service, but they are linked by the Internet or other technology. The provider may offer information directly to the patient or to another specialist who is directly treating the patient. In another instance, telepractice may be professionals talking on telephones to determine a specific course of treatment for a client.

Issues to Consider in Pursuing a Telepractice

1. *State licensure laws* will affect professionals providing services in a variety of states. It is imperative that telepractice practitioners be aware of, and adhere to, any licensure rules affecting their delivery of services.

2. *Protection of client confidentiality* may be more difficult to monitor with a telepractice. You will need to ensure that any information provided through the Internet or other technology is secure.

3. *Equipment is not always reliable* and "back-up" equipment may need to be readily available. For example, you may be scheduled to consult on a client through group conferencing via the Internet, yet just before the scheduled appointment, your computer equipment may fail and you may be unable to communicate with your colleagues or clients.

4. *The efficacy of telepractice* must continue to be investigated. Telepractice holds much promise for providing services in rural communities and for enhancing communication and collaboration among professionals. However, the efficacy of this type of service delivery needs to be researched before it can be embraced fully.

You should maintain current skills in the rapidly expanding use of technology. In your research of certain disorders, you will find articles about telepractice in treating children and adults who have communicative disorders. E-mail, lists, electronic publishing, and the Internet are only a glimmer of our technological future.

So far, you have learned about various structural and organizational aspects of clinical practicum. You know that you will have opportunities to learn the skills of the profession in a variety of clinical settings. In completing your clinical practicum or internship, you must follow many administrative and ethical rules, regulations, and guidelines.

Once you understand the structures and procedures of clinical practicum, you may concentrate on the clinical methods of speech-language pathology. You will have learned about these methods in various courses taken prior to enrolling in clinical practicum. In the second part of the book, we give you an overview of these methods that help you treat clients with communicative disorders.

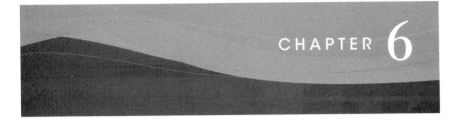

CHAPTER 6

Multicultural Issues in Clinical Practicum

Chapter Outline

- Student Clinicians with Multicultural Backgrounds
- ASHA Position Statements
- Multicultural Assessment Issues
- Treatment Issues
- Working with an Interpreter

Because of the rapidly changing composition of society in the United States, the issues of diversity and multiculturalism are currently in the forefront of government, business, and education. Historically, ASHA has had policies regarding nondiscrimination based on gender, race, linguistic background, and other factors. In 1998 the ASHA Joint Subcommittee of the Executive Board on English Language Proficiency published a position statement and technical report extending this nondiscrimination policy to students and professionals who speak English with nonstandard dialects or accents (ASHA, 1998). Over the past several years, ASHA has developed various other guidelines and position statements on effective and appropriate delivery of clinical services to people with diverse linguistic and cultural backgrounds. ASHA also has sponsored numerous workshops and conferences on multicultural concerns to educate the professionals. Furthermore, to coordinate its activities relative to minority populations, ASHA has an Office of Multicultural Affairs (OMA).

To effectively serve the growing culturally and linguistically diverse population of the United States, ASHA considers recruitment of individuals from diverse cultural, racial, ethnic, and linguistic backgrounds a priority in professional education. In 1992 ASHA published its *Multicultural Action Agenda 2000*, which included increased efforts to recruit individuals with multicultural backgrounds to the professions of speech-language pathology and audiology (Cole, 1992) and in 2001 ASHA developed the three-year *Focused Initiative: Culturally and Linguistically Diverse Populations*. ASHA continues to emphasize the importance of diversity through various avenues, including recruitment and retention of minorities. However, recruitment of minority students with diverse linguistic backgrounds has created some professional training issues.

Student Clinicians with Multicultural Backgrounds

Students from diverse cultural and linguistic backgrounds have much to offer to the profession of speech-language pathology, but they may face several challenges at the university level. These challenges include the possibility of having a weak academic background and dealing with an educational system dominated by white middle-class values and training structures, along with limited financial support. These are universal problems across disciplines and educational programs in the country. However, because of the obvious emphasis on speech and language proficiency in the field of communication sciences and disorders, nonnative English speakers or speakers who employ an English dialect other than *Standard American English (SAE)* sometimes are dissuaded from majoring in communicative disorders. It is important to remember that individuals should not be discriminated against because of race, ethnicity, language, dialects, or cultural differences. In fact, ASHA's Code of Ethics prohibits such practice. To emphasize its stand on this issue, ASHA published a position statement and technical report regarding students and professionals who use a nonstandard English dialect or accent (American Speech-Language-Hearing Association, 1998). This paper addresses people (a) who were not born in the United States and learned another language before they learned English; (b) who were born in the United States and learned another language before they learned to speak English; and (c) who were born in the United States and speak only English. It does not discuss the issue of students or professionals who have not yet become proficient in English as their second language.

As noted in this paper, student clinicians need not necessarily speak SAE. However, to succeed in clinical practicum and later in professional practice, all student clinicians should possess a certain standard of SAE linguistic competence. In the United States, student clinicians in communicative disorders may speak one of the several dialectal varieties of English. More importantly, the student clinicians should possess proficiency in English or an English dialect to achieve above average academic performance. For admission and matriculation to most graduate programs, students must earn a minimum grade point average of B.

ASHA has not yet developed a standard for English language proficiency for the practice of speech-language pathology in the United States (Campbell, 1994). ASHA's position statement refers primarily to students' knowledge of communication and its disorders, their skills in evaluating and treating these disorders, and their ability to model the speech or language target. In addition to ASHA's position, some training programs have found it essential for students' intelligibility to be evaluated. Most universities have established certain speech and language proficiency standards for all student clinicians, regardless of their language history. Some training programs may require all students majoring in communicative disorders to have their speech, language, and hearing screened. Following the screening, certain students may be referred for additional evaluation. Diagnostic testing may reveal the need for intervention and some individuals may seek elective clinical services.

In general, as a student clinician you should do the following:

1. Develop a thorough knowledge of normal and disordered communication and communication development.

2. Acquire effective diagnostic and intervention skills.

3. Learn to effectively communicate with clients from a variety of cultural, ethnic, racial, and linguistic backgrounds.

4. Develop the skill to model all target behaviors required of your clients. For example, for articulation therapy, you will need to be able to model each of the English phonemes or allophones.

5. Learn to write clearly and concisely, using correct grammar.

An issue that has not received much attention is that clinicians with multicultural backgrounds may or may not possess cultural sensitivity. They still may need to study the cultural and linguistic differences of other groups. Therefore, the recommendation that clinicians should study and understand the cultural and linguistic background of clients they serve applies to all clinicians.

If you have concerns regarding your oral or written communication skills, discuss them with your advisor. If you are a student clinician with a diverse cultural or linguistic background, you may encounter certain obstacles, but you also will encounter many rewards, such as excellent employment opportunities, many research questions to be investigated, and colleagues who are eager to share your unique knowledge and experiences.

ASHA Position Statements

Numerous articles about multicultural issues have been published in various ASHA journals. In addition, ASHA has published several position statements. These position statements reflect ASHA's philosophy regarding multicultural and bilingual issues and help guide today's service delivery to these populations. All student clinicians should have a basic knowledge of the various position statements. The following section gives an overview of several of them.

Bilingual Speech-Language Pathologists and Audiologists

ASHA does not certify an individual as a bilingual speech-language pathologist or audiologist. However, ASHA (American Speech-Language-Hearing Association, 1989b) defines certain competencies necessary for being identified as bilingual for the purpose of clinical service delivery. *A bilingual speech-language pathologist is one who speaks his or her own language proficiently and speaks (or signs) at least one other language with native or near-native proficiency.* Communication skills should encompass all parameters of oral or manual language, including the appropriate grammar, meaning, and social use.

In many geographic areas of the United States, there is an immense need for bilingual speech-language pathologists. ASHA strongly supports efforts of universities in recruiting bilingual students. There are many student clinicians who are bilingual. Before identifying yourself as a bilingual student clinician, examine ASHA's definition of a bilingual speech-language pathologist and your language skills. Some people who have grown up speaking two languages often use one language predominantly and, hence, the other language is forgotten or no longer used proficiently. A person may speak two languages well enough to engage in such communication as social exchanges, but may not be proficient enough to provide clinical service in both languages.

ASHA-Suggested Competencies Required of Bilingual Clinicians

1. The ability to describe the development of speech and oral (or manual) and written language for both bilingual and monolingual individuals.

2. The skill to differentiate communication differences from communication disorders in oral (or manual) and written language through the use of both formal and informal evaluation.

3. The ability to provide treatment in the client's primary language.

4. Knowledge of various cultural factors related to service delivery (American Speech-Language-Hearing Association, 1989b).

Review these ASHA-suggested competencies required of bilingual clinicians. You may already have proficient language skills in two or more languages or you may want to upgrade certain language skills. If you are bilingual, find out from your advisor if you may be certified as a bilingual speech-language pathologist in your state. This may be a part of the state's licensure or credential process. If you are not bilingual, you may want to take classes in a second language to enhance your knowledge of a different language and to gain some insight into what it is like to be a speaker of a minority language who is required to learn a new language in which to communicate. And, employment opportunities for bilingual speech-language pathologists are excellent.

Clinical Management of Minority Language Populations

Depending on your work setting and geographical area, you may be one of the almost 50% of ASHA members providing services to individuals who do not speak English as a native language (American Speech-Language-Hearing Association, 1993). In response to the needs of its members and as part of its service to minority populations, ASHA published a position paper entitled "Clinical Management of Communicatively Handicapped Minority Language Populations" (American Speech-Language-Hearing Association, 1985b). The paper discusses competencies you should have for evaluation and treatment of individuals with communicative disorders who are minority language speakers. These competencies include those listed in ASHA's other position paper entitled "Definitions: Bilingual Speech-Language Pathologists and Audiologists" (American Speech-Language-Hearing Association, 1989b).

The position paper on "Clinical Management of Communicatively Handicapped Minority Language Populations" (American Speech-Language-Hearing Association, 1985b) suggests methods that can be used when a competent bilingual specialist is not available. If you are a monolingual student intern at a clinical practicum site serving individuals who are bilingual or monolingual in a language other than yours, you may implement some of ASHA's (1985b) suggestions for serving minority language populations.

ASHA Guidelines for Serving Minority Language Populations

1. *Contracting with a bilingual speech-language pathologist* or audiologist to serve as a consultant

2. *Employing an itinerant bilingual speech-language pathologist* or audiologist to provide services for a specific language population

3. *Collaborating with university bilingual speech-language pathology* and audiology programs

4. *Developing an interdisciplinary team* that consists of at least one bilingual professional who also is proficient in language development and non-biased assessment procedures

5. *Creating SLPCF and practicum sites* for individuals from bilingual speech-language pathology and audiology programs (American Speech-Language-Hearing Association, 1985b).

The American Speech-Language-Hearing Association paper (1985b) also discusses the use of interpreters or translators. In working with multicultural populations, you may have to rely on interpreters or translators. Interpreters may be trained professionals, the client's friend, or one of the client's family members. Guidelines for the use of interpreters include training the interpreter, planning assessment sessions, using the same interpreter, and using natural assessment measures. For more specific information, refer to the "Clinical Management" position paper and to the section in this chapter, "Guidelines for Working with an Interpreter."

Social Dialects

The American Speech-Language-Hearing Association's (1983) position paper entitled "Social Dialects" and its 2003 paper entitled "Technical Report: American English Dialects" (American Speech-Language-Hearing Association, 2003b) clarify some of the confusion regarding the role of speech-language pathologists serving individuals who speak dialects other than SAE. Historically, some speech-language pathologists have considered dialectal variations as disorders to be treated. Some laypersons tend to make negative judgments about people who speak dialects that are influenced by a second language. ASHA's position on this matter is unequivocal. *The dialectical varieties of Standard English are not disorders.* To appropriately evaluate a communicative disorder, the clinician should differentiate between linguistic variation because of a dialectical difference and linguistic variation because of a speech, language, or hearing disorder.

You may work with individuals with linguistic variation because of dialectical differences when those individuals have chosen to receive treatment. For example, you may work with clients who wish to change or reduce their specific accents. Also, you may work with individuals who speak a dialectical variation of English (e.g., Black English) who wish to learn SAE. In this case, your clients may want to retain their native dialects, but, in certain situations, be able to code switch to SAE. For example, many clients are happy with and are proud of their dialects, which reflect their cultural heritage. However, they may find the acquisition of the standard dialect to have social or occupational advantage. In certain cases, individuals may speak in a dialectical variation of English and may have a language disorder unrelated to the dialect. Remember, except in the case of elective services, you can only recommend speech therapy for those individuals who exhibit a language disorder, not a language difference.

Provision of English as a Second Language Instruction by Speech-Language Pathologists in School Settings

The effectiveness of school-based speech-language pathologists is partially dependent on their ability to work collaboratively with teachers and other educational specialists. Speech-language pathologists include curriculum in the context of their treatment, teach sections of classes, and work with individual students in the classroom. Teachers provide opportunities for students to generalize skills learned in speech-language therapy and rely on the speech-language pathologist to help students who are having difficulty with comprehension or written and oral language. Because of the increasing demands on educators, the roles of the different personnel sometimes become blurred. The increasing diversity of the school population has added to the confusion of professional roles. According to ASHA (1998), speech-language pathologists with appropriate training in instructing students who have English as a second language may provide this service. Speech-language pathologists who have not received the necessary linguistic, theoretical, and methodological training should not provide direct instruction in English as a second language (ESL), but may collaborate with ESL instructors for assessment and treatment of appropriate students. As with other areas of professional practice, if you are not trained or prepared to provide a specific service, do not do it. Follow the ASHA's (1998) guidelines for collaborating in ESL instruction.

ASHA Guidelines for Collaborating in ESL Instruction

1. *Before an assessment*, discuss with the ESL teacher such issues as language development and code switching during second language acquisition, socialization, and language use in the classroom and community.

2. *As part of an assessment*, discuss with the ESL teacher such issues as the student's test performance, specific test results, and methods and strategies for maximizing the student's learning.

3. *During intervention*, continue to collaborate with the ESL teacher, discussing ideas and resources, and coordinating goals, objectives, and activities related to the communicative disorder connected to those of developing proficiency in English.

If there is no appropriate ESL program available, ASHA suggests that the speech-language pathologist act as a consultant to the teachers and other professionals and be an advocate for the child. In all cases, the speech-language pathologist should be aware of cultural and linguistic factors that affect a student's education and progress in speech therapy. Also, the speech-language pathologist should be sensitive to a student's and his or her family's cultural and linguistic differences. In the educational setting, it is important that a communicative disorder not be misinterpreted as acquisition of a second language, and that second language acquisition is not diagnosed as a communicative disorder.

Available Resources

There are many excellent resources available for second-language students as well as for professional clinicians. ASHA is a major source of information. As a member of the NSSLHA, you will have access to ASHA's various publications. The *ASHA Leader* typically contains information on professional issues, including those that affect multicultural clinical services.

An excellent source is a bibliography of publications on multicultural issues maintained and updated by ASHA's Office of Multicultural Affairs. The bibliography contains publications on almost all aspects of speech-language disorders that address multicultural issues. Your clinic director or supervisor may have access to the bibliography.

There are now several books and book chapters on multicultural speech-language pathology, special education, and general education (Battle, 2002; Brice, 2002; Cheng, 1991, 1995, 1998; Coleman, 2000; Goldstein, 2004; Hamayan & Damico, 1991; Kahmi, Pollock, & Harris, 1996; Kayser, 1995, 2007 Payne, 1997; Roseberry-McKibbin, 2002; Screen & Anderson, 1994; Seymour & Nober, 1998; Shekar & Hegde, 1995, 1996; Trueba, Cheng, & Ima, 1993; Trueba, Jacobs, & Kirton, 1990; Van Keulen, Weddington, & DeBose, 1998; Westby, 1994; Yavas, 1994). Make use of these and other resources to understand clients of diverse cultural backgrounds and to plan clinical and educational programs for them. There is also an extensive literature on alternative assessment strategies recommended for multicultural clients; consult the articles cited in the next section.

Multicultural Assessment Issues

In ASHA's 1993 Omnibus Survey (American Speech-Language-Hearing Association, 1993), 15.5% of the respondents reported specific graduate coursework related to communication disorders among multicultural populations, and 10.6% of the respondents reported specific graduate coursework related to limited-English-speaking populations. Avenues for obtaining information included on-the-job education, self-study, and continuing education. However, 49.8% of the respondents reported that they provided services for individuals who did not speak English as a native language. This means that practical exigencies demand that clinicians who do not have adequate training in multicultural speech-language pathology provide services anyway. Obviously, there is a need to have training at the university level for working with multicultural populations.

Because of the complexity of evaluations in general and evaluation of culturally diverse populations, this section does not attempt to give all the information you will need to evaluate each type of client you may encounter. Your university may offer a specialized class on multicultural issues or offer culturally relevant information in each of your classes. Nonetheless, you may have to independently gather additional information for specific clients. The following information provides a framework you can build and expand on, depending on your clients and their backgrounds.

Assessment is a multifaceted process that involves interactions between the examiner, the client, the client's family, and various educators, physicians, and allied professionals. To make comprehensive and accurate evaluations, the speech-language pathologist should possess knowledge of normal and abnormal communication development, knowledge of how tests are standardized, effective test administration skills, good observation skills, and interviewing skills. In addition, to make nonbiased assessment of nonnative speakers of English or individuals who speak dialectical variations, the clinician should have a knowledge of linguistic standards of the client's community, the client's culture and values, and sensitivity to cultural variations. The clinician should also be aware of any prejudices he or she may have that may contribute to biased assessment results. Equally important for assessing clients with varied cultural backgrounds is a thorough knowledge of the limitations of traditional assessment approaches and available alternative procedures that may be integrated with the traditional procedures.

Alternative and Integrated Assessment

Consider the following when evaluating a client from a minority or varied cultural background.

- Evaluate performance using specific criterion. Standardized tests of speech and language skills in children and adults play a major role in the traditional assessment approach. The main problem in relying on standardized tests is that they are not standardized on minority populations. Including an adequate number of minority children or adults in the standardization sample will not solve the limitations of standardized tests (Hegde & Pomaville, 2008). Instead of attempting to evaluate a client's performance using inappropriate normative data, evaluate performance by indicating the criterion of the client's performance on specific tasks (e.g., 80% or 90% accuracy). This will help evaluate the skill level without making inappropriate comparisons.

- Evaluate the results to determine what the client can and cannot do and whether the client can meet the social, academic, occupational, and personal communication needs; this will be more effective in developing functional and client-appropriate treatment targets than the results of standardized tests.

The **authentic assessment approach** advocates the necessity of measuring naturalistic and meaningful communication. Therefore, in this approach:

- Select skills to be assessed from the child's academic curricula (e.g., language structures, reading and writing skills required in the child's grade) as well as the home environment (words frequently used at home, language structures selected from the child's storybooks) and construct assessment items to specifically evaluate those skills.

- Select other assessment skills that are useful and functional in the child's milieu (e.g., conversational skills and narrative skills), and construct assessment strategies to evaluate them.

- Observe skills in natural settings (e.g., as the child talks to the teacher, a peer, a family member) and obtain information on the child's skills from adults who interact with the child (e.g., parents, teachers, peers).

- Evaluate the assessment results in terms of at least minimally meeting the communication demands placed on the child in academic and social contexts; note that the approach avoids comparison with norms.

The **dynamic assessment approach** is based on the concept that assessment may require some form of teaching to find out if the client can *learn* the missing skills. Therefore, in this approach, you do the following:

- Conduct trial treatment sessions to evaluate whether the client can learn the skills that are absent; this is similar to stimulability testing, but the efforts to teach the absent skills are much more extensive.

- During assessment, reinforce correct responses and give corrective feedback for incorrect responses while testing; this will also help evaluate whether the client can learn with the help of feedback.

- Ask the client to evaluate his or her responses to assessment items (whether and why a response is correct or incorrect).

- Modify test items and instructions as found appropriate for the individual client.

- Test, teach, and retest to complete the dynamic assessment.

The **portfolio assessment** approach requires the collection of a variety of items that represent a client's oral communication skills, literacy skills, and other items that reflect the client's strengths. The approach significantly expands the typical client file and requires additional storage capacity. In this approach:

- Add data to the client's file throughout the period of service, including treatment

- Obtain multiple measures of speech, language, writing, and reading skills; continuously update them

- Include in the portfolio a variety of items that help understand the client's strengths and weaknesses; invite other professionals to select items for the portfolio

- Include not only assessment and treatment reports but also transcribed speech and language samples; samples of writing, drawing, painting, audiotaped reading, math work, and oral narratives; videos of social or family interactions; academic work samples; clinician's and teacher's observational reports; interview data; and so forth

The main advantage of alternative approaches is that they minimize biased assessment, due mostly to inappropriate tests administered to minority children and adults. Each approach has its limitations, however. Criterion and client-specific assessment may not fulfill the requirement of school districts in qualifying students for services, which are often based on standardized tests. Authentic assessment (also a client-specific approach) requires extensive preparation, based on the characteristics of individual clients. Dynamic assessment requires teaching skills before completely assessing them. The portfolio assessment may pose storage of items collected and other practical problems. None can replace all elements of the traditional approach. For instance, a detailed case history, hearing screening, orofacial examination, and speech and language sampling need to be a part of each alternative approach. Therefore, what is needed is an integrated approach that retains the essential and useful elements of the traditional approach and selects and integrates the advantages of alternative approaches (Hegde & Pomaville, 2008). See the next two sections for this integrated strategy.

Before the Evaluation

Culturally sensitive planning is needed to conduct assessment that is appropriate for all clients, especially for clients of cultural diversity. Take the following steps in planning your assessment sessions.

1. *Know the cultural background of your clients.* Try to understand the client's dispositions, values, and expectations regarding communication and its disorders. This will assist you in establishing rapport with your clients and their families, which, in turn, will help you more efficiently and accurately evaluate your clients. Your interview will be more productive because you will know to whom to address your questions, what types of questions will be most effective, what types of questions should be avoided (or carefully worded), and what types of responses to expect. Knowledge of the cultural background of your clients also may influence the way you structure your assessment, your selection of tests, and your choice of materials for language sampling. Also, to work most effectively with your clients, you should know the dispositions and practices regarding such nonverbal communication modes as eye contact, smiling, handshake, and touching. Many miscommunications and misinterpretations can be avoided if you are aware of the meaning of these and other behaviors in specific cultural groups. Remember, what is desirable or acceptable in one culture may not be in another.

2. *Understand how your life experiences may influence your attitude toward a client.* It is almost impossible for one to be totally without prejudice. You have grown up in a community and culture that held certain values. When you encounter individuals who challenge those values through their own beliefs and lifestyles, you may react in a prejudicial manner. Because you view yourself as a person without prejudice, you may attempt to rationalize

behavior that is unacceptable but that you do not want to judge. In other cases, you may find yourself disliking a client for no apparent reason. You may hold such prejudicial beliefs as "people who wear white shoes after Labor Day have no class" or "people of color have less intelligence than white people." Regardless of the extent of your prejudicial beliefs, the more you can acknowledge them, the more you will be able to change them, and the less influence they will have on your evaluations. Try to use the self-analysis as an exercise in being nonjudgmental.

3. *Know the beliefs and behavioral dispositions toward communicative disorders.* It is important to understand your clients' beliefs regarding the origin of a communicative disorder. For example, Harris (1993) reported that in some Native American groups a child's disability might be considered a gift from the Creator. In such Southeast Asian communities as the Hmong, only disabilities that are physical or obviously mental are taken seriously. Knowing an individual's beliefs will affect the structure of your questions, evaluation tasks, counseling, and family involvement in treatment. Your treatment procedure for a disorder in a culturally diverse child may be the same as the one you use with other clients because of the demonstrated effectiveness of the procedure. Nonetheless, you may provide different types of counseling or activities for family involvement in treatment.

4. *Know phonological and linguistic differences.* You may not always know your client's primary language before the evaluation, but you may have some clues based on information in the case history or previous evaluations. As much as possible in advance of the assessment session, study the phonological and linguistic characteristics of your client's native language or dialectal variation. During the assessment session, you should be able to judge if certain behaviors are related to a difference or a disorder and whether in-depth evaluation is in order. For example, in the Hmong language the only final consonant is /ŋ/ (Cheng, 1991); therefore, evaluation of English morphological skills of the Hmong child learning English as a second language may need to place most emphasis on receptive morphological skills. This would be done with the understanding that expressive skills may be slow to emerge because of transition from a sound system different from English and not because there is a language disorder.

5. *Know health statistics.* The prevalence of certain diseases varies across race and culture. Therefore, you need to know health statistics that are relevant to an understanding of a particular client. For example, if you are working with children who are from a population that historically has a high incidence of otitis media, you may explore your clients' hearing history and health care treatment in greater detail than you would otherwise.

6. *Use an assessment approach that integrates alternative procedures of evaluating clients of varied backgrounds.* Be prepared to abandon standardized tests if none can be found that suit the individual client. If there are tests recommended

for a particular ethnocultural group, review each test item to ensure it is appropriate for the individual's culture (Mattes & Omark, 1991). For example, in certain rural agricultural areas of California, some children of migrant farm workers may never have seen an elevator or an escalator. A child's inability to identify one of these on a test might lead you to an inaccurate conclusion regarding the child's vocabulary. However, the same child may have an excellent vocabulary for various farm implements. Review the test norms; many do not have norms for various cultural groups. Therefore, to avoid biased test results, do not use tests that are not standardized on the particular group to which your client belongs. Also, avoid tests that sample only a small number of people representing the culture of the person you will be testing. Although some experts recommend that you modify an existing test to use with your client, try to avoid this strategy. Rely on spontaneous speech samples, observation of behaviors, and interview information. Consistent with criterion-referenced, client-specific, and authentic approaches, prepare assessment stimulus materials that are from the client's home and school environment (e.g., a child's storybook, play materials); select functional and useful assessment targets based on the child's educational curricula, storybooks, social communication demands, and family communication needs (e.g., names of family members). Consistent with the portfolio assessment, request parents to bring language samples recorded at home and the child's writing, drawing, painting, or math work samples. In accordance with the dynamic assessment strategy, plan on spending additional time on teaching a few skills, either in the initial assessment session or more likely in a subsequent session.

7. *Choose material that is culturally appropriate.* Use materials that are culturally appropriate for such activities as vocabulary sampling and spontaneous speech sampling. Avoid materials that depict stereotypes of cultures. If possible, use materials that accurately reflect the client's culture. To obtain the best speech sample, attempt to select materials the client relates to and is comfortable with.

8. *Determine if you will need to use the services of an interpreter.* Before the evaluation session, judge the need for an interpreter. You may judge this through information from the client's case history form, from speaking with the clinic administrative assistant, or by telephoning the client. If you are unsure of the need for an interpreter, plan to use one. It is easier to excuse an unneeded interpreter than to locate one at the last minute or to have to postpone a session because an interpreter cannot be found.

9. *Train your interpreter.* After you have selected an interpreter, discuss the evaluation session with him or her. Review the format of the session, discuss specific interview questions, and provide training for any tests to be administered. Also discuss your expectations regarding the interpreter's behavior during and after the evaluation session. Include in your discussion

such professional issues as maintaining client confidentiality, not guaranteeing treatment outcome, and so on. If possible, use an interpreter with whom you have worked before whose skills you know and who knows what you expect. If you are working with a new interpreter, find out what the interpreter's experience is and what type of additional training he or she needs. Role-play different testing situations in training your interpreter. For additional information, refer to the section in this chapter entitled "Working with an Interpreter."

During the Evaluation

In evaluating multicultural clients, you need to take such special steps as the following:

1. *Be sensitive to cultural issues.* Before your session, you will have reviewed information related to your client's culture. During the session, be aware of and respect cultural communication practices. For example, in the client's culture it may not be acceptable to touch the top of an individual's head. Know what behaviors are considered rude and which are considered polite. For instance, in Asian cultures, maintaining a constant eye contact with a teacher or an authority figure is considered rude. Also, students are encouraged to listen more and talk less. Therefore, silence and lack of eye contact on the part of an Asian child may not suggest a pragmatic language disorder. Such understanding not only will help you establish better rapport with your clients, but it will also help you evaluate their communicative performance more accurately.

2. *Talk to the client, not the interpreter.* At the beginning of the session, through the interpreter, introduce yourself and the interpreter to the client. Explain what the interpreter's role is and what your role is. For example, "I am Julie Smith, and I will be evaluating your son's speech and language today. This is Mr. Yang, and he will be interpreting for us during this session." Although it is important to acknowledge the interpreter's presence, you should always look at the client or family members when you are talking to them.

3. *Explain why you will be asking questions.* Certain ethnic and cultural groups may not be used to responding to direct questions. It may be considered threatening or rude. At the beginning of the evaluation, explain that you will be asking some questions and why. When you ask specific questions, explain why they are necessary. Often, you will be able to tell from clients' and family members' body language if continued use of such questions is necessary.

4. *Use the appropriate title of the cultural group.* Find out in advance what the acceptable title is for the individual's cultural group and use the title appropriately during the assessment (Battle, 2002). Also determine how different

family members and significant individuals are referred to. For instance, in Asian cultures, it is not common to address older relatives by their name; they typically are addressed in terms of the relation. If an Asian boy is accompanied to the clinic by his uncle and you are talking to the child, it is preferable to use the phrase "Your uncle" and not "Mr. Kapoor." If possible, find out how the family hierarchy affects interaction. For example, are there certain titles for the maternal grandmother and the paternal grandmother? Does one have more interaction or influence with the family? If you are unsure of an appropriate title, ask your client. You may feel slightly embarrassed to ask, but it will make your client more comfortable to know you are concerned about using correct terms, and it is much better than finding out at the end of an hour-long session that you have used certain names and titles inappropriately or incorrectly.

5. *Find out the client's primary language.* During the interview you will find out the client's primary language. Remember to determine whether different languages are used at home, school, or work. Also, if clients have acquired disorders (e.g., aphasia), find out what language they used premorbidly and what language is used now.

6. *Conduct an* **ethnographic interview.** An ethnographic interview is one that focuses on the client and his or her interactions within the family. The ethnographic interview is directed by the responses a family member provides to such questions as, Who is the primary person whom children talk to in your family? What do the boys talk about? What do the girls talk about? How do they learn to speak? (Tomblin, Morris, & Spriestersbach, 1999). There are many other questions that would be appropriate for the ethnographic interview. Basically, you are trying to learn about the dynamics of the culture and of the particular family and how your client fits within that culture and family. This will help you identify if there is a disorder and assist you with future intervention.

7. *In a naturalistic context, obtain an adequate sample of your client's speech.* If possible, obtain more than one speech sample, in different settings, and with different individuals; obtain a sample in which the client and a family member converse with each other. Obtain samples from home and work or school. *For many of your clients the speech sample will be your best source of information.* You can judge various parameters of language, articulation, voice, and fluency from an adequate sample. You can also gain an understanding of which antecedents enhance linguistic performance, which diminish performance, or which seem to have no impact. You may obtain a speech sample with your client talking with different members of the family. This will give you additional diagnostic information and possibly give you information for future treatment sessions. For example, you may determine which family member seems most appropriate for working with the client at home.

8. *Sample social and cognitively demanding language.* In both simple and complex language, people discuss familiar events, share personal experiences, and answer simple questions about stories to which they have listened. To succeed in educational programs and in many businesses, individuals must learn to use complex and technical language. The skills needed to succeed include such abilities as telling or writing imaginary stories, making persuasive arguments, describing complex ideas or events, and following directions (Tomblin et al., 1999).

9. *In administering standardized tests that are indeed normed on the particular cultural group to which the client belongs, reject the temptation of modifying the test items.* If you did modify the test stimuli, test targets, instructions, and so forth because of the demands of your professional setting, realize that the results cannot be interpreted in terms of the test norms. Consider the modified test results as only suggestive, and seek more valid information through naturalistic sampling of communication skills, teacher or family interview, criterion-referenced assessment, client-specific procedures, and a portfolio of relevant items. In administering appropriate bilingual tests, administer each test separately; do not mix the two language items. If you are administering a test that has been normed for two languages, completely administer the test in one language before administering the test in a second language.

10. *Be aware of individual differences within each culture.* Do not stereotype your client based on information you have about his or her background. Regardless of ethnicity, culture, age, or gender, each client and his or her family are unique.

11. *Use a variety of methods to evaluate performance.* Do not rely on standardized test scores as the only method of assessing a client's communicative performance. Obtain information about performance in the home through interviewing family members, speech samples audiotaped in the home, or home visits. If possible, determine how the client communicates with different individuals, including various family members, friends, or colleagues. With school-age children, obtain information about their communicative and academic performance in school.

12. *Obtain case history information orally.* You may obtain some preliminary case history information in writing. However, review and verify this information with the client (Terrell & Terrell, 1993). Allow the client to expand on the information during the interview. Some clients may not have the reading and writing skills necessary to respond to written questions through writing. In some cases, clients may avoid writing information that they think is sensitive but may report the same information verbally. Therefore, during the interview, give your clients and their family members the opportunity to discuss the client's medical history, developmental history, and so on.

13. *When assessing a child, ask parents to compare the performance of that child with that of other children who are at home.* It may be difficult to find developmental or normative data for certain clients. Also, if the child has limited English skills and potential for evaluation in the native language is limited, sometimes comparing communicative development with like children yields useful information. Parents often can describe how older or younger siblings communicate. They know generally how much language their children use, what sounds they do and do not produce, what kinds of directions they follow, and what types of communicative interaction they engage in.

14. *When assessing a school-age child, ask teachers to compare the performance of that child with that of other children in the same classroom.* Classroom teachers are an excellent source of information on children's pattern of communication. For example, you may have a 5-year-old client who is from a linguistic population for which there is little normative data on speech and language development. However, the child's teacher may have in her or his classroom several other children from the same linguistic and cultural background. The teacher can report observed speech and language behaviors of your client and how those behaviors compare to those of children of similar age and culture in the class.

15. *If necessary, train test-taking skills. Most tests provide opportunities to practice required responses (e.g., pointing to a picture or naming a picture).* Individuals from certain cultural and linguistic backgrounds may need additional time and opportunities to learn the required response. For example, some individuals may be reluctant to point, whereas others may not be used to responding to direct questions from strangers. When you have gathered background information on your client's typical communicative behaviors prior to the assessment session, you will have an idea of what types of responses will be easier to evoke and which will require additional time and practice.

16. *If necessary, complete the evaluation during a subsequent visit or visits.* As with all your clients, familiarity with the clinician and the clinical setting will help evoke more valid communicative behaviors. In addition, some cultures do not view time as a perimeter in which a task must be completed (Tomblin et al., 1999). Also, multiple samples of your client's speech and language will increase the reliability of your assessment results. During your initial evaluation session, your client may be hesitant to speak, responding to questions with only short answers, thus giving the impression of a limited mean length of utterance or restricted vocabulary. A sample obtained in the client's home, on a second occasion in the clinic setting, or during interaction with another family member might yield different information. Other activities, such as the initial interview and administration of standardized tests, may take more time with certain populations. As they meet with you

on repeated occasions, your clients will begin to feel more comfortable with you. They then are more likely to accept such intrusive activities as the oral examination.

17. *Find out what the home, school, or occupational environments are like.* If possible, schedule a visit to the client's home. If your client is in school or day care, schedule a visit to that setting. In the case of adult clients, schedule a visit to their occupational setting. Observe the client in the extraclinical settings. Find out how the client interacts with different individuals. If appropriate and practical, interview key people in your client's life. Try to understand the types of activities your client enjoys during the course of a day. If your client is a child, observe what types of toys are available at home and what types of play activities are attractive to him or her. In the case of all young children, observe the home literacy environment. Are there books and writing materials that are appropriate for the child? Is there evidence of parental literacy role models? Because of time and supervisory constraints and distance from the clinic, home or school observation is not always possible. If direct observation in natural settings is not possible, seek detailed information on verbal, nonverbal, literacy, and recreational activities in which the client engages at home, school, work, and other nonclinical settings.

After the Evaluation

Multicultural factors affect how you analyze and interpret your assessment data. Therefore, after the evaluation is completed, take the following steps to make appropriate analyses and recommendations:

1. *Talk with your interpreter.* Let your interpreter give his or her impressions of the session. The interpreter from the same cultural background as the client's may have certain insights or knowledge that you do not. If a sample was obtained in the client's native language, analyze the results with the interpreter. Although you may not be able to obtain a complete analysis of all language structures, you should be able to obtain information regarding speech intelligibility, general vocabulary use, and basic pragmatic skills. Make as complete an analysis of language structures as practical. Review any information in need of clarification. Discuss modifications you would like the interpreter to make in future sessions.

2. *Analyze your results.* Determine if your client exhibits a language disorder in his or her primary language. Remember, a speech or language difference because of second-language acquisition or dialectical variation is not a disorder. Treatment in such cases is purely elective.

3. *Schedule a follow-up session.* Find out if the client's status has changed since the last session. If it has, make a reassessment of the child's communicative

performance. Review the assessment or reassessment results with the client and his or her family. If the client needs help understanding what you are saying, rephrase it. Invite the client to ask questions and allow sufficient time for response. Pay attention to body language and questions asked to help determine if the client understands what you are saying. Vocabulary and concepts you take for granted may be new to someone outside the field of speech-language pathology and especially to someone not familiar with your communication patterns.

4. *Understand how what you are saying may be interpreted by your clients and their family members.* Remember the importance of understanding the values of a particular culture. Your clients may be members of a group that does not believe that humans should intervene when there is a disability. Therefore, they may accept your diagnosis but be unwilling to follow up with treatment. Other clients may believe a disability is a disgrace and not want to acknowledge its existence. Still others may believe the disability is caused by their lack of trying. In all these instances, you will encounter roadblocks that you must deal with in providing effective treatment.

In essence, flexibility in conducting an assessment, knowledge of alternative approaches, and sensitivity to the client's unique background are the key concepts in assessing clients of multicultural backgrounds. Collection of resources on the different cultural groups that you serve will be important in offering appropriate services. For instance, if you serve a particular cultural group in your area (e.g., the Hmong from South East Asia), it will be important to gather information on their cultural and linguistic background. Such information building on different minority groups is time consuming; it cannot be done overnight when a client of a particular cultural group applies for help. It should be a continuous and careful effort to have updated information on clients the clinician serves. In some cases, you may need to devise your own assessment procedures to suit your clients. When you see a need to devise client-specific procedures, consult with your supervisor to ensure reliability and validity of your procedures.

Treatment Issues

There is little research on treatment efficacy for multicultural populations. Most clinicians use treatment procedures that are known to be effective or are based on their personal experiences. When research has not specified unique procedures needed to treat clients of specific cultural backgrounds, you only can use the standard procedures that are known to be effective. However, you should use such techniques with a great deal of caution. You should modify treatment procedures if the data collected during treatment warrant changes. You also should maintain clear descriptions of modifications and document the effects of modified procedures. In planning your treatment sessions for culturally diverse clients, consider the following suggestions and consult other sources (Battle, 2002; Cheng, 1991, 1995, 1998; Hamayan & Damico, 1991; Kahmi et al., 1996; Kayser, 1995, 2002; Langdon & Cheng, 1992; Mattes & Omark, 1991; Payne, 1997; Roseberry-McKibbin, 2002; Seymour & Nober, 1998; Shekar & Hegde, 1995, 1996; Trueba et al., 1990, 1993; Van Keulen et al., 1998; Westby, 1994; Yavas, 1994).

1. *Ask the client, parents, or other family members if selected target communication skills are acceptable.* Much has been written about the cultural differences in communication patterns found across ethnocultural groups. Such differences can create dilemmas for the clinician who wants to select appropriate treatment targets for clients of different cultural backgrounds. For instance, it is often reported that children of Asian background do not maintain eye contact with such authority figures as clinicians and teachers during conversation. Should the clinician teach or not teach eye contact as an accepted conversational skill? Similarly, should the clinician teach or not teach plural morphemes to an African American child who omits them because of Black English? The solution is simple: Ask caregivers or clients themselves. Most caregivers or clients will consider them as socially, educationally, and occupationally useful or even necessary skills in the mainstream American society. Do not teach skills the clients or their families do not want.

2. *Note that some multicultural questions relevant to assessment may not be relevant to treatment.* Multicultural issues are critical in assessment, perhaps less so in treatment. One should not draw conclusions based on culturally inappropriate assessment tools. For instance, you should not conclude that the child does not have language concepts because he or she did not name certain unfamiliar stimulus pictures. Nonetheless, unfamiliar stimulus pictures are fine to teach new concepts. For instance, if a recent immigrant child from a tropical country did not name ski lifts or snowmobiles, you should not conclude that the child is deficient in some aspect of language. Terms or concepts related to ski lifts and snowmobiles, however, may be excellent language targets for a Hmong child who now lives in Minnesota.

3. *Initially, use culturally appropriate stimulus materials.* Review stimulus items you have selected to ensure they are not offensive to your clients. For example, if your client is a vegetarian Hindu, you may want to omit stimulus pictures that show individuals eating meat, especially beef. If your client is a Muslim, you may want to avoid pictures that depict the consumption of pork. As much as possible, pictures of people should include a sample of people from your clients' culture or ethnic background. For example, if you are working with African American clients, you will want to have pictures depicting that ethnic background. However, do not use materials that depict stereotypes of the culture. Furthermore, expand the stimulus material and target responses gradually to include events and objects present in the wider social milieu of the client; most clients and families would want this.

4. *Use activities that reflect your client's environment.* Because treatment sessions that are relevant to the client's culture may best hold his or her interest, use activities that are culturally relevant. For instance, if you plan to use certain kinds of games as backup reinforcers in treatment, find out what games are popular at home. In general, choose activities that can be replicated in the client's environment. This will make treatment more meaningful and will assist with generalization and maintenance. Once again, expand the activities that may be found in the client's larger social milieu; it is likely that the educational, social, and personal communication needs would require them anyway.

5. *Provide treatment in the client's natural environment.* Of course, this is not always possible or realistic. But duplicate your client's natural environment as much as possible by using appropriate language, activities, and materials.

6. *Note that there exists very little treatment research suggesting that people of different ethnocultural backgrounds react differently to the same treatment procedures.* In all likelihood, treatment procedures described in the subsequent chapters of this book are effective with clients of all ethnocultural backgrounds. Also note that individual differences regardless of ethnocultural backgrounds are an important consideration to modify treatment procedures. No research suggests that the principles of positive reinforcement, modeling, shaping, prompting, corrective feedback, extinction, and differential reinforcement described in Part II of this book are not effective with a particular ethnocultural group.

7. *Modify treatment procedures to suit the client.* As noted before, practical exigencies may force you to initially select a standard treatment method with your culturally different client. However, as you learn from the initial treatment sessions, you are likely to modify the treatment sessions to suit the individual client. For instance, a particular potential reinforcer you selected may not be effective; you may have to change it. Some of these modifications may be dictated by the cultural background of the client. In all cases, be alert to the possibility that the methods may need to be changed because of the cultural and linguistic background of the client. Note also that you do this with all clients, regardless of their cultural background.

8. *Keep accurate and detailed records of treatment methods and their outcome.* You are required to keep detailed records of treatment sessions with all clients. However, with clients of culturally diverse backgrounds, this requirement is more pressing because even a method with demonstrated effectiveness may fail. You may have to make constant modifications in treatment methods. As noted before, it is important that you document these modifications and their effects so that future treatment of clients with similar cultural background may be facilitated.

9. *Do not schedule appointments on religious or cultural holidays.* Individuals who practice Christianity do not typically go to the dentist on December 25.

Citizens of the United States do not usually attend speech therapy on July 4. Similarly, you may anticipate that clients of different religious and ethnic backgrounds may observe different holidays and events. You may not be aware of all the religious ceremonies or celebrations your clients participate in. In advance, ask your clients what days and dates are unacceptable for clinical appointments.

10. *Collaborate with family members and other professionals.* Engage other people in your clients' treatment. In the educational setting, work closely with the classroom teacher and other educational specialists. In the medical setting, collaborate with other health care professionals. Involve family members in treatment and train them to work appropriately with your client in the home and community.

11. *Learn to appreciate your clients' culture and language differences.* As you work with clients with multicultural backgrounds, it is hoped that you will learn new information about different cultures and languages. Although evaluation and treatment are individualized for each client, your knowledge of linguistic differences and varying cultural practices will be useful across clients and will enrich you as a person. You will become more sensitive to clients' beliefs and more observant of behavioral variations and how they all affect assessment and treatment variables.

12. *Share your experiences with clients of differing cultural backgrounds with other clinicians.* The profession is still learning about assessing and treating clients with different cultural and linguistic backgrounds. Eventually, your professional experience in assessing and treating clients of varied backgrounds will be valuable to other clinicians as well. Therefore, when you gain experience in working with varied clients, share it with your colleagues.

There is a great need to conduct treatment efficacy research involving clients of varying linguistic and cultural backgrounds. Although some attention has been paid to assessment issues in multicultural speech-language pathology, little attention has been paid to the potential need for unique treatment procedures for multicultural populations. Therefore, it is essential that clinicians employ empirically supported treatment procedures and make careful measurements to document their effectiveness. Dissemination of treatment outcomes with multicultural populations is equally important.

Working with an Interpreter

Earlier we noted situations that require the use of an interpreter. The interpreter helps obtain information, assists with evaluation, and helps report information to clients and family members. There are two basic types of interpreting: **consecutive interpreting** and **simultaneous interpreting.** In consecutive interpreting, an individual talks, pauses, and then the interpreter translates. In simultaneous interpreting, the interpreter translates as the individual talks. As with all aspects of assessment and treatment of communicative disorders, you will learn to use interpreters effectively as you gain more experience and knowledge. As a starting point for learning to work effectively with an interpreter, follow these suggestions:

1. *Use the same interpreter as much as possible.* If you are able to use the same interpreter on a number of occasions, both you and the interpreter can benefit (ASHA, 1985b). You will not need to spend as much time training the interpreter. Your interpreter will know your expectations and thus is likely to assist you most effectively.

2. *Use an interpreter from the same ethnic background as the client, if possible.* A qualified interpreter from the same cultural or ethnic background as your client may help you establish rapport more quickly, provide more accurate interpretation, and give valuable insights into your client's culture (Cheng, 1991).

3. *Meet with the interpreter in advance.* It is important that you know in advance your interpreter's communication style and level of competence in the minority language and in English. Even if you are working with an interpreter you have used before, arrange to meet with him or her a few minutes before the scheduled assessment time. Schedule sufficient time so you can review the planned assessment and discuss the unique aspects of the client to be evaluated. Review confidentiality policies. You also can clarify your expectations of the interpreter's performance. The interpreter may offer information on the client's cultural background that may be helpful in selecting assessment procedures. The extra time also may be used to provide any needed training to the interpreter.

4. *Train the interpreter to administer any new tests you will be using.* Review tests the interpreter will be administering or assisting with. After you have explained the test administration guidelines, role-play test administration to help the interpreter gain experience with the test. This will give you an opportunity to correct any problems, such as improper prompting or cueing. Also, your interpreter will have a chance to ask questions and clarify any misunderstanding of your instructions.

5. *Discuss the testing format with the interpreter.* Give your interpreter an overview of the planned assessment schedule. Tell the interpreter that you may alter the assessment plan if necessary. Describe potential modifications.

6. *Describe what you want the interpreter to do in clear and simple language.* Allow time to discuss the expected skills. Include information regarding client confidentiality. Remind your interpreter that you will be the only one to make evaluative comments and diagnostic statements.

7. *Let the interpreter ask questions or make comments before meeting with the client.* You will want your interpreter to have enough time to clarify any needed

information. Also, as noted before, your interpreter may have valuable information to provide about your client's culture or language.

8. *Arrange a comfortable environment.* All participants in a session (e.g., you, the client, and the interpreter) should be able to make eye contact with each other. As you know, when talking to a client through an interpreter, you should maintain eye contact with the client. Consider that in some cultures, direct eye contact is a sign of rudeness or aggression, so adapt the intensity of eye contact as necessary.

9. *When you meet with the client, introduce yourself and the interpreter to the client.* When communicating with the client, you, not your interpreter, should take the lead. To introduce your interpreter correctly, find out in advance how he or she wants to be addressed.

10. *Describe your role and that of the interpreter to the client.* Do not assume that the client will automatically distinguish your role from that of your interpreter. In simple language, tell the client what you will be doing and how the interpreter will help.

11. *Talk to and look at the client, not the interpreter.* Although you will not ignore the interpreter's presence, most of your comments and questions will be made while looking at the individual they are addressed to. To show your interest (and gain information through observation), maintain appropriate eye contact with the client and the accompanying persons when you talk. When the client or the accompanying persons talk, continue to maintain eye contact, even when you must wait for interpretation to understand what has been said.

12. *Use brief sentences or paragraphs.* Remember, to accurately translate information, your interpreter must be able to recall everything you say. Try to keep your utterances short, but do not omit any critical information. If you routinely work with the same interpreter, you may be able to increase the length of your comments because he or she will become familiar with the structure of your clinical sessions and with the vocabulary used.

13. *Use a normal rate of speech and allow sufficient pauses.* Do not speak too rapidly. Again, the interpreter must be able to remember and understand what you have said (Cheng, 1991).

14. *Do not allow others to talk during the interpreting process.* You may be in a meeting with several other professionals. Even though they may not understand the client's language, during the interpreting process, everyone should be listening to the speaker and not engaging in side conversations.

15. *After the session, discuss the session with the interpreter.* Get unclear or confusing information clarified. Also, give the interpreter an opportunity to make comments and ask questions. Learn as much as possible from the interpreter about the client's culture and communication. If you will use the

interpreter again, add any suggestions you have for enhancing his or her skills in administering tests or translating questions and answers.

16. *Thank the interpreter for assisting and pay for the service.* The interpreter is a professional. Treat your interpreter with respect. Acknowledge his or her help. If appropriate, pay your interpreter.

As our discussion so far suggests, working with clients of differing cultural backgrounds requires more than the usually required technical competence in the traditional assessment and treatment procedures. The core competence in working with diverse populations is a broader cultural understanding. This core competence serves as a foundation for you to learn other skills. For instance, when you have the basic multicultural competence, you can modify your professional behavior and techniques to suit individual clients with differing linguistic and cultural backgrounds.

A broader cultural understanding requires more than studying linguistic differences. Although it is necessary to understand how Black English or Spanish-influenced English differs from Standard English on phonologic, syntactic, morphologic, and pragmatic variables, such knowledge in itself is not sufficient to develop cultural sensitivity and understanding. Literature on multiculturalism in speech-language pathology tends to be overly concerned with linguistic differences. As a student clinician, you should go beyond the linguistic differences. An understanding of people requires a basic study of history, geography, religion, and literature. Minimally, you should read a few books from the culture you are trying to understand. An excellent means of cultural education is to read a few literary classics from the culture.

A more personal means of learning about other cultures is to foster friendship with persons of varied cultures. Students have an excellent opportunity to do this as many programs in communicative disorders now have both students and faculty who are from diverse cultural backgrounds. If you see diversity around you as an opportunity to broaden your cultural understanding and educational base, you will be enhancing your skills in working with people of different cultures.

PART II

Clinical Methods in Speech-Language Pathology

In Part I you learned how clinical practicum in speech–language pathology is organized. You also learned some of the rules and guidelines a student clinician must follow.

In Part II you will find an overview of how to treat adults and children who have various communicative disorders. Selection of target behaviors, treatment procedures to increase desirable communicative behaviors, procedures to decrease undesirable behaviors, and methods to promote maintenance of communicative skills are described.

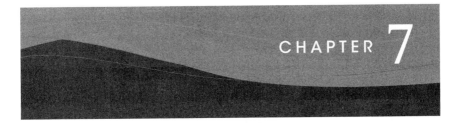

CHAPTER 7

Target Behaviors across Disorders

Chapter Outline

Typically, you start treatment only after you have selected target behaviors for your client. Occasionally, you may experiment with a few different targets before you finalize them. In either case, formal treatment begins only after the skills you want to teach your client have been carefully selected.

Your starting point for selecting target behaviors depends on what you find out about your clients. You must first determine if the clients assigned to you have been assessed or treated at your clinic or have received services at another clinic.

If the clients have received services at your clinic, you should carefully read the reports in the files. The files may contain an initial assessment (diagnostic) report, treatment reports, progress notes, and reports from other professionals. These reports help you make a rough evaluation of each client's status.

If the clients were newly referred to the clinic, you should assess them before starting treatment. Assessment procedures are described briefly in Chapter 5. In this chapter, you learn about selecting target behaviors for clients of all ages who have many types of communicative disorders.

Selection of Target Behaviors

A **target behavior** is a generic term that means any skill or action—simple or complex—you teach a client or a student. The term is applicable to educational and medical settings. Anything a clinician teaches regardless of the professional setting is a target behavior. Therefore, it includes the whole range of skills from the normal pattern of swallow for clients with dysphagia to the appropriate use of morphological skills by a child with language delay.

You need to select target behaviors for several reasons: *First, you need to teach multiple targets to most clients.* If clients need to learn only one or a few targets, there probably is no reason to choose. However, most persons with communicative disorders are unable to produce many target behaviors. A child with an articulation disorder, for example, may not produce several phonemes. Another child with a language disorder may not produce many classes of verbal behaviors, including grammatic, semantic, or pragmatic features. Similarly, adults with aphasia, people who have had a laryngectomy, persons who are dysarthric, and children with cerebral palsy or hearing loss are unable to produce multiple target behaviors that are essential for everyday communication.

Second, most clients cannot learn multiple targets at once. You need to select a few behaviors for the initial treatment and continue to teach only a few behaviors at a time. You teach more complex behaviors to clients as they master simpler behaviors. Therefore, to teach most of the missing communicative behaviors, the clinician must make some initial choices and select target behaviors.

Third, multiple targets should be sequenced. Again, this requires careful selection of behaviors. You must design a logical sequence of treatment. A sequence is necessary, because some behaviors best serve an immediate purpose of improving communication, whereas other behaviors may be deferred to a later stage in treatment. For example, it is better to teach children who are nonverbal such words as *Mommy, Daddy, juice,* or *hungry* than it is to teach *red, sofa,* or *triangle.* For an adult man with aphasia, it may be better to teach the forgotten name of his wife than it is to teach the name of the local football team in which he never had interest.

Fourth, some behaviors need to be taught before others. This, too, means selection of target behaviors. For persons who are nonverbal, it is necessary to teach a basic set of words before teaching word order or other syntactic features. Many morphologic or syntactic features are useless for a child who does not produce even the simple words. Nouns and verbs need to be taught before many grammatic morphemes can be taught. For example, you cannot teach prepositions (*in, on, under*) to a child who does not name anything. You cannot teach the auxiliary verb *ing* to a child who does not produce main verbs (*walk, eat*). Similarly, for children who do not produce certain speech sounds, it may be necessary to teach them at the word level before teaching them at the phrase or sentence level. Therefore, the clinician must choose target behaviors at all stages of treatment.

Approaches to Target Behavior Selection

The two main approaches to selecting target behaviors are normative and client specific. In the well-established **normative approach**, you select target behaviors that are appropriate for the client in view of his or her age and the age-based norms. For example, if a 4-year-old child does not produce language behaviors appropriate for 4-year-olds, then those behaviors are the targets.

In the more recently developed **client-specific approach**, the targets that make an immediate and significant difference in the client's communication are selected regardless of the norms. In this approach, you do not necessarily follow the table of norms to select target behaviors. You teach behaviors that best serve a client's communicative, educational, and social needs. A study of the client's environment and the educational and social demands made on that client is likely to suggest relevant and useful target behaviors.

The client-specific approach is suitable for choosing targets that are *culturally and linguistically appropriate* for the individual client. Because this approach requires a careful study of each individual client, the cultural and linguistic backgrounds of the client can be assessed for the relevance of target behaviors. As we noted in Chapter 6, choosing a culturally and linguistically appropriate service model is important in the practice of speech-language pathology.

In some cases, the normative and the client-specific approaches may suggest the same target behaviors for a given client. However, in many other cases, the targets may be different. The client-specific approach is more demanding than the normative, because it requires a greater study of the individual client and his or her family and cultural background.

The two approaches contrast more for children than for adults and more in the case of speech and language targets than for other targets. More research is needed to find out the best approach to selecting target behaviors. This means that clinicians cannot automatically assume that norms are the best targets for children. Some evidence suggests that target behaviors that are especially relevant for a client may be better generalized and maintained than those that are selected with no particular regard to the needs of the client (Hegde, 1998a). The client-specific approach makes clinical sense because it takes into consideration the uniqueness of each client. The following guidelines on selecting target behaviors are based on the client-specific strategy.

Guidelines on Selecting Target Behaviors

To select target behaviors, use the following guidelines that apply to various disorders of communication.

1. *Select behaviors that will make an immediate and socially significant difference in the communicative skills of the client.* Select target behaviors that will improve the client's social communication, academic achievement, and occupational performance. Note that target behaviors that make a socially and personally meaningful difference when learned are known as **functional targets**. In treating a child with misarticulations, select those sounds that are most frequently used in conversation and misarticulated by the child and whose correct production will most improve intelligibility. In treating clients with language disorders, select words that will immediately help the client achieve basic communication. In treating clients with vocal abuse, select the most frequently exhibited abusive behaviors for reduction. Note that behaviors or skills that immediately improve communication effectiveness also are those that fulfill the needs of the client, are produced in socially appropriate situations, and are reinforced by family members and others who interact with the client. Such skills are more likely to be sustained over time.

2. *Select the actual target behaviors, not their surrogates.* Do not select processes that are presumed to underlie a directly observable target skill, a theoretical prerequisite not experimentally shown to be necessary to learn the skill in question, or a skill supposedly related to the missing skills. Unfortunately, many clinicians select some other, unrelated skill in the hopes of instilling a skill that can be taught directly. This practice wastes time, as teaching an unrelated or presumably underlying skill may not have any effect on the actual missing skill. In teaching writing (literacy skills) to children, select alphabet printing, copying printed letters and words, writing to dictation, and so forth; avoid selecting fine motor coordination—even if it is a related or essential skill—in writing. In treating a child with an articulation disorder, select the production of sounds in error, not blowing whistles or chewing gum in the hopes of strengthening speech muscles. In treating children and adults who stutter, select dysfluencies or stuttering (as defined) for reduction, not a presumed mental problem (e.g., poor self-image).

3. *Select behaviors that help expand communicative skills.* Teach words that can easily be expanded into phrases and sentences. Although all words can be expanded, some expansions may be more significant for a client than other expansions. For instance, persons with language impairment who learn such adjectives as big and little and such nouns as cup and car can expand them into big car, little cup, and so forth. Such expandable words provide more meaningful communication than what is possible with triangle or refrigerator.

4. *Select behaviors that are linguistically and culturally appropriate for the client.* Find out what kinds of vocabulary, language structures, and pragmatic communication patterns are valued in the client's culture and the family. For instance, in teaching a set of basic words to a child who lives in an extended family, kinship terms may be more important than a set of words that name objects. For bilingual children, select language targets that will help them succeed academically. Talk to teachers and family members before you finalize the target behaviors for a client from an unfamiliar cultural background.

Potential Target Behaviors across Disorders

In this section, you will find a range of potential target behaviors that may be appropriate for clients of all ages and disorders of communication. Keep in perspective, though, that the suggested behaviors generally are appropriate, but the final selection depends on several factors, including a client's (a) environment; (b) communicative level before starting treatment; (c) communicative needs and demands in the client's social, educational, or occupation settings; and (d) associated clinical conditions (e.g., autism spectrum disorders, hearing impairment, intellectual disabilities, or neurological deficits).

Frequent shifts are common in the theory and clinical practice in all areas of speech–language pathology. Therefore, you must read articles in various journals to find out current trends and recent advances in both what to teach and how. Also, note that student clinicians select target behaviors for their clients only after consulting with their clinical supervisors and finalize them after consulting with family members.

A practical consideration is that each supervisor has his or her views on what to teach and how. Because you want to learn various approaches, find out your supervisor's approach. Read the books or articles your supervisor recommends. A more advanced student clinician always can discuss with the supervisor a different approach that she or he wishes to try. Most supervisors welcome novel suggestions from student clinicians and will readily approve the use of a different approach, provided the suggestions are based on evidence. But a good start is to first learn what the supervisor has to offer.

Sometimes, student clinicians wonder whether they should use an approach learned in an academic course that may not agree with what the clinical supervisor recommends. Generally, supervisors would like you to apply your academic knowledge to clinical practice. However, some supervisors may have strong opinions about certain approaches. Therefore, discuss the different approaches with the supervisor, including the one you learned in an academic course.

If your supervisor also has taught your academic course on a disorder, review the class notes and the text used in the class. When you discuss the potential target behaviors for your client with a disorder of articulation, for example, you should review your course information. If it is still current, review the textbook you used.

If it is not, read a more recently published book on articulation and phonology. When you discuss your client with your supervisor, you should be knowledgeable about the disorder under discussion and its assessment and treatment.

Articulation and Phonological Disorders

The first few clients assigned to most student clinicians may have articulation or language disorders; in the typical undergraduate academic sequence, courses on articulation disorders and language disorders are likely to precede courses on other communicative disorders. Therefore, you may initially treat clients with disorders of articulation or language.

Obviously, a client with an articulation disorder does not produce or only inconsistently produces certain speech sounds. Equally obvious is that the treatment targets are those sounds that are not produced correctly. Nonetheless, as you have found out from your academic courses, the nature of articulation disorders makes the process of selecting treatment targets a bit more complicated.

Most of the complications are due to theoretical shifts in the study of articulation and its disorders. Because of changing theories, the treatment targets for clients with articulation disorders have changed dramatically over the past few years, although some fundamentals have remained the same. Some of the changes may not be as substantial as they initially appear, but shifts in theories have suggested apparently dissimilar treatment targets for clients with articulation disorders (Peña-Brooks & Hegde, 2007). Student clinicians need to understand different approaches that are supported by treatment research data.

An overview of assessment of articulation is described in Chapter 5, where it is pointed out that an analysis of your assessment or reassessment data will show the types and variety of speech sound errors a client makes. You summarize the number of sounds in error, the frequency of those errors, and the types of errors. Further analysis may be made of the patterns of errors. The pattern analysis may depend either on distinctive feature theory or phonological theory, although many clinicians currently make phonological analysis, rather than the distinctive feature analysis. This analysis sets the stage for selecting treatment targets.

Selection of Individual Sounds for Training

Most experts agree that a mild disorder of articulation involving only a few sounds does not require a pattern analysis. Patterns may be discovered when the child misarticulates many phonemes, thus forming classes of misarticulations that are handled more efficiently as error groups. When this is not the case, the traditional sound-by-sound approach will be adequate.

Select individual sounds for training when one or more of the following conditions are met:

- The child's speech is generally intelligible.

- Only a few sounds are in error.

- The errors of articulation are caused by such organic factors as cleft palate, velopharyngeal insufficiency (VPI), and neurological involvement.

The meaning of *only a few sounds in error* is not always precise. The critical point is that the phonemes in error do not form significant patterns based on distinctive features or phonological processes. A few errors, even if they share distinctive features, may be handled efficiently within the sound-by-sound approach. Patterns or relations are unlikely in case of just a few misarticulations. Also, the analysis of a negligible pattern that may underlie misarticulations of a few phonemes may not add much to treatment economy or efficiency.

Treatment Targets Based on the Sound-by-Sound Analysis

1. Find out if each phoneme is produced correctly or not.

2. Classify errors as substitutions, distortions, or omissions.

3. Find out the word positions in which the sounds are misarticulated.

4. Select the initial target sounds for training, and write your target behavior statements in objective and quantitative terms.

5. In the case of a child who is bilingual or multicultural, or both, select the phonemes based on a clear understanding of the phoneme use in the client's language.

The following is an example of a target behavior statement for a child who substitutes /w/ for /r/ in all word positions:

The target is the correct production of /r/ at 90% accuracy in conversational speech produced at the clinic and the child's home. The correct productions should be observed in all word positions and in at least three consecutive speech samples, each containing a minimum of 20 opportunities for producing the target phoneme.

Note that the example of target behavior description specifies the following:

1. Quantitative criterion of performance (*90% correct*)

2. Response mode (*conversational speech*)

3. Response setting (*clinic and the child's home*)

4. Number of speech samples in which the target behavior productions are documented (*three samples*)

5. Number of opportunities for producing the target phoneme in each sample (*20*)

The quantitative criteria mentioned in the example of target behavior description are only suggestive. Each of those criteria may be modified. A different response setting may be specified. For example, depending on the client, classrooms or workplaces may be the settings in which the target phoneme productions are documented. Discuss these criteria with your clinical supervisor, who may suggest alternatives.

In writing target behavior statements, avoid such phrases as *the client will produce /s/ in conversational speech*. Whether the target behavior will be learned or not will depend on many variables, some not under the clinician's control. For instance, the client may be chronically absent from treatment sessions. Such statements as *the client will do this or that* may be construed as a promise to the client or family members, which is unethical. Also, state when the client will meet the goal in probabilistic terms, not by a certain date. It is acceptable to make such probabilistic statements as *the phoneme or phonemes are expected to be learned in 3 months of therapy given twice weekly in 30-minute sessions*.

Selection of Sound Patterns for Treatment

Theories of normal and disordered sound production have described several patterns, clusters, or classes. When a theory describes patterns of misarticulations, the treatment goal is their elimination. When a theory describes patterns of normal sound production, then the treatment goal is to teach the missing patterns to a client. Three patterns are available for selection: (1) patterns based on place-manner-voice analysis; (2) patterns based on distinctive features; and (3) patterns based on phonological processes.

Patterns Based on Place-Manner-Voice Analysis

This older method of classifying speech sounds into patterns is based on how the sounds are normally produced. This older method is not discarded because the newer approaches of distinctive features and phonological processes do incorporate some of its basic concepts. In the place-manner-voice analysis, errors of substitution are classified according to similarities in the place of articulation, manner of articulation, or in the presence or absence of voicing. In this method, you find patterns in multiple substitutions that are based on the place of articulation, manner of articulation, or the feature of voicing.

Target Patterns Based on the Place-Manner-Voice Analysis

1. Find out all substitution errors of the client.

2. Group substitutions that are based on place of articulation. For instance, a child may substitute lingua-alveolars for linguadentals

(e.g., d/ð); or linguavelars may be substituted for lingua-alveolars (e.g., k/t; g/d).

3. Group substitutions that are based on manner of production. Sounds produced in one manner may be substituted for sounds produced in another manner. For instance, a child may substitute stops for fricatives (e.g., b/v; t/s; p/f) and glides for liquids (e.g., w/r; w/l).

4. Group substitutions that are based on voicing features. A child, for instance, may substitute voiced sounds for voiceless sounds (e.g., b/t; g/k).

5. Teach one or more sounds from each group. Probe to find out if untrained sounds in the group are produced without training (generalization). For example, teach a few fricatives to a child who substitutes stops for fricatives; teach a few voiceless sounds to a child who uses voiced sounds instead. Find out if the untrained fricatives or untrained voiceless sounds are produced. If not, teach them as well. Generalization may or may not occur; if it does, you will save clinical training time. Still, you should extend treatment to nonclinical settings for maintenance.

6. In the case of clients who are bilingual–bicultural, make this analysis with a firm knowledge of the phonology of the clients' language.

See Chapter 8 for training procedures and how to probe for generalization.

The following is an example of a target behavior description for a client who substitutes voiced sounds for voiceless sounds:

> The target is the correct production of voiceless sounds [specify them] in all word positions at 90% accuracy in conversational speech evoked at the clinic and at the child's home. The correct productions should be observed in at least three consecutive speech samples. Each speech sample should have at least 20 opportunities for producing the target phoneme.

When you write a target behavior statement for a pattern of misarticulation, you must *list the individual sounds* as well. Just saying that you will teach voiced sounds or fricatives will not be specific enough. It is likely that not all sounds in a category are in error. Even if they are, you do not teach a category or a pattern directly. You teach concrete individual sounds that belong to a conceptual category or pattern.

Patterns Based on Distinctive Features

In the 1970s, the distinctive feature approach to articulation training was researched frequently. Although researched less frequently in recent years, you may wish to learn this approach by using it with a client or two (Peña-Brooks & Hegde, 2007).

Distinctive features are unique characteristics that distinguish one speech sound from another. A feature system proposed by Chomsky and Halle (1968) has been used widely. Using a binary system of pluses and minuses, Chomsky and Halle have described 11 distinctive features of English consonants.

The distinctive feature analysis is not much different from the traditional place-manner-voice analysis (Elbert & Gierut, 1986; Peña-Brooks & Hegde, 2007). What is new about it—the binary system—is only a superficial application of a quantitative method with little mathematical meaning. However, clinical training is the only way to test the validity of distinctive features. If they are valid, untrained sounds with the same features as the trained sounds should be produced on the basis of generalization. Therefore, you can do some informal clinical experimentation while using this approach. A client who is trained on a few sounds that share a set of features should begin to produce, without training, other missing sounds that have the same features. Reliable baselines and continuous treatment data will help you determine if this happens in treatment.

Target Patterns Based on Distinctive Features

1. Find out all the errors of your client.

2. Determine the distinctive features shared by the phonemes in error.

3. Group misarticulated sounds on the basis of shared (common) distinctive features.

4. Teach a few sounds from each group. Probe to see if untrained sounds within the group are produced without training. If they are, reinforce them and implement a maintenance procedure.

5. Make a distinctive feature analysis of a bilingual client's misarticulations with a firm knowledge of the linguistic and phonological features of the relevant language.

The following is an example of a target behavior description for a client who substitutes nonnasal sounds for nasal sounds (d/n; b/m; g/n). The assumption is that the client has not mastered the distinctive feature *nasal* or has not mastered the contrast between nasal and nonnasal sounds:

The target is the correct production of nasal sounds (/n/ and /m/) in all word positions at 90% accuracy in conversational speech evoked at the clinic and at the child's home. The correct productions should be observed in at least three consecutive speech samples. Each speech sample should have at least 20 opportunities for producing the target phoneme.

Note, again, that you should specify the sounds that you plan to teach. Do not write *I will teach the nasal feature* or *I will teach stridency*. Instead, list the sounds that share the feature stridency. You cannot teach a distinctive feature directly. You only can teach some sounds that have certain features. The value of the method, as pointed out, is in monitoring potential production of untrained sounds. The system simply makes it easier to track the effects of treating some sounds on other, untrained, sounds.

Patterns Based on Phonological Processes

Most experts now recommend a phonological approach to organize target behaviors for persons with multiple misarticulations resulting in limited speech intelligibility (Bernthal, Bankson, & Flipsen, 2009; Peña-Brooks & Hegde, 2007). There are several phonological process analyses that are not totally compatible with each other. Ultimately, your systematic clinical work will help you select the one that has worked the best. Eventually, you may modify an approach in light of your experience and use it consistently. Meanwhile, clinical research may show that a particular approach is better than others. During your clinical practicum, you may experiment with different approaches or follow your supervisor's suggestion.

You should know the basic phonological processes to select the appropriate processes for a given client. Though there is no full agreement among experts on the total number of processes, the following are most frequently described in the literature and are categorized as shown (Bernthal, Bankson, & Flipsen, 2009; Peña-Brooks & Hegde, 2007).

Frequently used phonological processes include the following:

1. **Syllable Structure Processes.** In these processes, the structure of syllables is changed.

   Final consonant deletion. Certain final consonants are omitted.

   [ba] for *ball;* [da] for *Daddy.*

   Unstressed syllable deletion. An unstressed initial or medial syllable is omitted.

   [medo] for *tomato;* [tefon] for *telephone.*

   Reduplication. A syllable, part of a syllable, or a monosyllabic word is repeated.

   [wawa] for *water;* [gogo] for *go.*

   Epenthesis. Addition of an unstressed sound, often the vowel [ə].

   [bə lak] for *black;* [lukə] for *look.*

   Cluster reduction. Most frequently, omission of a sound in a cluster of sounds; sometimes, one of the sounds of a cluster may be deleted and another may be substituted.

   [bu] for *blue;* [cod] for *cold;* [no] for *snow;* [fi] for *tree.*

2. **Substitution Processes.** In these processes, target sounds are replaced by other sounds. These processes often involve changes based on place of articulation or manner of articulation.

The following two processes are based on a *shift in place of articulation*:

Fronting. A sound typically produced in the back is replaced by the one produced in the front of the oral cavity.

[ti] for *key*; [su] for *shoe*.

Backing. A sound typically produced in the front is replaced by the one produced in the back of the oral cavity.

[gu] for *do*; [kæn] for *tan*.

The following processes are based on a *shift in the manner of articulation*:

Gliding of liquids. A glide is produced instead of a liquid; this is observed also in consonant clusters.

[wʌn] for *run*; [bwo] for *blow*.

Stopping. A stop is produced instead of a fricative or an affricate.

[tʌn] for *sun*; [du] for *zoo*.

Affrication. An affricate is produced instead of a fricative.

[tsu] for *shoe*; [tsʌn] for *sun*.

Deaffrication. Affricates are replaced by sounds of other kind.

[sɑp] for *chop*; [dɑb] for *job*.

Vocalization. A vowel, typically [o] or [u], is produced instead of a syllabic liquid.

[nudu] for *noodle*; [zipu] for *zipper*.

Denasalization. A nonnasal sound is produced instead of a nasal sound (the manner of production may be similar for the target and the substituted sound).

[bud] for *moon*; [deis] for *nice*.

Glottal replacements. The glottal stop is produced instead of a sound in the final or intervocalic position.

[ba/l] for *bottle*; [tu/] for *tooth*.

3. **Assimilation Processes.** In these processes, one sound becomes more like another sound. In progressive assimilation, a sound is assimilated to a previous sound, as in [bup] for *boot*; in regressive assimilation, a sound is assimilated to a subsequent sound, as in [bʌmp] for *jump*. Several kinds of assimilation processes are described:

Velar assimilation. A nonvelar sound changes into a velar sound.

[kok] for *coat* (progressive); [kek] for *take* (regressive).

Nasal assimilation. A nonnasal sound changes into a nasal sound.

[mani] for *bunny*; [non] for *nose*.

Labial assimilation. A nonlabial sound changes into a labial sound.

[pIp] for *pit*; [bup] for *boot*.

Prevocalic voicing. A voiceless consonant in prevocalic positions is voiced.

[dam] for *Tom*; [bai] for *pie*.

Devoicing of final consonants. A voiced consonant in final word positions is devoiced.

[bæk] for *bag*; [nos] for *nose*.

Metathesis is an additional phonological process in which sounds are transposed.

[eflənt] for *elephant*.

[æminəl] for *animal*.

[bæksIt] for *basket*.

Target Phonological Processes

1. Select one phonological analysis procedure, because there are several somewhat incompatible approaches.

2. Following the procedure prescribed by the selected approach, record continuous speech samples, transcribe the samples, and make a process analysis.

3. Select processes and the involved target sounds for intervention. Take note that you teach specific sounds to eliminate a process.

4. In the case of a client who is bilingual, make phonological process analyses only with a firm knowledge of the client's two languages and their phonological features.

Your initial targets should be the elimination of those phonological processes that:

• Reduce intelligibility the most;

• Include sounds from different classes;

- Are outgrown soonest by normally developing children; and

- Tend to persist in children with multiple misarticulations.

When you have selected a process for remediation, write target behavior descriptions that specify what sounds will be taught. Do not simply state that the "goal of treatment is to eliminate final consonant deletion." It is both abstract and negative. Also, the reader would not know what you do to eliminate a process. Instead, specify the process to be eliminated and the sounds to be taught. For example:

> The treatment goal is to eliminate the final consonant deletion process by teaching the correct production of the following consonants in word final positions: [list the phonemes]. The final criterion is at least 90% accuracy in the production of the target phonemes in three conversational speech samples recorded in nonclinical settings.

Note that no phonological process is eliminated without training certain individual phonemes. Also, phonological processes are theoretical ways of grouping errors; they should not be confused with treatment methods. Therefore, you should not write that *I will be using the phonological process treatment.*

Language Disorders

What to teach children with language problems was controversial during the times when theories of language were changing rapidly. When speech–language pathologists began to study Chomsky's transformational generative grammar in the 1960s and 1970s, other language targets seemed inappropriate. Some years later, when the semantic theory of language became popular, teaching vocabulary or grammar was considered a dated practice. Finally, when the pragmatic theory was hailed as the latest revolution in the study of language, teaching anything other than pragmatic rules was considered passé.

Theoretical diversity still persists, but the magnitude of theoretical shifts has diminished. Although we are always looking over our shoulders for that next revolution, we have learned in recent years that new theories did not eliminate the need to teach the skills the old theories specified. New theories only listed additional behaviors to teach. Obviously, it would be foolish to claim that we do not have to teach vocabulary or grammatical morphemes or syntactical features just because of an emphasis on pragmatic aspects of language. **Pragmatics,** or the *study* of social use of language, suggests that clients should be taught such pragmatic language skills as conversational turn taking and topic maintenance. However, a client who does not produce words, phrases, and sentences has no use for pragmatic skills; you cannot use what you do not have. Clinically, pragmatic concerns are especially important at an advanced stage in therapy. Having established certain language behaviors, including words, phrases, and sentences, you promote their naturalistic production in social contexts (Hegde, 1998a; Hegde & Maul, 2006; Paul, 2007; Reed, 2005).

In treating most, if not all, disorders of communication, you shape the final target behaviors from simpler behaviors. Clinicians continuously build more complex behaviors by integrating simpler ones. This is especially true of language because it is the most integrative of all communicative behaviors. Clinicians build this complex, integrative structure by teaching simpler, concrete responses.

Student clinicians need not wonder about the final target behavior for people with language impairments. It is always the same: *personally significant and socially useful verbal skills.* This final target is ideal and sometimes not achieved. Each client reaches a certain level of proficiency in learning those skills. But there is no question that we would like to take clients with language disorders to the highest level of performance in naturalistic settings that can be achieved with the best possible techniques.

Student clinicians often wonder about the starting point. A general rule that applies to all clients is that it depends on the client. The initial selection of targets depends mostly on the existing language repertoire of a client. This is true of children and adults with language problems that may have varied etiology or associated conditions. In many children, the diagnosis may be language disorder with no significant associated clinical conditions. In other children and most adult clients, it may be a language disorder associated with neurological disease, brain injury, intellectual disabilities, hearing impairments, genetic syndromes, autism spectrum disorders, and other clinical conditions. In each case, you should find out the client's communicative repertoire and build on it. A careful analysis of your assessment data will help you select the initial target behaviors.

Language Targets I: Basic Vocabulary

For many infants and children with language delay, the initial verbal targets are a set of words. Although you should not select some standard set of canned target words for all clients, you can use a few general guidelines to select words that give a good starting point for language treatment.

Basic Target Words

1. *Concrete words that name specific things or actions.* For the initial targets, do not select generic or abstract words. For instance, do not try to teach such words as *toys, food,* or *clothes*. Instead, teach specific words such as *car, milk,* and *sock*.

2. *Names (nouns) of manipulable objects.* Teach names of toys (*car, truck, ball, balloon, train, choo choo*) the child plays with. Also, teach words that name food items (*milk, juice, cookie*), clothing and personal belongings

(continues)

(*shirt, sock, shoe, hat*), kinship terms (*brother, sister, mommy, daddy, grandma, grandpa*), and proper names of family members.

3. *Names of animals and pets.* Teach these names—especially the names of the child's (or family's) pets—and later integrate them into short stories to expand vocabulary and teach sentence structures.

4. *Verbs.* Select commonly used verbs (*run, jump, hop, walk, push, laugh, smile, eat, drink*). Represent them by action that might help keep the child's interest in therapy. Once taught, use the verbs to teach basic sentence structures.

5. *Adjectives to describe objects and people.* Teach simple adjectives (*big, small, tall, short, red, green*) that can be used later to expand the client's utterances.

6. *Culturally and linguistically relevant words.* For all clients, select words that are appropriate for the cultural and linguistic background of the client (e.g., names of food items, festivals or celebrations that are specific to the child's family and culture).

Language Targets II: Phrases

Teach phrases when the child can produce several single words. Initially, teach two-word phrases. As the child learns more phrases, increase the number of words in utterances until the child is ready to learn morphological and syntactic elements of language.

Target Phrases

1. *Simple phrases.* Combine already learned words to form the initial target phrases to teach. For example, teach two-word utterances that are a combination of adjectives and nouns the child reliably produces (*big ball, little car, red sock*).

2. *Two-word utterances.* Combine nouns and action verbs you already have taught the client. You may teach such phrases as *boy run, kitty jump, baby eat.*

3. *Two- or three-word utterances.* Form these by combining already learned and yet to be learned words. Requests or mands are excellent for this kind of target responses. For example, teach such combinations as *want milk, more juice, cookie please,* and so forth. Other targets may include nouns and verbs: *ball hit, boy hit ball, push car.*

Language Targets III: Morphologic and Syntactic Elements

Start morphologic training when a child can produce phrases. While teaching morphologic elements, you may continue to teach new words and multiword phrases to expand the child's verbal repertoire. Before you can teach syntactic structures, you need to teach several grammatic morphemes.

Morphologic Treatment Targets

1. *Morphologic features that help build a language repertoire.* See what features may be integrated into the existing language responses. You know the selected responses should be useful to the individual client so they are likely to be produced and reinforced at home.

2. *The present progressive ing.* This is one of the early morphologic features to teach. Use the already taught noun and verb combinations to teach the use of the present progressive. For example, you could teach *boy running, Daddy coming, frog jumping, kitty eating*, and so forth.

3. *Other morphologic features.* Prepositions (*car in box, book on table*), regular plurals (*two cups, my cookies, give me marbles*), possessives (*Daddy's hat, Mommy's coat, Kitty's tail*), articles (*I want a cookie, give me the ball*), regular past tense inflections (*I missed it, he jumped, she smiled*), irregular plurals (*two children, three men, many women, several fish, five deer*), and irregular past tense words (*he went, I ate, she broke*).

4. *Morphologic features that help expand the multiword utterances into syntactically more correct utterances or complete sentences.* Expand the previously taught phrases into longer utterances by adding additional grammatical features. For example, by adding the auxiliary verb *is*, you can expand the multiword utterances into such sentences as *the boy is running, the man is working, the girl is smiling*, and so forth. Copula also will help expand phrases into sentences (*the man is nice, the lady is beautiful, the dog is big, the cat is small*). Expand phrases used to teach prepositions into sentences (*car is in the box, book is on the table*).

5. *Pronouns.* Teach them by using other, already taught sentence structures (*she is walking, he is eating, it is coming; this is my coat, that is your hat*).

6. *Additional grammatic morphemes and syntactic structures.* Select those that help form complex sentences. For example, teach questions involving *who, what, where, why, how*, and *when*. Also, teach negative sentences involving *no, not, nothing*, and so forth.

(continues)

7. *Grammatic morphemes and syntactic structures that are culturally and linguistically relevant.* For clients who are bilingual and bicultural, select grammatic morphemes and syntactic structures with a clear knowledge of the clients' primary language and cultural background. For instance, if the omission of plural *s* is apparently due to the influence of the child's primary language, treat this as a language difference, although treatment may be necessary for mainstream English usage in classrooms and in formal writing. Discuss this with the family members who, in most if not all cases, will request treatment.

Language Targets IV: Functional Units and Their Social Use

So far, we have described various structural elements of language that are appropriate for early and intermediate training. In the more advanced stages of language treatment, you should teach broader functional or pragmatic language skills. Always remember that the final goal of language intervention is to promote appropriate conversational speech in natural settings.

In speech-language pathology, *functional units* have two different meanings. In pragmatics, **functional units** mean language structures that have different speaker intentions and listener effects. Sometimes also called speech acts, functional units may express needs or feelings, control other persons, establish communication, and so forth. Other functional units include utterances that call for attention, request information, give information, request action, and respond to requests. Pragmatic structures especially relevant to conversational speech include topic initiation, topic maintenance, turn taking, and conversational repair (McLaughlin, 2006; Owens, 2008). As you can see, pragmatic (functional) units are not based on the structure of language as morphologic or syntactic units are. Instead, they are based on what they do for both the speaker and the listener.

Functional units that have another meaning are described in the behavioral analysis of language. Like pragmatics, behavioral analysis also describes language in functional units. These units are not based on the structure of language. However, the *functional units in behavioral analysis* are based on a cause–effect analysis. That is, verbal behaviors are divided into different groups because the responses belonging to those groups have different causes. In a general sense, this is what pragmatic units are supposed to be but may or may not be. From the beginning, behavioral analysis has emphasized functional units as against structural units of language. Although initially rejected by both linguists and speech-language pathologists alike, the basic logic of the behavioral analysis is especially applicable in language intervention (Hegde & Maul, 2006).

The basic logic of the behavioral analysis is that meaningful units of language are not structures but cause–effect (functional) units that describe what a speaker said, why it was said, and what effects it had on the listener (Skinner, 1957; Winokur, 1976). Therefore, a functional unit specifies not just an utterance but the circumstance under which it is produced and the effects that follow. A functional unit of verbal behavior is defined as a causal relation between an utterance, its antecedent, and its consequence. The utterance may be described structurally—it may be a word, a phrase, a sentence, and so on. The antecedent may be either an event in the environment or an internal, typically motivating state of the speaker (hunger or pain, for instance). The consequence is the effect the utterance has on a listener or listeners.

Although there are important differences between them, both pragmatics and behavioral analysis have drawn attention to meaningful units of speech as they are produced in specified conditions to produce specified effects. If speech is useful, it is precisely because it affects the behavior of other persons. Language is a tool only in this sense: You can produce it to accomplish something; it is not a tool you pick up and "use," because language defined as verbal behavior is simply certain kinds of actions. Children with language disorders lack those powerful social actions that produce effects on others. Therefore, in language intervention, you eventually must teach conversational skills that the children can produce to influence others.

Research continues to be done on teaching behavioral and pragmatic functional units. These units will be refined as clinical data emerge. Also, you will find new targets as researchers describe and evaluate them.

Pragmatic Language Treatment Targets

1. *Requests or mands.* In pragmatics, requests are subdivided into requests for action, information, objects, and so on. In the behavioral analysis, all requests, commands, demands, and similar utterances are classified into single functional response units called *mands*. It is possible that when a client learns to make certain kinds of requests, other kinds of requests will be made without further training. Obviously, this can happen only when the client produces the basic words to make any kind of request. If not, you must first teach selected words. As you do with any other response category, teach one or two types of requests or mands and probe to see if the client begins to produce other kinds of requests or mands.

2. *Tacts or descriptive statements.* Children and adults with limited language do not readily describe or talk about events in their environment. They may not comment on things and objects that evoke speech from most people. Statements that describe and comment on things, events, and persons are called *tacts* in the behavioral analysis. Such statements are excellent pragmatic targets to teach. In teaching them, you should often include the conversational skills described next.

3. *Topic initiation.* This skill is emphasized in pragmatic research. Persons with language impairment do not readily start talking about a topic.

(continues)

Topic initiation requires that the speaker be the first one to introduce a new topic for conversation. However, with most clients with language impairment, you will have to say something to have the child begin conversation on a topic. For example, you may have to ask questions on a topic to prompt the client to begin talking.

4. *Topic maintenance.* Once the client begins to initiate conversation, topic maintenance becomes an appropriate target to teach. Again, persons with language impairment tend not to stay on a topic of conversation. They may shift from one topic to another without saying much about any of them. To overcome this problem, you can work with progressively longer durations of speech on targeted topics of conversation.

5. *Turn taking in conversation.* Conversational speech requires that two or more individuals take turns in speaking and listening. Each person engaged in conversation is both a speaker and a listener. A person who plays only one of these roles is not a good conversational partner. Therefore, it is necessary to teach persons with language impairment to talk and to listen in an alternating manner.

6. *Conversational repair.* This is another conversational skill described in pragmatics. Many persons with language impairment fail to do something when they do not understand what is said to them. This may be why they do not continue a conversational topic. Normally, the listener who does not understand a speaker suggests this in some way to the speaker. The listener may say, "Tell me more about it," "I don't understand," "Please speak louder," and so forth. Such statements prompt the speaker to simplify, change words, expand, and repeat to modify the utterance in these and many other ways. Both the listener actions and the speaker modifications are involved in conversational repair. Teach clients to request more information, to ask for clarification, or to say, "I don't understand."

7. *Narrative skill.* A more complex language skill is to narrate events, stories, and experiences in a cohesive and chronologically correct manner. Obviously, before you target narrative skills, you must have taught many other skills, including vocabulary, morphologic features, and syntactic aspects of language.

8. *Culturally appropriate pragmatic communicative behaviors.* Pragmatic communicative behaviors are heavily culturally determined. Therefore, select pragmatic features for training only after you have made a clear analysis of the cultural communication patterns of a multicultural client. Discuss these target behaviors with family members. For instance, if eye contact during conversation is not a part of the child's verbal culture, find out if parents still want this taught to the child. Most parents would.

Literacy Skills

Promoting literacy skills in children is an important area of professional practice within speech-language pathology (American Speech-Language Hearing Association, 2001a, 2001b, 2001c). Because literacy skills are language based, speech-language pathologists have valuable contributions to make (Haney, 2002; Hegde & Maul, 2006; Justice, 2006; Justice, Chow, Capellini, Flanigan, & Colton, 2003; Lawhon & Cobb, 2002; Pence, 2007). Literacy skills include reading and writing.

Emergent literacy skills include some of the earliest skills that precede or are presumed to be prerequisites for reading and writing skills that develop later. These skills include a preschooler's recognition of the letters of the alphabet, sight reading of words, understanding the meaning of everyday symbols (e.g., a stop sign), printing the letters of the alphabet and simple words, and so forth (Hegde & Maul, 2006; Justice, 2006).

Preschool children with oral language disorders have a high risk of developing reading and writing problems later in grade school (Hegde & Maul, 2006; Justice, 2006; Pence, 2007). Therefore, to develop literacy skills in children, speech-language pathologists should:

- Develop emergent (early) literacy enrichment programs that parents implement at home;

- Offer early intervention for language disorders to prevent later language as well as literacy problems; and

- Offer literacy intervention, either integrated with language treatment or as an independent program.

Use the following guidelines in selecting treatment targets. Note that the target behaviors include the children's skills as well as the parent behaviors.

Treatment Targets in Literacy Intervention

1. **Emergent literacy skills and parental behaviors that promote early literacy skills in preschoolers.** Children of parents who exhibit certain kinds of behaviors are more likely to develop literacy skills than those whose parents exhibit opposite behaviors. Therefore, to promote emergent and full-fledged literacy skills in their children, target the following parental behaviors:

   a. *Storybook reading to children.* Counsel and train parents to regularly read storybooks to preschool and school-age children, at least until

(continues)

the children are independent, regular, and proficient readers. Ask parents to jointly look at the text and point to the words as they read. This will help promote an understanding of printed words and their names. Also ask parents to periodically ask questions about the text that they have just read. The questions can range from such simple questions as "Who said they were tired?" to more complex questions, such as "What do you think he will do after he has rested?"

b. *Literacy-rich home environment.* Ask parents to have books and writing materials (crayons, pens, pencils, papers, child-size desks and chairs, good lighting to read and write) freely available to their children. A home rich in literacy materials is likely to promote literacy skills in children.

c. *Modeling literacy skills at home.* Ask parents and older siblings to model such good literacy skills as frequent reading and writing. Parents and others who engage in literate behaviors are likely to stimulate such behaviors in children.

d. *Getting children involved in literacy skills practice.* Teach parents to have their children participate in such common literacy skills as writing a letter; addressing a letter; signing or writing a birthday greeting card for another child; writing the name of a teacher on a note to the teacher; preparing a grocery list; looking up words in a dictionary; and reading together, or helping a child to read, instructions for putting together a puzzle, a toy train track, a vacation route on a map, and so forth.

2. **Oral language skills.** We know that children with oral language disorders tend to have difficulty learning literacy skills. Therefore, effective treatment of oral language skills, including appropriate phonologic, morphologic, syntactic, and pragmatic skills in children with oral language disorders, is one of the best methods of promoting later literacy skills in such children. Follow the guidelines given in the previous sections on the selection of language target behaviors for children.

3. **Literacy skills.** Integrate literacy skills (traditional reading and writing) into language treatment. When such integrated intervention proves insufficient, target more reading and writing skills in independent treatment sessions.

4. **Reading skills.** In the absence of evidence contradicting this, the best strategy is to target the skills directly, instead of presumed underlying processes (e.g., cognitive processes or phonological awareness) or theoretically linked precursors or predictors (e.g., reading readiness,

fine motor coordination). Literacy skills may be integrated with speech and language training or treated independently.

a. *Integrating printed letters of the alphabet in all oral speech and language training.* For example, as you model a speech sound, show the representative letter of the alphabet; as you teach a word during language training, point out the letters of that word.

b. *Integrating printed word stimuli during oral speech and language training.* For example, while modeling or evoking the target speech sounds or morphologic features at the word level, show the printed word as well.

c. *Integrating printed phrases and sentences into oral speech and language training.* For example, while training speech sounds or grammatical elements, present corresponding phrases and sentences along with your oral models or evoking questions.

d. *Reading the letters of the alphabet, simple and functional words, phrases, and sentences selected from the child's family environment and academic curricula.* Consult with the teachers; start with teaching the names of each letter of the alphabet.

e. *Reading during advanced language training.* For example, while training such language skills as storytelling, help the child read a short story and then narrate it.

f. *Reading as independent target.* For example, time and resource permitting, teach reading directly; begin with name reading, especially the name of the child and those of family members; subsequently, include such advanced oral language features as different forms of sentences and short stories.

5. **Writing skills.** Again, the best strategy is to target the writing skills themselves, instead of theoretical precursors or processes. Actual writing skills may be a part of language treatment or independent targets.

a. *Writing the letters of the alphabet during oral speech and language training.* For example, manually guide the child to write the letter of the alphabet that represents the speech sound, the first and the subsequent letters of the words under training, and so forth.

b. *Writing words during oral speech and language training.* For example, manually guide the child to write the target words used in speech and language training.

(continues)

   c. *Writing phrases and sentences during speech and language training.* For example, teach the child to write the phrases and sentences used in teaching oral speech and language skills.

   d. *Writing during advanced language training.* For example, while teaching such pragmatic language skills as narration, storytelling, and story element sequencing, teach the child to write a short story to dictation.

   e. *Writing as independent target.* For example, time and resources permitting, teach writing directly; begin with name writing, especially the name of the child and those of family members; subsequently, include such advanced oral language features as different forms of sentences and short stories.

Voice Disorders

Voice disorders are generally classified as aphonia and dysphonia. Aphonia is lack of voice, whereas dysphonia is any kind of voice disorder except for aphonia and includes disorders of pitch, loudness, vocal quality, and resonance (Hegde & Pomaville, 2008). Some voice disorders are related to abnormal vocal fold actions, others to oral and nasal resonance problems, several to physical diseases, and many to undesirable vocal behaviors of the client. After a medical examination and a careful voice assessment, you determine the nature of the disorder and the desirable target behaviors to be trained and the undesirable vocal behaviors that should be modified or eliminated (Andrews, 2006; Boone, McFarlane, & Von Berg, 2005; Case, 2002; Hegde, 2008c).

Target Behaviors in Aphonia

The treatment target for clients with aphonia is phonation (laryngeal sound production), because the main problem is lack of phonation. Aphonia may be a behavioral disorder (functional with no organic pathology) or a neurologic or structural disorder. Bilateral vocal fold paralysis or a severely injured or surgically removed larynx may result in aphonia, but the approach is often medical (Teflon injection) because of serious swallowing problems. In unilateral vocal fold paralysis, effortful closure of the folds is a treatment target (by pushing or pulling exercises).

Treatment Targets for Clients with Functional Aphonia

1. Reflexive phonation that may be shaped into voluntary voice production (e.g., coughing, laughing, throat clearing)

2. Reduced tension in the laryngeal area (through relaxation or gentle laryngeal massage)

3. Prolonged vocalization inherent in laughing, coughing, or throat clearing

4. Progressive vocal production from faint phonation to loud phonation to produce words, phrases, and sentences

Target Behaviors in Dysphonia

Some forms of dysphonia are caused by physical problems or diseases. Among these are paralysis and ankylosis, carcinoma, varieties of laryngeal tumors and lesions, infections, and papilloma. Other forms are caused by structural changes in the larynx (e.g., nodules and polyps) associated with abuse or misuse of the vocal mechanism.

In treating dysphonia that has a physical cause, the necessary medical or surgical treatment is first carried out. Then the voice therapy techniques are used to improve the functioning of the vocal mechanism. When surgery removes the laryngeal structures, as in laryngectomy, you should integrate new ways of phonation or new sources of phonation into the voice therapy. In treating disorders of phonation attributable to vocal abuse or misuse, you must change the vocal and general behaviors of the client. Because a majority of voice disorders are related to vocal abuse or misuse, a major task of the voice clinician is to change vocally abusive behaviors and to modify patterns of misuse.

Treatment Targets for Clients with Dysphonia

1. **Respiration training.** Use this target when there is evidence of faulty use of the airstream during phonation and continuous speech. A specific target is a deep enough inhalation to sustain utterances of typical length. Sustained exhalation while prolonging certain vowels is a common target.

2. **Muscular effort.** Some clients have difficulty in approximating their vocal folds because of unilateral cord paralysis, general fatigue, and myasthenia. Such clients need to exert muscular effort in achieving vocal fold approximations. A specific target is to teach the client to push on the arm of the chair on which he or she is sitting and phonate simultaneously. Hard glottal attacks also have been targeted for such cases.

(continues)

3. **Esophageal speech.** This is a target for clients who have undergone a laryngectomy. In teaching esophageal speech, target either the injection or inhalation of air; in some cases, the two may be combined. In injecting air into the esophagus, the client is asked to first impound some air in the oral cavity and then push it back. The production of plosive consonants is especially helpful in this process. In inhaling air into the esophagus, the client rapidly takes in air while keeping the esophagus relaxed and open. The air passing through the esophagus produces vibrating sound that is articulated into speech sounds.

4. **Phonation with artificial larynx.** An alternative target for the laryngectomee, phonation with artificial larynx, involves the use of mechanical devices to produce sound that is articulated into speech sounds.

5. **Relaxation.** When there is evidence of excessive muscular tension affecting the voice of the client, muscular relaxation might be a useful target. Systematic relaxation of specific muscle groups is targeted.

6. **Vocal rest.** This is a target for clients with infectious or traumatic laryngitis. The client is asked to refrain from speaking and whispering.

7. **Altered head positions.** Changing the head position while speaking often results in better voice. You must try different head positions to find a position that promotes best voice quality. Extended, flexed, or tilted head positions have all been noted to change the voice.

8. **Elimination of vocally abusive behaviors.** Find out the client-specific vocally abusive behaviors and target their reduction; they generally include such behaviors as the following:

   a. Yelling and screaming

   b. Smoking

   c. Coughing and frequent throat clearing

   d. Excessive talking, singing, crying, or laughing

   e. Talking too much with allergic reactions and upper respiratory infection

   f. Talking in noisy situations

9. **Elimination of vocal misuse.** Reduce the following:

   a. Frequent use of hard glottal attack

   b. Excessively loud speaking

    c. Habitual speaking with inappropriate pitch levels

    d. Continuous speaking or singing for extended durations

10. **Culturally appropriate vocal behaviors.** In selecting specific vocal behaviors for your multicultural voice client, consider cultural patterns of communication. For instance, an artificial larynx may or may not be culturally acceptable to certain clients. Discuss your treatment strategy with the client or family, or both, to place it within the cultural context.

Target Behaviors in Disorders of Loudness and Pitch

Disorders of loudness include excessive loudness or insufficient loudness of voice. Disorders of pitch include too high or too low a pitch for a given person.

Treatment Targets for Clients with Loudness and Pitch Disorders

1. **Increased loudness.** This is a target for clients who speak excessively softly. Select a client-specific level of loudness.

2. **Decreased loudness.** This is a target for those who speak with excessive loudness. Again, select a loudness level that is appropriate for the client.

3. **Higher pitch.** In the typical case of a high-pitched male voice, target a client-specific lower pitch.

4. **Lower pitch.** In the low-pitched female voice, target a higher pitch. The target pitch is relative to the client's typical pretreatment pitch.

Target Behaviors in Disorders of Resonance

Disorders of resonance include hypernasality, hyponasality, and reduced oral resonance.

Treatment Targets for Clients with Resonance Disorders

1. **Reduced nasal resonance on nonnasal speech sounds.** This is a target for many clients including those with hearing impairment,

(continues)

velopharyngeal incompetence, cleft palate, and paralysis of the velum associated with cerebral palsy, stroke, and other neurological problems. A predominant voice problem in these clients is hypernasality.

2. **Increased nasal resonance on nasal speech sounds.** This is a target for clients with hyponasality (denasality). People with hearing impairment, among others, may need this target.

3. **Increased oral resonance.** In some cases of resonance disorders, lack of oral resonance is a dominant problem. In them, you increase oral resonance.

Disorders of Fluency

Historically, the targets in stuttering treatment programs have varied because of the numerous definitions of stuttering. Among other targets, increased self-confidence, reduced anxiety, resolution of social role conflict, reduction of parental concern for normal nonfluencies, improved self-image, fluent stuttering, acceptance of stuttering, modification of negative attitudes, and resolution of repressed psychological conflicts have all been targeted. That these targets may not be appropriate is suggested by lack of documented evidence for their effectiveness in reducing stuttering (Bloodstein, 1995; Hegde, 1998a, 2007).

As with all disorders, consider the clients' cultural backgrounds to assess their or the family members' dispositions toward fluency and its disorders before planning a treatment program. Discuss the clients' and their family members' views of stuttering, its origin, and remediation. Your overall intervention strategy may partly be dependent on what you learn from them. For instance, if the parents believe that stuttering is not modifiable, you may have to counsel them and offer scientific and professional information before attempting direct intervention.

Currently, many effective treatment programs exist. Treatment targets, however, depend on the specific treatment program. Generally, three effective treatment approaches exist. First, there is the fluency shaping technique—an indirect method of reducing stuttering by teaching skills that enhance fluency. Second, there is the direct stuttering reduction strategy—a collection of two specific techniques of pause-and-talk (time-out) and response cost. In both pause-and-talk and response cost, the treatment involves placing a direct behavioral contingency on dysfluencies or stutterings (see Chapter 9 for procedures). Third, there is the fluency reinforcement technique—suitable especially for young children. Fluency reinforcement strategy is also a direct strategy; the reinforcement contingency is placed on fluent productions to increase them. Note that the target behaviors in direct stuttering reduction strategy and fluency reinforcement strategy are opposite each other (incompatible behaviors; stuttering is directly reduced in the former and fluency is directly increased in the latter). Target behaviors are specific to these two general strategies. Typically, no fluency shaping skills are taught in direct stuttering reduction or in fluency reinforcement. Therefore, these two techniques do not affect speech rate or other prosodic features.

Treatment Targets in Fluency Shaping

1. **Management of airflow.** This target behavior has two components. The first is a slightly exaggerated inhalation of air. The second is a slight exhalation of air through the mouth before starting phonation. It is important that the client does not impound the air in the lungs. A small amount of air must be exhaled as soon as the peak of inhalation is reached. You may use this target for most persons who stutter, but especially with those whose stutterings are associated with mismanaged airflow (e.g., dysfluent speech during inhalation or exhausting the air supply while still attempting to produce speech).

2. **Gentle onset of phonation.** Teach the client to initiate phonation gently after the slight exhalation of air through the mouth. The phonatory onset should be relaxed, soft, and easy.

3. **Reduced rate of speech through syllable prolongation.** Reduce the rate of speech to a level where speech is free from stuttering. Note that the slowed target speech rate is client specific. Some have to slow down more than others to maintain a stutter-free speech. Do not reduce the rate by pauses between words or phrases; reduce it by syllable (vowels that follow the initial consonants) prolongation. Teach the production of phrases and sentences without gaps between words. The client should produce words as though they were a string of prolonged syllables without word boundaries.

4. **Normal prosody.** The rate reduction and explicit management of airflow and phonatory onset result in an unnatural fluency. Therefore, in the final stages of treatment, shape normal prosody, including a near-normal rate, intonation, and rhythm.

5. **Maintenance of fluent conversational speech in natural settings.** This is the final target. Make sure that at the time of dismissal, the client is close to 98% fluent in the clinic. This high rate of fluency is not expected to be maintained in the natural settings. A minimum of 95% fluency must be maintained over time across natural settings.

Treatment Targets with Direct Stuttering Reduction Strategy

1. All forms of dysfluencies or stuttering as defined by the clinician

2. Any associated motor behaviors if they need to be specifically manipulated (normally they do not)

Treatment Targets with Fluency Reinforcement Strategy

1. Fluently produced words, phrases, and sentences

2. Fluent conversational speech

Cluttering is another disorder of fluency, characterized by an excessively fast rate of speech, reduced speech intelligibility due to this fast rate, increased frequency of dysfluencies, possible language deficiencies, and lack of concern about the problem. Cluttering is often associated with stuttering. Therefore, stuttering treatment procedures also need to be used with people who clutter. Controlled experimental treatment research on cluttering is limited. Teaching maintenance of intelligible and fluent speech in people who clutter still is a major clinical challenge.

Treatment Targets for Clients with Cluttering

1. **Slower rate of speech.** Target a slower rate of speech and more deliberate articulation to increase speech intelligibility.

2. **Slight syllable prolongation.** Target slightly prolonged syllable durations to increase speech intelligibility and to decrease dysfluencies.

3. **Pauses between phrases and sentences.** Target deliberate pausing at appropriate junctures to control the runaway rate of speech.

4. **Deliberate stress on syllables.** Target syllables produced with deliberate stress to improve articulation, slow the rate, and enhance intelligibility.

5. **Reduced dysfluency rate.** In addition to the slower rate, target dysfluencies for reduction through time-out (pause-and-talk) or response cost.

6. **Language skills.** Target language skills if the client exhibits deficiencies; use standard language treatment procedures.

7. **Increased awareness of the problem.** Increase the client's awareness of his or her speech difficulty by giving contingent feedback.

8. **Self-monitoring skills.** Teach self-monitoring skills to promote maintenance of treatment gains.

Neurogenic Communicative Disorders in Adults

Several types of communicative disorders are associated with neurological disease or damage. These types of communicative disorders include aphasia, apraxia, dysarthria, and dementia, along with those associated with right hemisphere syndrome and traumatic brain injury.

Varied neurological conditions are associated with communicative disorders. Consequently, the clients in this group are similarly varied. There are subgroups within each diagnostic category. Individual differences in subgroups are also significant as they are in all groups of persons with (or without) communicative problems. Therefore, a comprehensive description of target behaviors for adults and children with neurogenic communicative disorders is beyond the scope of this book. There are several books that you may read to understand the full range of target behaviors that may be selected for clients with neurogenic communicative disorders (Brookshire, 2007; Collins, 1991; Cummings & Benson, 1992; Davis, 2000; Duffy, 2005; Freed, 2000; Hall, Jordan, & Robin, 2007; Hegde, 2006, 2008a, 2008b; Helm-Estabrooks & Albert, 2004; LaPointe, 2005; Murdoch & Theodoros, 2001; Murray & Clark, 2006; Myers, 1999; Payne, 1997; Vogel & Cannito, 2001; Yorkston, Beukelman, Strand, & Bell, 1999).

For neurologically affected persons who are bilingual or bicultural, it is important to have a general understanding of the first language and the cultural patterns of communication before a treatment plan can be developed. As with all disorders of communication, target behaviors selected for neurologically involved clients should be culturally appropriate. To do this, it is necessary to analyze the premorbid levels of education, cultural experience, and family interaction. In the case of bilingual persons, you will have to determine the language in which the treatment should be offered (Payne, 1997).

Target Behaviors for Clients with Aphasia

Aphasia is an impairment in understanding, formulating, and expressing language caused by brain damage (Hegde, 2006; Hegde, 2008a). Before selecting target behaviors, the complex pattern of neurological and verbal deficits must be evaluated carefully. The individual client's pattern of deficits will determine the selection of target behaviors. Therefore, select target behaviors only after a careful assessment of the type of aphasia, the client's predominant problems, his or her communicative needs, and chances of some immediate success at communication. Select behaviors that are meaningful and pragmatic for the client (Hegde, 2006, 2008a, 2008b).

Treatment Targets for Clients with Aphasia

1. **Auditory comprehension of spoken language.** Initially, ask clients to point to named pictures, objects, or body parts. Ask yes/no questions. Later, ask for correct responses to phrases and sentences. Ask them to follow instructions. Gradually increase the complexity of speech presented to the clients.

2. **Naming responses.** Select names of objects, persons, and actions that are of immediate use to a client. Besides synonyms and antonyms, rhyming words, spelling selected words, and completing sentences with target words may all be useful targets.

3. **Phrases and sentences.** Select as initial targets useful phrases and simple sentences. Subsequently expand the repertoire by adding a variety of sentence forms or functional units including mands (requests, commands, demands), tacts or declarative statements, *wh* questions, yes/no questions, passives, and other forms. Include specific morphologic features necessary for these verbal expressions.

4. **Pragmatic aspects of language.** Teach such conversational skills as turn taking, topic maintenance, and narration as found appropriate.

5. **Gestures paired with verbal expressions.** If it improves communication, pair ordinary gestures or a formal system of gestures (e.g., AMERIND) with words and sentences.

6. **Writing.** Select such writing skills as copying letters, words, and sentences; and writing from dictation and spontaneous writing. Teach them in that order.

7. **Reading skills.** First, teach reading isolated words that are useful to the client. Next, teach silent reading (and comprehension) of materials of high interest and pragmatic value. Select reading passages from graded materials. Target more complex and longer reading passages as the client's comprehension of read information improves.

Target Behaviors for Clients with Right Hemisphere Syndrome

A constellation of symptoms associated with disease or damage to the right hemisphere of the brain is known as the right hemisphere syndrome (Brookshire, 2007; Hegde, 2006, 2008a, 2008b, 2008c; Myers, 1999). Clients with this syndrome exhibit a variety of deficits in perception, attention, emotional expression, abstract reasoning, and communication. A special feature of right hemisphere syndrome is left neglect: The client tends to ignore stimuli in the left visual field, including people, objects, and printed material. Unlike clients with aphasia, those with right hemisphere syndrome do not exhibit serious linguistic deficits; nonetheless, they communicate poorly because of their other deficits.

Treatment Targets for Clients with Right Hemisphere Syndrome

1. **Denial of illness and deficits in awareness.** Increase client's awareness of deficits by providing contingent corrective feedback on deficit behaviors. Provide videotaped feedback of errors. Give positive feedback for appropriate behaviors to develop discrimination between acceptable and unacceptable behaviors. Teach self-monitoring skills. Teach family members and others to give corrective as well as positive feedback.

2. **Impaired attention.** Target attending behaviors during communication training. Reinforce the client for paying attention to treatment stimuli and instructions given, and for following directions and staying on task. Integrate attention training with pragmatic communication training.

3. **Visual neglect.** Target improved attention to speakers on the left; reduce left neglect during reading, writing, and drawing.

4. **Abstract reasoning.** Teach correct inferences drawn from read or narrated stories, understanding proverbs and metaphors, and detection of absurdities in statements.

5. **Pragmatic communication skills.** Target such skills as topic maintenance, turn taking, narrative skills, maintained eye contact during discourse, and so forth. Target the reduction of such deficits as confabulation and impulsive and inappropriate responding.

6. **Functional reading and writing skills.** Target basic reading and writing skills necessary for everyday functioning (e.g., making a grocery list, reading a newspaper).

(continues)

7. **Impulsive behavior.** Teach clients to wait before responding to stimuli.

8. **Compensatory strategies.** Train such strategies as writing down appointments to compensate for residual memory deficits; self-monitoring one's own speech errors to correct them; evaluating one's own actions' social appropriateness.

Target Behaviors for Clients with Apraxia of Speech

Apraxia of speech is a motor speech disorder involving difficulty in initiating and executing movement patterns necessary to produce speech, even though there is no paralysis, weakness, or incoordination of speech muscles. It is a disorder of both articulation and prosody. The difficulty is thought to be due to impaired motor planning of speech (Duffy, 2005; Freed, 2000; Hegde, 2008a, 2008b, 2008c).

Presumably, damage to the motor programmer in the brain may cause apraxia of speech. The disorder also may result from edema or damage to tissue surrounding the motor programmer. Apraxia of speech may be associated with aphasia and dysarthrias as well. In such cases, treatment targets include those that are appropriate for clients with aphasia and dysarthrias.

Treatment Targets for Clients with Apraxia of Speech

1. **Nonspeech movements.** Target these for clients who cannot imitate speech sounds and syllables. Select those movements that are related to speech: tongue protrusion, blowing, biting the lower lip, pressing the two lips together, tongue tip movements, and so forth. These often are appropriate initial targets for clients with severe apraxia of speech. However, generally, do not start with nonspeech movements unless attempts at starting treatment with speech movements have failed.

2. **Misarticulated but correctly imitated speech sounds.** The initial speech sounds to be treated may be those that are imitated or correctly produced with fewer trials.

3. **Sounds that are produced with visible movements of the articulators.** Such targets may lead to initial success in treatment. These also are good initial targets.

4. **Singletons and clusters.** Generally, treat them in that order, but consider the pattern of errors of individual clients.

5. **Most frequently occurring sounds.** Treat them first. Target less frequently or rarely used sounds for later treatment.

6. **Stressed syllables.** Select these for treatment, if your client's performance on them is better than that on unstressed syllables. This is true of some clients.

7. **Gesturing and writing.** These are targets especially in the case of severely apraxic clients.

8. **Rhythm.** Use it as in the Melodic Intonation Therapy in which speech is taught with musical intonation (see Helm-Estabrooks & Albert, 2004, for details).

9. **Normal prosody.** Teach normal sounding intonation by systematically varying it during sentence production and continuous speech.

10. **Nonverbal or augmentative means of communication.** For clients with severe apraxia of speech, teach augmentative and alternative means of communication.

Target Behaviors for Clients with Dysarthrias

A group of speech disorders that are caused by impaired speech muscles is called **dysarthrias.** This impairment, in turn, is caused by brain injury or various neurological diseases; both the central and peripheral nervous systems may be involved. Besides muscular control problems, symptoms include respiratory, phonatory, resonatory, articulatory, and prosodic problems. There are different types of dysarthrias, although they share many common characteristics. Targets selected for a client depend on the predominant type of dysarthria and the pattern of difficulties (Duffy, 2005; Freed, 2000; Hegde, 2008a, 2008b, 2008c).

Treatment Targets for Clients with Dysarthrias

1. **Appropriate posture and tone and improved strength of muscles.** Target relaxation when there is hypertonia. Induce postural adjustments that facilitate improved speech. Improved strength of the

(continues)

general musculature may be targeted by the physical therapist, but the speech–language pathologist's target is improved tone of muscles involved in speech production.

2. **Improved respiratory management for speech.** Improved muscle strength and appropriate postural adjustments are interrelated with this target. Teach controlled and sustained exhalation that helps produce sustained and louder speech.

3. **Improved phonatory behaviors.** Treat hyperadduction through relaxation training and hypoadduction through increased muscular effort by such means as pushing exercises.

4. **Improved articulatory skills.** Achieve improved intelligibility of speech through articulation training. Target a slower rate of syllable and word production rather than the production of specific sounds.

5. **Improved resonance characteristics.** To achieve this target, reduce hypernasality and increase oral resonance.

6. **Improved prosody.** Teach improved rhythm, stress, and intonation of speech. You may have to teach speech rate control as well.

7. **Nonverbal or augmentative means of communication.** For severely impaired persons who do not benefit from verbal communication training, teach nonverbal means of communication. For others, teach augmentative means to supplement oral speech.

Target Behaviors for Clients with Dementia

An acquired neurological syndrome associated with persistent or progressive deterioration in intellectual functions and behavior is called **dementia** (Bourgeois, 2005; Brookshire, 2007; Hegde, 2006, 2008a, 2008b, 2008c). Dementia is frequently associated with such neurological diseases as Alzheimer's disease, Pick's disease, and Parkinson's disease. Dementia is diagnosed when at least three of the following five functions show evidence of impairment: (1) memory; (2) visuospatial skills; (3) emotion or personality; (4) language; and (5) intellect (cognition). Symptoms across individuals may vary; variations are especially marked at different stages of dementia. Therefore, the target behaviors selected will depend on the kinds of impairment a client exhibits. In the advanced stages of dementia, treatment often is limited to clinical management, which may include efforts to slow down the progression of physical and intellectual deterioration by such means as regular exercise and social involvement (Mahendra & Arkin, 2003). Clinical management is a team effort, and often implemented in a healthcare setting where all aspects of the client's behavior are managed.

Treatment Targets for Clients with Dementia

1. **Simple and predictable daily routines.** Design a daily routine in which the client has no surprises and sudden changes; teach clients to keep their belongings in the same place.

2. **Memory skills.** Design various reminders (alarms, written instructions, staff reminders, signs that remind activities, written lists of activities or appointments, use of electronic devices that remind tasks, keeping personal belongings in a specific place, etc.) and teach the client to use such reminders.

2. **Orientation.** Teach the client to consult signs and directions, local area maps, calendars, digital clocks with large displays, and other environmental cues to maintain orientation.

3. **Maintenance of daily living skills.** Target such skills as cooking, eating, dressing, bathing, and so forth. Initiate a program of physical exercise and social involvement (getting together with friends or family members as long as possible).

4. **Maintenance of communication skills.** Teach the client to:

   a. Make various kinds of requests (e.g., request to be given written directions, repeat information, simplify messages; request more time to respond, etc.)

   b. Use gestures, facial expressions, and signs to convey messages

   c. Describe objects and persons when naming fails

   d. Use self-cueing techniques

   e. Initiate conversation

   f. Reduce inappropriate, irrelevant, or vulgar verbal behaviors by ignoring them

   g. Interact socially with family members and friends; tell stories, maintain topic of discussion, take conversational turns

   h. Achieve effective communication, not linguistic accuracy

In all cases and especially in the advanced cases of dementia, the treatment targets are the behaviors of family members and other caregivers.

Treatment Targets for Family Members and Other Caregivers of Clients with Dementia

1. **Understanding dementia.** Provide systematic information to promote a better understanding of dementia, its course, and its effects.

2. **Understanding the particular client.** Provide information on the strengths and limitations of the client in communicative skills and general behavioral self-management.

3. **Understanding community resources.** Provide information on resources available to the family members in their communities.

4. **Structuring the living environment.** Ask the family members to:

   a. reduce variability in the arrangement of living conditions and such daily routines as eating and bathing; schedule such activities at the same time of the day

   b. reduce sensory stimuli (noise and visual distractions)

   c. use different rooms for specific purposes

   d. limit access to hazardous material

   e. balance the needs of security and freedom

5. **Sustaining the client's personal care habits.** Ask the caregivers to support and reinforce independent living skills as long as possible.

6. **Exhibiting nonprovoking behaviors.** Ask them to be calm and exhibit nonprovoking behaviors to reduce the client's emotional outbursts.

7. **Minimizing effects of negative factors.** Ask the family members and caregivers to analyze situations that lead to disturbed behaviors in the client and teach them to minimize or eliminate such situations.

8. **Reducing the demands made on the client.** Teach them to minimize the demands they make on the client. Ask them to provide adequate help and support when they do make reasonable demands.

9. **Providing respite care.** Arrange for respite care so the family members and professional caregivers have periods during which they are free from the constant demands of care.

10. **Effective ways of communicating with the client.** Teach the family members and caregivers to:

    a. use gestures, facial expressions, posture, and other cues to supplement their verbal expressions

    b. establish eye contact, gain the client's attention, and address the client directly

    c. ask *yes* or *no* questions instead of open-ended ones

    d. speak in clear, simple, redundant speech with short sentences

    e. keep all instructions simple and repeat them

    f. engage the client in conversations on familiar and simple topics

    g. specify the referents of speech

Target Behaviors for Clients with Traumatic Brain Injury

Individuals who sustain traumatic brain injury exhibit a variety of behavioral deficits that include impaired communication (Hegde, 2006, 2008a, 2008b, 2008c; High, Sader, Struchen, & Hart, 2006; Murdoch & Theodoros, 2001; Silver, McAllister, & Yudofsky, 2005). **Traumatic brain injury** typically results from physical trauma or external force and excludes such other causes of brain damage as stroke and progressive neurological diseases (e.g., Alzheimer's disease). Injury with an open wound in the head, crushed or fractured skull, torn meninges, and damaged brain tissue is called *penetrating brain injury*. Injury associated with intact meninges is called *nonpenetrating brain injury*. Both adults and children may be treated with traumatic brain injury. Major symptoms include confusion, disorientation, memory problems, slurred speech, seizure and other neurological symptoms, attention deficits, impaired thinking and reasoning, auditory comprehension problems, initial mutism and subsequent confused language, naming problems, perseveration, reading and writing deficits, dysarthria, and a variety of pragmatic language problems.

Treatment Targets for Clients with Traumatic Brain Injury

1. **Orientation.** Target orientation to time, place, and person. Design questions that test orientation (e.g., "Where are you now?" and "What time is it?")

(continues)

2. **Attention.** Target increased attentiveness to surroundings, people and events, and conversational partners.

3. **Use of augmentative and alternative communication devices.** Target the use of such devices as a communication board in the initial stages of rehabilitation.

4. **Memory for daily routines.** Prepare lists of daily routines and written signs and instructions that may be used to improve memory for daily routines.

5. **Improved naming skills.** Make a list of names of significant people in the client's life and of caregivers to be used in treatment.

6. **Comprehension of spoken language.** Target increased attention to communication partners and conversational topics to improve comprehension.

7. **Reduction in inappropriate, irrelevant, or tangential responses.** Target these behaviors for reduction by using appropriate behavioral contingencies.

8. **Improved speech production.** Target the reduction of symptoms of dysarthria (respiratory, phonatory, articulatory, resonatory, and prosodic problems).

9. **Improved pragmatic language skills.** Target such pragmatic skills as turn taking, topic maintenance, cohesive narration, eye contact, and so forth.

10. **Self-monitoring skills.** Teach self-monitoring skills to help maintain the treatment gains.

11. **Compensatory strategies.** Target compensatory strategies (e.g., requesting information, writing down instructions, asking others to speak slowly, use of electronic devices, etc.) to reduce the negative effects of residual deficits.

12. **Family support.** Target the behaviors of family members such that they provide support and encouragement to the client.

Neurogenic Communicative Disorders in Children

A major group of children with neurogenic communicative disorders are classified as having **cerebral palsy,** which is brain injury suffered in the prenatal and perinatal period. However, brain injury suffered later in childhood may not be classified as cerebral palsy; instead, such older children belong to the group with traumatic brain injury.

Brain injury in children is different from that in adults mainly because of their still-developing neuromuscular system and communicative behaviors. Even so, many common effects are seen in adults and children with neuropathologies. Children with neuropathologies are a diverse group, with varied etiological factors, symptoms, and subgroup classifications (Hegde, 2008a; Love, 2000; Mecham, 1996). Target behaviors selected for a child depend on these factors. Therefore, you should select target behaviors after a careful assessment of both the neurophysiological status and communicative behaviors. Neurologically affected children typically need physiotherapy to improve muscle functioning. Some speech-language pathologists with special training in techniques that promote neuromotor development may combine some of those techniques with communication training methods. Because neuropathologies affect all aspects of speech, treatment targets include the fundamental processes of speech.

Treatment Targets for Children with Neuropathologies

1. **Respiratory management for speech.** Teach the client to inhale a sufficient amount of air for speech, then exhale in a controlled manner to sustain phonation and speech, and to maintain a rhythmic pattern of inhalation and exhalation.

2. **Appropriate phonatory behaviors.** Target appropriate loudness, pitch, and voice quality.

3. **Improved resonance with or without surgical or prosthetic treatment.** Reduce hypernasality and nasal emission, and increase oral resonance.

4. **Improved articulation and intelligibility.** Teach specific speech sounds that are difficult for the individual client. Teach visible sounds, correctly imitated sounds, and sounds that are correctly produced in some contexts before other sounds. You also may consider speech muscle training to improve your client's strength, tone, and range of motion.

5. **Improved prosody.** Target appropriate stress and intonation to reduce monotonous speech.

Target Behaviors for Children with Childhood Apraxia of Speech

In some children, a form of articulation disorder is diagnosed as **childhood apraxia of speech,** formerly called *developmental apraxia of speech* (American Speech-Language-Hearing Association, 2007; Hall et al., 1993; Love, 2000). Although adults with apraxia of speech show evidence of brain injury, children with a diagnosis of childhood apraxia of speech may not. Clinicians do not agree on the criteria to be used in diagnosing this disorder. Therefore, this diagnostic category is controversial (Forrester, 2003).

Treatment Targets for Children with Childhood Apraxia of Speech

1. **Speech-related movements of oral structures.** Target only speech-related movements. Note that targeting oral movements that are unrelated to speech is a questionable practice.

2. **Imitation of speech sounds.** Initially, target visible sounds and use massed trials. But do not linger on these targets, because isolated sound productions are not a problem for the person with developmental apraxia.

3. **Syllables and words in which the articulatory breakdowns occur.** If the breakdowns occur only in phrases and sentences, start treatment at this level. Use words that require back-to-front and front-to-back articulatory placement (e.g., *back/cab*).

4. **Reduced rate of speech.** Target slower articulatory rate and even stress to achieve improved intelligibility.

Target Behaviors for Persons with Hearing Impairment

Hearing impairment varies from a minimal loss to profound deafness. The degree of effect on communication depends on various factors, including the age of onset, the type and degree of loss, the quality and the time of initial intervention, and many others. Even mild hearing impairment in infancy is a potential cause of speech and language problems. Severe to profound loss almost always creates significant problems of speech, language, resonance, prosody, and intelligibility.

Complete audiological and otological examinations and a thorough assessment of all aspects of communication are essential before you select target behaviors for your client who is hearing impaired. Compared to those who are hard of hearing, the deaf require a more intensive as well as extensive treatment program. The deaf who seek oral communication need training on all aspects of speech and language production. Also, these speech and language targets are part of a carefully developed program of aural rehabilitation whose major components are the use of amplification, auditory training, and working with the family members.

Treatment Targets for Persons with Hearing Impairment

1. **Oral language.** For the infant with hearing impairment, an early, home-based, language stimulation is started first, and formal language training is initiated as soon as practical. Basic vocabulary and morphologic, syntactic, and pragmatic aspects of language are all targets.

2. **Speech production and improved articulation.** For the infant, the period of language stimulation is also the period of speech stimulation. The child constantly hears the speech sounds in syllables and words. Later, formal speech training is started. Teach all misarticulated target sounds; among these, fricatives, affricates, and those that are produced at the back of the mouth are especially important to teach. Also, teach correct productions of distorted vowels.

3. **Improved voice quality.** Children and adults who are deaf need extensive training in improving their voice quality. You may target reduced hypernasality, improved oral resonance, improved nasal resonance on nasal sounds, reduced nasal emission, and overall improved voice quality.

4. **Improved prosody.** With or without the help of biofeedback devices, teach improved rhythm and intonation of speech. Also teach modified speech rate, smooth flow of words, and appropriate pitch and loudness.

5. **Nonoral means of communication.** For clients who cannot benefit from oral speech-language training, target nonoral means of communication, including American Sign Language.

Target Behaviors for Persons with Limited Oral Skills

Many children and adults with multiple physical and sensory disabilities may not master the skills of oral language needed for social communication. Although people with limited oral skills are sometimes referred to as *nonverbal individuals*, people are rarely nonverbal. Most often, they are *minimally verbal* in the sense that their verbal skills are inadequate to meet academic, occupational, social, and personal communication needs. These people benefit from various means of communication that either enhance their limited oral communication skills or replace them altogether.

Nonverbal or minimally verbal persons may be taught several modes of communication, but most learn some oral speech. Therefore, in many children and adults, the selected nonverbal modes *supplement* oral speech and language. For this reason, these modes of communication are called *augmentative*; they augment (enhance, expand) oral speech. In persons with severe disabilities, the nonverbal means may be the primary mode of communication. When that is the case, the mode of nonverbal communication is called *alternative communication.*

There are many modes of augmentative and alternative communication (AAC). Each has its advantages and limitations. Select the one that suits a client after a careful assessment of his or her physical potential and limitations, communicative needs, cost of the system, and practicality (Beukleman & Miranda, 2005; Beukleman, Yorkston, & Reichle, 2000; Glennen & DeCoste, 1997; Hegde & Maul, 2006; Hegde & Pomaville, 2008). Note that the earlier view of assessing eligibility criteria for AAC is no longer valid and there is no insistence that clients should be offered extensive oral communication training that fails before offering AAC; in fact, nonoral means of communication may promote oral communication in infants and young children. Furthermore, there are no prerequisite skills, especially presumed cognitive skills for AAC use, whose absence precludes such means of communication (Romski & Sevcik, 1993). No matter how severe the disability, a carefully designed and implemented AAC system can help.

The two major means of nonverbal communication are unaided and aided. **Unaided** means of communication do not require the use of equipment and include gestures, signs, mime, and facial expression. Incidentally, speech is also unaided communication, but our focus here is nonverbal means. **Aided** means of communication use graphic or physical symbols and equipment of various sorts, including mechanical and electronic devices. There are several unaided and aided systems of communication.

Unaided Systems of Communication for the Nonverbal

1. **Gestures.** Teach a set of basic gestures (e.g., specific gestures for *yes, no, hungry, hurts, bathroom,* etc.).

2. **Patterns of eye blink.** Teach these to communicate specific messages (e.g., a single blink for drink, two blinks for food).

3. **Pointing.** Teach finger pointing, pointing by gaze, or both.

4. **Pantomime.** May be an independent target or a target combined with minimal speech.

5. **American Sign Language (ASL).** Considered a separate language with its own rule system, ASL is the most sophisticated and widely used system of nonverbal communication. You may teach this system to deaf persons, because most prefer it.

6. **Left-hand manual alphabet.** This is a target for individuals whose right hand is paralyzed.

7. **Signed English.** In this system, signs stand for words and morphologic features. The signs parallel the word order of spoken English.

8. **Signed Exact English.** Another set of signs that closely follows the spoken and written forms of English.

9. **Amer-Ind Gestural Code.** This is not a linguistic or sign system; it is also known as American Indian Hand Talk. It has been used by peoples of various North American tribal bands to communicate with each other. It has been an excellent means of intercultural communication.

10. **Fingerspelling.** In this system, words are spelled by fingers; letters are represented by various handshapes.

Because some of the aided systems are based on computer technology, new systems are likely to emerge in the near future. You should keep in touch with recent developments and select the one that is most useful and practical for a particular client. Among the aided systems, some use symbols, pictures, and graphic devices whereas others involve electronic devices.

Aided Systems of Communication for the Nonverbal

1. **Object display.** Teach the client to communicate by pointing to various objects displayed in front. Use real or miniaturized objects.

2. **Pictures, photographs, and line drawings.** Select commercially available packages or prepare them for individual clients.

(continues)

3. **Traditional orthography.** English (or any other language) may be represented on a communication board. You may design boards with the letters of the language and some commonly used words and phrases. The display may be electronic.

4. **Blissymbolics.** These are a collection of semi-iconic and abstract symbols printed and pasted on a communication board. Teach individual symbols for single words and combination of symbols to form phrases and sentences. Because the symbols are not language specific, they may be read by speakers of any language.

5. **Rebuses.** In this system, words or parts of words are represented by pictographic drawings. Some of the drawings are combined with letters of the alphabet; others are more like pictures of the objects or persons.

6. **Abstract symbol systems.** There are several symbol systems that use abstract, geometric shapes whose meaning is established only by training; examples are Carrier symbols (Premack-type) or Yerkish Lexigrams. The Premack-type symbols are plastic shapes that may be arranged into phrases and sentences. The Yerkish Lexigrams contain nine geometric figures that may be combined to form messages.

7. **Braille and International Morse Code.** These use traditional orthography. Braille contains a set of tactile symbols (raised dots) traditionally used by persons who are blind. Morse code is a system of dots and dashes. Messages expressed in Morse code may be printed in English. You may use computerized electronic devices to translate and print Morse code messages.

8. **Speech generators or synthesizers.** These are electronic devices that store messages. The speaker can retrieve these messages and display them on small screens or deliver them through built-in speakers. A computer monitor may be used to display messages.

9. **Neuro-assisted devices.** Use these with the most severely disabled individuals who cannot use their hands or feet to point or type messages or activate switches by movement to deliver messages electronically. These devices do not require the speaker to move or act on the switching mechanism to generate messages. The body's electrical signals activate the device and generate messages. Both muscle action potentials and brain waves have been used to activate specially designed electric typewriters, teletypewriters, and computers. Currently, this technology is expensive and of limited use, but improvements and lower cost may be expected.

Target Behaviors for Clients with Swallowing Disorders

Swallowing disorders, also known as dysphagia, may be experienced by children and adults but are generally more common in older individuals with neurological diseases and disorders, including strokes and degenerative neurological diseases (e.g., Alzheimer's disease and AIDS dementia complex). In younger as well as older people, traumatic brain injury, spinal cord injury, injury to the laryngeal structures, and surgical or radiation treatment for oral, laryngeal, pharyngeal, and esophageal cancer are among the varied causes of swallowing disorders (Corbin-Lewis, Liss, & Sciortino, 2005; Hegde, 2008a, 2008b, 2008c; Logemann, 1998).

Swallowing food and liquid may be impaired in the oral, pharyngeal, and esophageal stages of swallow. Speech-language pathologists limit their assessment and treatment to disorders of the oral and pharyngeal phases of swallow because the esophageal stage of swallow is involuntary and its disorders are treated medically. Regardless of the nature of the swallowing disorder evident in individual clients, the final treatment target for individuals with swallowing disorders is always the same: safe swallowing of food and liquid to meet the nutritional needs of individuals and maintain their physical health. Consistent with this main and general target, however, clinicians design specific treatment targets to control the pattern of swallowing disorder an individual experiences. Because of varied conditions and their unique effects on swallowing, the treatment targets for individual clients vary to a great extent; we have listed only some of the major treatment targets. Treatment targets are grouped into four categories: *compensatory treatment, swallowing maneuvers, direct treatment,* and *indirect treatment.* Student clinicians should consult other sources on dysphagia to select specific targets for individual clients (Groher, 1997; Hegde, 2008c; Logemann, 1998).

Selected Treatment Targets for Individuals with Swallowing Disorders

1. **Compensatory treatment targets.** Target skills that help compensate for the existing difficulty in swallowing so that the client can still swallow liquids and solid foods in spite of the difficulty.

   a. **Postures that promote safer swallow.** These include the *chin-down posture* (holding the chin down while swallowing) that widens the valleculae; the *chin-up posture* that helps drain food toward the back of the mouth; the *head rotation toward the weaker side,* which

(continues)

helps direct food to the more efficient side of the pharynx; *combined chin-down and head rotation* that may promote better laryngeal closure during swallow; *head tilt to the stronger side*, which helps direct food to that side; and *lying down on one side*, which helps control diffuse residue in the pharynx.

b. **Increased oral sensory awareness.** Improved oral sensory awareness may help better the swallow and the target is to apply a sensory stimulus prior to swallow; specific targets include the *application of a downward pressure on the tongue* with a spoon; presentation of a *sour bolus* (50% lemon juice, 50% barium) before presenting the regular bolus of food; presentation of a *cold bolus*; presentation of a *bolus that needs chewing*; and presenting a *large volume bolus*.

c. **Modification of volume and speech of food presentation.** Larger or smaller bolus, depending on the individual; slower rate of smaller bolus presentation in some individuals.

d. **Modification of food consistency.** Presentation of thin liquids for individuals with oral dysfunction, among other conditions; presentation of thickened liquids for individuals with delayed pharyngeal swallow; presentation of purees and thickened liquids for individuals with reduced laryngeal closure.

e. **Use of intraoral prosthesis.** Use of artificially fashioned devices that help compensate for physiological deficiencies; include *palatal lift prosthesis, palatal obturator,* and *palatal augmentation* or *reshaping prosthesis.*

2. **Swallowing maneuvers.** Certain ways of swallowing that promote safer swallow of solid and liquid food; there are four commonly used maneuvers.

a. **The supraglottic swallow,** which involves holding the food in the mouth, taking a deep breath and swallowing while holding the breath, and coughing soon after swallowing; helps protect the airway at the level of the vocal folds.

b. **The super-supraglottic swallow,** which involves inhaling and holding the breath while bearing down, and swallowing while bearing down and holding the breath; minimizes the chances of aspiration.

c. **The effortful swallow,** which involves squeezing as hard as possible during swallow; promotes the posterior motion of the tongue base.

d. **The Mendelsohn maneuver,** which involves holding the larynx up for several seconds during swallow; improves laryngeal movement.

3. **Direct treatment targets.** Involves placing food in the client's mouth and shaping and reinforcing a safe swallow; targets are specific to the swallowing phase in which the disorder is evident; targets include postural adjustments described previously.

a. For clients with **mastication disorders,** the targets include putting pressure on the weak cheek; putting food on the normal or stronger side of the mouth; head tilt toward the stronger side; use of a palate reshaping prosthesis.

b. For clients with **preparatory phase disorders,** the targets include tilting the head forward to keep the food in front of the mouth until swallowing it; tilting the head back to promote swallow; holding the bolus in the anterior or middle portion of the mouth.

c. For clients with **oral phase disorders,** the targets include placing food in the posterior part of the mouth, placing a straw (to drink) at the level of the faucial arch; tilting the head back; using the supraglottic swallow maneuver, holding the bolus against the palate, swallowing with a strong, posterior tongue movement.

d. For clients with **pharyngeal phase disorders,** the targets include tilting the head forward, presenting small boluses, alternating liquid and semisolid swallows, initiating dry swallow after each food swallow, the supraglottic swallow maneuver, and tilting the head forward.

4. **Indirect treatment targets.** These targets include exercises to improve swallowing without presenting food during exercises. They include a variety of exercises, but only a few are mentioned here.

a. **Oral motor exercises** to improve the strength of the muscles involved in swallowing; include such tongue exercises as raising and holding the anterior or posterior tongue portions, pushing the tongue against a tongue depressor; stretching, rounding, and puckering the lips, closing the lips tightly, and alternating between the production of "o" and "e"; keeping the jaw wide opened for as long as possible, sideways or circular motions of the jaw.

b. **Stimulation of the swallowing reflex** include such targets as placing an ice water–cooled laryngeal mirror at the base of the anterior faucial arch and asking the client to swallow (without food).

(continues)

c. **Lifting and pushing exercises** to improve laryngeal adduction and prevent aspiration; include such targets as sitting in a chair and holding the breath as tightly as possible; pushing down or pulling up on the chair arm with both the hands; pushing down or pulling up with a single hand and try to produce clear voice; production of a hard glottal attack; inhaling, holding breath, and coughing.

It is important to stress that the targets listed should be tailored to the specific patterns of disorders and disabilities an individual exhibits. A thorough assessment of the kinds of swallowing problems an individual exhibits is essential before selecting the target behaviors. The clinicians should know why each target is used and what to do if a selected target does not work.

Target behaviors described in this chapter should help you get started with most clients. In all cases, remember that the final treatment target is effective communication or safe swallow in natural settings. Throughout the treatment phase, periodically assess your client's status to find out what additional target behaviors must be taught to enhance communication or improve swallow. Follow the logic of moving from simple behaviors to more complex behaviors and from clinically controlled speech or swallow to speech or swallow controlled by natural events in the client's environment.

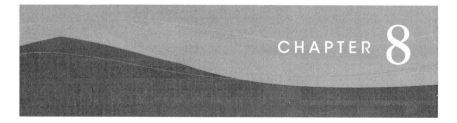

CHAPTER 8

Treatment in Speech-Language Pathology: Concepts and Methods

Chapter Outline

· ·

- Basic Methods of Treatment
- How to Evoke Communicative Behaviors
- Creating New Responses
- Increasing the Frequency of Responses
- Strengthening and Sustaining Target Behaviors
- Sequence of Treatment

In speech-language pathology, the term *treatment* includes medical and educational connotations of treating and teaching persons with communicative disorders. Most importantly, the term is used in its basic scientific sense. Treatment is an agent of change. To effect change is the main job of clinicians and educators. Any time you teach a new communicative behavior to someone or alter an existing one, you will have changed that person. Therefore, you will have treated that person.

The terms *intervention* and *remediation* also mean effecting changes in some undesirable situation. Therefore, in this book, we use the terms *treatment, teaching, intervention,* and *remediation* interchangeably. They all refer to what speech-language pathologists do to effect positive changes in people's communication skills. In medical contexts, specialists may prefer to use the term *treatment,* and in educational contexts, the terms *teaching, intervention,* or *remediation* may be preferred. As a student clinician, you should follow the established practice in using the preferred terms.

All treatment methods are means of creating something that did not exist or changing something that did. We create or alter communicative behaviors. In speech-language pathology, **treatment** is rearranging communicative relations between speakers and their listeners. Success in treating communicative disorders depends on how effectively the clinician changes the way certain speakers and their listeners react to each other.

The rearrangement of the listener-speaker relation begins with the new ways in which the speech-language pathologist organizes his or her interaction with the client (Hegde, 1998a, 2008c). The clinician manipulates stimuli and creates new stimuli that might increase the probability of appropriate communicative behaviors. For example, in a case of a child with a language delay, the clinician may bring and manipulate various objects, toys, pictures, and other stimuli that might set the stage for speech and language. The clinician may model the correct responses, ask the child to imitate those responses, prompt the child to say something, and perform other acts that might lead to a desirable response.

The rearrangement continues when the clinician responds to the child's attempts at communication in ways that are different from what the child has been accustomed to. Although the family members may have responded favorably to a nonverbal child's gestures, the clinician may not. Instead, the clinician may proceed quickly to teach words to replace gestures. When a child begins to reliably produce those target words, the clinician will expect the child to use words in communication, instead of gestures. The clinician may reinforce only the word productions. In this manner, the clinician may change the results of a child's communicative attempts. Words produce more favorable results than gestures. Consequently, the child's communicative attempts change for the better.

The final and probably most important part of rearranging a communicative relation is to change the ways family, friends, and others in the life of a client react to the client. In the case of a child with a language delay, the clinician teaches family members new ways of interacting with the child. These are the ways the clinician will have used to change the communicative behaviors by the child. Family members, teachers, and friends are taught to react the way the clinician reacted. These persons now should react differently to the child's gestures and words. These differential (discriminated) reactions help support and sustain the newly learned communicative behaviors and help eliminate old, undesirable behaviors.

Basic Methods of Treatment

To treat disorders of communication, you should:

1. *Evoke communicative behaviors.* Normally, no special procedures are required to evoke speech from speakers. Speech itself is a powerful stimulus. Also, events surrounding us and our internal body states provide additional stimuli to speak. However, these typical stimuli may be ineffective with persons who have a communicative disorder. Therefore, we need special stimuli to evoke speech.

2. *Create nonexistent communicative behaviors.* Many clients who seek treatment do not produce certain desirable communicative behaviors. The task of the clinician is to create those behaviors. For example, a clinician who treats a child who has not acquired language must create verbal behaviors the child did not previously produce.

3. *Increase existing communicative behaviors.* Many other clients who seek treatment do have certain communicative behaviors in their repertoire, but the behaviors are not produced frequently enough. In such cases, the clinician's task is to increase the frequency of those behaviors. For instance, a person who stutters does speak fluently but not often enough.

4. *Strengthen and sustain communicative behaviors.* Communicative behaviors created in the clinic or increased to a higher frequency may not be produced in the natural environment. Also, newly learned behaviors may not last. Therefore, before dismissing clients from treatment, the clinician must use procedures that help strengthen and sustain newly taught behaviors.

5. *Control undesirable behaviors.* Treatment also includes procedures that help decrease certain behaviors. These include undesirable communicative behaviors and such inappropriate behaviors as uncooperative behaviors, distracted or competing behaviors, crying, and other behaviors that interfere with treatment.

In this chapter, we describe procedures to create, evoke, increase, strengthen, and sustain communicative behaviors. In Chapter 9 we describe procedures to decrease undesirable and uncooperative behaviors.

How to Evoke Communicative Behaviors

Evoking procedures are special stimulus events needed to have clients in treatment produce speech. The frequently used evoking procedures include instructions, modeling, prompts, and physical stimuli.

Instructions

Instructions describe the skill to be learned. Technically, instructions set up the target behaviors. Therefore, instructions are the starting point of treatment. We often have to tell the young and the old what we want them to learn. Various instructions are used in treating disorders of articulation, language, voice, and fluency.

Instructions in Treating Articulation Disorders

In teaching the correct production of speech sounds, give instructions on how to produce them. Describe tongue positions, lip configurations, direction of airflow, mouth opening or closing, and other actions necessary to produce the target sounds. Also, describe the articulatory movements and contacts needed to produce the target sounds. While giving these instructions, model what you describe.

What follows is a sample of instructions given in treatment sessions designed to correct certain kinds of articulation disorders. You might find other examples in textbooks on articulation disorders.

Instructions to Correct an Interdental Lisp

1. I want you to say /ʃ/(sh). While you are saying it, smile so your lips go like this (*demonstrate lip retraction*). Then, push your tongue toward your front teeth, like this (*demonstrate*). Let us see if your /ʃ/ (sh) changes for an /s/.

2. Let me hear you say /i/. Okay, now make a long /i/ and as you make it, raise the tip of your tongue to blow the air through the teeth.

Instructions to Teach the Correct Production of /l/

1. Put the tip of your tongue here (*demonstrate the correct tongue position for /l/*). Now say /ɑ/ as you lower the tip of your tongue. Did you hear [lɑ]? Good. Repeat that for me.

2. Look at the mirror. Open your mouth like this (*demonstrate a slight mouth opening to show the tongue placement*). Now say /l/.

Instruction to Teach the Correct Production of /f/

Bite gently on your lower lip like this (*demonstrate*). Now as you do it, blow air like this (*demonstrate*).

Many other kinds of instructions are used in teaching the correct production of various speech sounds. When you select target sounds for a client, give some thought to how you might give instructions to produce them. Write the instructions down and practice their delivery along with demonstrations.

Instructions in Treating Language Disorders

Various aspects of language may be treatment targets for children with language delay or disorder, adults with aphasia, and children and adults with inappropriate language. In treating language disorders, instructions may be given about when to use the selected target language feature or element.

Children who have not learned language typically do not begin to produce elements of language when instructed about the rules of usage. For example, a child who does not produce the plural morpheme correctly will not produce it solely because the clinician has described the rules of plural usage. However, simplified descriptions of certain rules may be helpful when combined with other treatment procedures.

Different kinds of instructions may be equally effective in teaching various elements of language. Therefore, the following examples are only suggestive. You may experiment with other kinds of instructions for the same target behaviors.

Instructions to Train the Irregular Plural Morpheme

When you see one of these (*show a picture*), you say: woman. Now you say: woman. Good. But when you see two like these (*show a different picture*), you say: women. Now you say: women. Good.

Instructions to Train the Regular Plural Morphemes *s*

When you see one of these (*show a picture*), you say: cup. Now you say: cup. Good. But when you see two of these (*show a different picture*), you say: cups. Now you say: cups. Good.

Instructions to Teach Appropriate Greeting Responses

Look at the picture here. They are eating breakfast. When it is breakfast time, you say: good morning. Now you say: good morning. Good. And look at this picture here. They are going to bed. When it is time to sleep, you say: good night. You say: good night. Excellent.

> ## Instructions to Teach Correct Recall of Names to an Aphasic Person
>
> When I show this picture (*the client's daughter*) and ask you who is this, say: Nina. Now you say: Nina. Very good. But when I show this picture (*the client's son*), and ask who is this, say: Tom. Now you say: Tom. That was correct!

In preparing instructions for a client in language treatment, do not describe grammar rules in linguistic terms, although you will be teaching behaviors that may seem to follow such rules. It is not helpful for a client to hear you say that "Gerunds are special forms of verbs that end in *ing*." The clients (and all speakers of any language) do not have to know the name or definition of a grammatic feature to use it correctly.

In some cases, you may describe the conditions under which a feature is used. For example, instead of describing the rules of verb usage, you may demonstrate actions and describe them to show when certain verbs are used. Whenever possible, make the conditions of usage concrete and use pictures and arranged situations; when you instruct in rules of conversations, engage in conversations to demonstrate them.

Instructions in Treating Voice Disorders

Treatment of voice disorders in adults and children requires many instructions. Mostly, treatment targets in voice therapy include changes in vocal quality, pitch, loudness, or resonance. In all cases, first you must instruct your clients about the particular target and how to achieve it. Once the target behavior is established in the clinic, you need to implement additional procedures to document its reliable occurrence in the natural environment and to sustain it over time. These procedures, too, require the use of instructions.

> ## Instructions to Treat Vocal Hyperfunction with Altered Head Position
>
> The position of your head while talking affects your voice. A change in head position may improve your voice. Let us try. (*Experiment with different head positions while the client produces prolonged vowels to see if a desirable change occurs.*) Now it sounds like your voice improves when you flex your neck downward so that your chin almost touches your chest. Keep your head in that position and say /i/. Does your voice sound better? Good.

Instructions to Increase Oral Resonance with Greater Mouth Opening

When you talk with closed mouth, your voice sounds muffled. It sounds better if you keep your mouth open while talking. Let us try. Say /ɑ/ while you open your mouth widely. Drop your jaw and make the sound. Now close your jaw and make the same sound. Do you hear a difference? Good. Let us now practice making sounds and saying words while keeping the mouth open.

To reduce a child's *vocally abusive behaviors*, first you have to establish the frequency of those behaviors. For example, a child may spend much time playing with toy guns. While playing, he or she may also produce tensed and loud phonation.

Instructions to Establish Baselines of Vocal Abuse

During the next week, I would like you to chart how often your son plays with the toy guns making the loud sounds you have described to me. Also, chart how long he played each time. Record the date and the beginning and ending time of each episode. Once we know how often he engages in this behavior, we can design a plan to reduce it.

Instructions to Document Maintenance of Treated Voice Characteristic

I would like you to keep a record of how often you used your new pitch (*loud voice, or any other treated characteristic*). Any time you talked in your old pitch, make a note on this card (*give the client a recording sheet or card*). Also, any time you talked with your new pitch, make a note. Make this kind of record for a week and bring it to the next session.

In preparing instruction for clients with voice disorders, first select the target vocal behavior and find out how that behavior may be facilitated. Make sure the selected facilitating technique works; experiment informally. Find out more about this approach in the section on shaping voice characteristics.

Instructions in Treating Fluency Disorders

In treating disorders of fluency, including stuttering and cluttering, instructions and demonstrations play a major role. Experimentally supported treatment procedures include fluency shaping, pause-and-talk, response cost, and fluency reinforcement. Fluency shaping includes airflow management, gentle phonatory onset, and rate reduction through syllable stretching. Response cost and fluency reinforcement are especially effective with younger children. Pause-and-talk may be equally effective with adults and older children.

Instructions to Teach Airflow Management

I would like you to breathe in a bit more air than usual. Like this. (*Demonstrate a deeper than the usual inhalation.*) Then, immediately let a little bit of air through your mouth. Like this. (*Demonstrate a slight exhalation through open mouth.*) You try it. Make sure you do not hold the air in your lungs. As soon as you breathe in, breathe out a little bit of air.

Instructions to Teach Gentle Phonatory Onset

Sometimes you start your sound abruptly and harshly. Your vocal cords work too hard when you do this. You experience too much muscular tension and effort when you start sounds abruptly and harshly. Instead, you should start your sound softly, easily, and with less effort and tension. Let us practice that.

Instructions to Teach Rate Reduction through Syllable Stretching

You may have noticed that when you speak slowly, your fluency improves. Practicing a slower rate of speech is part of our treatment program. You don't want to slow down your speech by pausing between words. (*Demonstrate this.*) Instead, I would like you to reduce your overall rate by stretching the syllables of words. I want you to stretch most syllables, but the first syllable of the first few words in a sentence must be stretched more than the other syllables. Like this. (*Demonstrate syllable stretching.*)

Instructions for Pause-and-Talk

In this procedure we call pause-and-talk, I want you to stop talking for 5 seconds when you stutter. Anytime you stutter, I am going to say "stop." You should immediately stop talking. I will be looking at my watch, and after 5 seconds, I will look at you and you can then talk.

Instructions for Response Cost

In this procedure, I will give you a token for fluent speech. (Substitute *smooth speech*, *easy speech*, or some other term if the client is a child.) Every time you stutter, I will take a token back from you. You will earn a token for fluency and lose one for stuttering. At the end, you can exchange your tokens for this gift you have selected.

Instructions for Fluency Reinforcement

In this procedure, I will be paying close attention to your fluent speech. Even though you stutter (*have bumpy speech*) you still have lots of fluent speech. I will praise you for your fluent (*smooth, easy*) speech. Keep that high praise coming your way! (*Add additional instructions if you also give some tangible reinforcers along with verbal praise.*)

A reduced rate also improves the fluency and intelligibility of a speaker with cluttering. In general, stuttering treatment procedures may be modified in treating cluttering.

Instructions in Treating Swallowing Disorders

In treating swallowing disorders, clinicians make extensive use of instructions. Whenever practical, modeling follows instructions so the patients can better understand what is required of them. It is not practical to list all the instructions given to patients in swallowing therapy because there are dozens of actions, maneuvers, exercises, and procedures, each requiring detailed and often-repeated instructions. Several sources give verbatim instructions the clinician may repeat to patients (Logemann, 1998; Provencio-Arambula, Provencio, & Hegde, 2007a, 2007b). A few examples will illustrate the nature of instructions given during swallowing therapy sessions.

Instructions to Teach Selected Swallowing Skills

1. In teaching the exercise to improve gross manipulation of material in the mouth:

   a. "Please grasp and then hold this piece of gauze between your tongue and your hard palate."

   b. "Please move the gauze from one side of your mouth to the other."

   c. "Please move the gauze slightly back and forth in your mouth."

2. In teaching the exercise to hold a cohesive bolus in the mouth:

   a. "I am going to place this paste—we call it a bolus—on your tongue, and I want you to move it around in your mouth. You shouldn't swallow it or lose it or spread it out around your mouth. Are you ready?"

   b. (*The clinician places the bolus on the patient's tongue*) "Cup your tongue around the bolus and move it around in the mouth. Make sure you don't lose it."

3. In teaching the *supraglottic swallow maneuver:*

   a. "Take a deep breath and hold it."

   b. (*If a tracheostomy is present*) "While still holding your breath, gently cover your tracheostomy tube."

   c. "Continue to hold your breath as you swallow."

   d. "Cough as soon as you have finished swallowing."

4. In teaching effortful swallow:

   a. "If you swallow with a great deal of muscular effort, you may swallow more safely."

   b. "Squeeze your muscles hard as you swallow."

How to Prepare Effective Instructions

The client understands the target behaviors only through your instructions and demonstrations. Unless you give effective instructions, the rest of the treatment procedures may be difficult to implement. Therefore, use the following general guidelines in preparing and delivering your instructions:

1. Select the target behavior.

2. Make an analysis of the target behavior. What topographic features distinguish the behavior? In other words, what is the shape or the form of the target behavior? How does it look, feel, or sound?

3. Find out how the target behavior can be evoked. Generally, simplify it so it can be produced by the client.

4. Write out instructions that help evoke the target behavior. Write them in simple, clear, and unambiguous words; whenever possible, use ordinary language. Especially for children, write instructions in words they can understand.

5. Instruct at the client's level of education and sophistication. Do not talk down to the client. Modify your presentation depending on the judged level of the client's education and sophistication.

6. Rehearse the instructions. Once you gain experience, you can give instructions spontaneously. In the beginning of your clinical practicum, you should practice giving instructions before you give them to your client.

7. Deliver instructions in a natural, conversational manner. Do not read instructions to your client; do not deliver instructions too formally.

8. Test the client's understanding of your instructions. Ask the client to repeat your instructions. See if the client can do what you ask him or her to do. If not, repeat your instructions, change words, add gestures, and demonstrate.

9. Repeat all or portions of your instructions whenever the client makes mistakes that suggest that the instructions are not remembered.

10. Give new instructions whenever you change the target behavior or you shift training to a higher level.

Modeling

Modeling, like instructions and other stimulus events, is a necessary part of treatment in communicative disorders. When the client does not respond correctly with instructions and other stimuli, you have to model the target response. Thus, **modeling** is the clinician's production of a client's target response. Clinical research has shown that modeling is an effective procedure in establishing many kinds of target behaviors. Therefore, modeling is one of the widely used methods of teaching new behaviors (Hegde, 1998a, 2008c).

In some language treatment programs, the clinician may model target responses but may not necessarily expect the child to imitate them. In most other treatment sessions, the clinician expects the client to imitate the modeled response. Note that modeling is the special stimulus provided by the clinician and imitation is the response given to this stimulus. Because imitation is a client's response, it never should be described as a treatment procedure. Modeling is a treatment procedure because the clinician provides it to evoke the imitated response.

Normally, a stimulus and its response are topographically different. For example, the stimulus "How are you doing?" is topographically different from the response "Fine, thank you." When the stimuli and their responses are topographically different, the response is spontaneous. To be called **imitation,** a response should meet two criteria. First, *imitated response should be topographically similar to the modeled stimulus.* Ideally, the stimulus and the response should be identical. But in clinical training, modeling and imitation may not be identical, especially in the beginning stage. Yet, an acceptable imitation and its stimulus (modeling) should have a similar form. In case of vocal and verbal behaviors, the two should sound similar. If not, there is no imitation.

Second, *imitated response should immediately follow the modeled stimulus.* Although delayed imitation sometimes is described in the literature, the most clinically useful imitation is immediate. This is because the clinician can reinforce the immediately imitated response. Obviously, the clinician cannot reinforce the client who repeats the modeled response at another time and place. Possibly, no individual may reinforce that response.

Modeling in the Treatment of Articulation Disorders

Probably, modeling is most frequently used in the treatment of articulation disorders. When the sounds are taught in words or in isolation, modeling is most useful. Most models are "live" in the sense that the clinician produces them in front of the client. However, taped models may be just as good. They provide standardized stimuli; a collection of such stimuli may be useful in treating articulation disorders.

How to Model in Treating Articulation Disorders

1. First, give instructions as described.

2. Model the articulatory movements or positions and the target sound while giving instructions (e.g., lip closure for bilabial sounds, tongue tip position for /t/).

3. Ask the client to imitate the sound you modeled. Prepare a collection of taped models and use whenever necessary.

Modeling in the Treatment of Language Disorders

Modeling is necessary also in the initial stages of language teaching. In teaching words, grammatical morphemes, and various pragmatic behaviors, the clinician should model the target behaviors. A special feature of modeling language targets is that you should first ask a relevant question and then model the target (Hegde, 1998a, 2008c). For example, in teaching the regular plural morpheme with the help of pictures, you should not just show the picture of two books and model "books" for the client to imitate. You should ask a question and then model the correct response. In the same example, you should ask a question such as "What do you see?" or "What are these?" and immediately model the response: "Say books." Similarly, in teaching words to children with language delay, you should show a picture or an object, ask a question, and immediately model the response. For example: "What is this? Say cat."

How to Model in Treating Language Disorders

1. Instruct the client about the modeling and imitation sequence.

2. Show a picture or object.

3. Ask a relevant question (e.g., "What do you see?" "What is the boy doing?").

4. Model the target response (e.g., "Say, I see two books." "The boy is running.").

5. Fade or withdraw modeling (but not the relevant question) as the imitative response is reliably produced.

When a question reliably precedes modeling, the correct response may be maintained later when modeling is withdrawn and only the question is asked. For example, assume a child consistently imitates "books," when you say "What are these? Say *books*." Then, you stop modeling and ask, "What are these?" The child may say "books." If you did not ask the question before modeling the response, the question, introduced later, may not evoke the correct response because it is a new stimulus to which the child previously has not responded.

When the client imitates the target response consistently, you should stop modeling. Yet, when the modeled stimulus suddenly is stopped, even after the client has been imitating the target response, the response may not be produced. This is likely to happen especially when the modeled target responses are long, as they often are when the targets are grammatic features. Therefore, in many cases, you should *fade the modeled stimulus*.

In **fading** a modeled stimulus, progressively withdraw parts of it. Withdraw additional parts as the correct response is maintained. For example, in teaching the preposition *on*, you may have asked the question "Where is the ball?" and modeled "Say the ball is on the table." Note that the modeled stimulus is a long sentence that included other syntactic elements. In fading this modeled stimulus, first you should drop the last word. After asking the question, you model "Say the ball is on the . . . ," and wait for the correct response. Ask the child to start with "The ball" as the likely response is just "table." If the child gives the correct response (the entire sentence), then on the next trial, drop another word by modeling only "Say the ball is on. . . ." Make sure the child repeats the whole target sentence. On each of the subsequent trials, drop one additional word of the modeled phrase until you ask only the question "Where is the ball?"

Modeling in the Treatment of Voice Disorders

Various voice qualities and characteristics also need to be modeled before the client can fully understand them. For example, the desired pitch, loudness, vocal quality, and resonance characteristics must be modeled for the client. In some cases, the clinician may be unable to model a desired voice characteristic. For example, an adult male may not be able to model a target vocal pitch for a child or a woman. In such cases, the model voice may be tape recorded from another child or woman and played for the client to imitate. Also, clients themselves may provide voice models. A client with too high a pitch may be able to produce a lower pitch with some help from the clinician. This desired pitch may be tape recorded and used as a model for the client to imitate. With appropriate software and such instruments as Visi-Pitch, many voice characteristics may be displayed on computer monitors.

How to Model in Treating Voice Disorders

1. Instruct the client in the modeling–imitation sequence.

2. Model the vocal target behavior.

3. Use taped models when necessary.

4. Tape record the client's correct imitations.

5. Use the client's productions as models.

6. Fade modeling by asking the client to produce the target behavior; do not model.

Modeling in the Treatment of Fluency Disorders

In teaching such fluency skills as management of airflow, reduced rate of speech, and gentle phonatory onset to persons who stutter, you should first model each skill separately and then in combination. For example, you may start with inhalation and a slight exhalation before saying a word or two. Therefore, model as you describe inhalation and exhalation. You then add rate reduction by describing and modeling it. Model each of the subsequent targets that were described in Chapter 7. Note that pause-and-talk, response cost, and fluency reinforcement do not need modeling of any target behaviors.

How to Model in Treating Fluency Disorders

1. Instruct the client in the modeling–imitation sequence.

2. Model each of the specific fluency skills separately, especially in the beginning stages.

3. Model a new skill when the earlier skill is correctly imitated.

4. Model the combined skills in the sequence they are taught (e.g., air-flow management and gentle phonatory onset).

5. Model the entire fluency skills in words, phrases, and sentences.

6. Fade modeling by asking the client to produce the target behavior; do not model.

Modeling in the Treatment of Swallowing Disorders

Most exercises or specific actions prescribed to improve the muscle action involved in swallowing can be modeled for the patient. For instance, the clinician can model the breath holding, maintaining lip closure, various kinds of tongue movements, head tilt, chin down, chin up, dry swallow, holding the bolus in the mouth, and so forth for the patient. As it is done in treating disorders of communication, instructions precede modeling. Obviously, motoric actions described to the patients and required of them may be modeled, but not sensory enhancement techniques (e.g., presenting a sour bolus).

How to Model in Treating Swallowing Disorders

1. Instruct the client in the modeling–imitation sequence.

2. Model each skill separately, especially in the beginning stages.

3. Model a new skill when the earlier skill is correctly imitated.

4. Model the combined skills in the sequence they are taught (e.g., model the chin down first, head rotation next in the combined chin down and head rotation exercise).

5. Fade modeling by asking the client to produce the target behavior; do not model.

How to Model Effectively

A clear model, produced by the clinician or a mechanical device, is effective in treatment and often necessary with most clients. With some clients, repeated modeling is indispensable. Use the following guidelines to provide effective modeling and to determine when to model, how much to model, and when to stop modeling.

1. Decide whether you will model the target response or whether a taped or otherwise mechanically represented model will be used. Possibly, as clinical instrumentation becomes more sophisticated and more commonly used, mechanical models will be used more frequently. If your clinic has such instruments, use mechanical models.

2. Use a client's own correct response as a model, if that is acceptable.

3. Model often in the early stages of treatment, because it is needed to establish the target behavior.

4. Model consistently and continuously in the beginning until the imitated responses are produced reliably. Use such objective criterion as production of five consecutively correct imitated responses before terminating modeling. Do not terminate modeling prematurely; this will unnecessarily increase the error rate.

5. Model judiciously. Do not overuse modeling and do not continue modeling when the client meets an objective criterion (such as five correctly imitated responses). Remember that the final target is not imitated responses but responses given to more natural stimuli.

6. Reinstate modeling when the client fails to give the correct response without it. Do not continue to evoke wrong responses by not providing the needed modeling. Reinstate modeling when two to four wrong responses are given on trials without modeling.

7. Fade a complex and lengthy model, instead of stopping suddenly. If the wrong responses return the instant you stop modeling, then drop the final element first and work your way backward until all elements of the modeled stimulus are faded and only the question is asked.

8. Model every new target response when first introduced.

9. Model the same target response when training is moved to a higher level. For example, model the /s/ in words when you shift training from syllable to word level. Model the phoneme in phrases, and again in sentences when the training is shifted to these higher levels.

10. Reduce the frequency of modeling in the final stages of treatment. Use it least frequently when the target response is stabilized in conversational speech.

11. Ask the client to imitate your model promptly.

12. Reinforce the imitated responses. In the beginning, reinforce approximations of the model, but reinforce only promptly produced responses. On subsequent trials, reinforce progressively better approximations until the response matches the model.

Prompting

Prompts and models are similar in one important respect: Both are special stimuli that precede the target response. In all other respects, models and prompts are different.

A prompt is often a partial stimulus, whereas a modeled stimulus is full-fledged. For example, when you model, you might say "Jimmy, say *the cat is jumping*"; but when you prompt the same response, you might say "Jimmy, *the cat is* . . . ." and wait for the response. All models are direct stimuli; they display the full response. *Some prompts are indirect stimuli*; they only suggest the target response instead of displaying it. For instance, to model a slower rate of speech for a person who stutters, you have to speak slowly to fully display it. But to prompt it, you may give a hand signal to suggest a slower rate. Some prompts may contain parts of the target response while others may contain no part of it. For instance, your prompt "Jimmy, *the cat is* . . ." contains some parts of the target response. But a hand gesture to slow down the rate of speech contains no part of the target response.

Some prompts are a special feature of modeled responses. For example, you might place an extra vocal emphasis on the target preposition *on* when you model: Say, *the ball is on the table.* This vocal emphasis is a prompt within a modeled stimulus. Such an emphasis makes the target response more distinct than without the emphasis. Other ways of making a target response embedded in a string of responses distinct include increased vocal intensity, varied pitch, slower delivery than the rest of the words in the string, and injecting a pause just before its production (Hegde, 1998a, 2008c).

Several other kinds of prompts are nonverbal. Gestures and motor behaviors, while suggesting the target response, can prompt responses. When you teach verbs, you can demonstrate action to prompt the correct word response. For example, a hopping motion you demonstrate with your hand may prompt the word *jump.* You may prompt the correct production of a phoneme by showing the correct articulatory posture without saying the sound or the word. For example, you can prompt the correct production of /m/ in "Mommy" by pressing a client's lips together.

Prompts should be strong enough to evoke the desired response but not unnecessarily strong, loud, or long. A prompt is a gentle hint. It is a minimal clue sufficient to evoke a response. Most clients find subtle prompts more acceptable than boisterous prompts. If a brief and quiet hand gesture can prompt a slower rate of speech in a person who stutters, do that and avoid lengthy verbal prompts or exaggerated nonverbal prompts.

Clients can maintain their target responses better if their family members learn to prompt. The clinician teaches the family members to provide such prompts. These prompts used in natural settings are especially subtle. Clients are likely to find loud and lengthy prompts in these natural settings unpleasant or embarrassing, because such clues are obvious to other persons.

Like modeling, prompts also should be faded. When you observe a few consecutively correct responses to prompts, stop prompting to see if the responses will be maintained. If not, reinstate prompts. Fade prompts by reducing their topography. For example, make a particular hand gesture progressively smaller until it is completely faded out. A lengthy verbal prompt (e.g., "What do you say for this?") may be reduced by using only some of the words or by word substitutions (e.g., "You say . . ." or "This is . . .").

How to Prompt in Treating Articulation Disorders

1. Prompt initially by naming the sound (*this word starts with an es*).

2. Use emphasis on the target sound to prompt it.

3. Prompt later by showing only the silent articulatory positions.

4. Fade the prompts as the client becomes proficient in producing the target sounds.

How to Prompt in Treating Language Disorders

1. Use prompts as partial modeling to stimulate language structures.

2. Use questions as prompts: What do you say for this?

3. Use such nonverbal prompts as movements and gestures that suggest verbs and other language targets.

4. Fade the prompts.

How to Prompt in Treating Voice Disorders

1. Give a brief model to prompt a vocal quality or characteristic.

2. Give various hand gestures to prompt higher or lower pitch.

3. Give other hand gestures to prompt increased or decreased vocal intensity.

4. Provide such nonverbal prompts as touching nose to suggest nasal resonance.

5. Fade the prompts.

How to Prompt in Treating Fluency Disorders

1. Give prompts for each of the specific skills separately.

2. Provide such nonverbal prompts as hand gestures to suggest reduced rate of speech.

3. Suggest airflow management by such nonverbal prompts as touching your nose or the chest.

4. Prompt gentle phonatory onset by touching your laryngeal area.

5. Fade the prompts.

How to Prompt in Treating Swallowing Disorders

1. Give prompts for each of the specific skills separately.

2. Withhold verbal instructions and provide nonverbal prompts; for example, bear down on the arms of the chair to prompt similar action, or show your own sealed lips to suggest holding lip closure; make your manual prompts progressively subtle.

3. Show sideways or back-and-forth hand movements to suggest similar tongue movements; make your hand movements progressively subtle.

4. Instead of asking the patient to tilt the head toward the left or right side, tilt your own head; in progressive steps, reduce the degree of tilting.

5. Instead of asking the patient to hold the breath, show breath holding, and make this prompt progressively more subtle.

6. Fade all prompts you give by making them progressively subtle.

How to Prompt Effectively

Prompting at the right time with the right clue will reduce the frequency of wrong responses. Use the following guidelines in using this technique effectively.

1. Use partial modeling to prompt the target responses if this would work. This will help fade modeling and will keep the correct response rate high.

2. Give your prompts promptly. Delayed prompts may promote delayed responses. The earliest sign of a hesitation or a wrong response is your clue to prompt.

3. Prompt more frequently in the beginning stages of treatment. Gradually reduce frequency as the correct responses become more stable and the responding becomes faster.

4. Prefer a subtle or short prompt over a loud or lengthy prompt. Prefer a silent, gestural prompt over a verbal prompt.

5. Fade prompts by making them progressively subtler or shorter.

6. Teach family members to prompt the target behaviors in a subtle manner.

Physical Stimuli

Instructions, modeling, and prompts can help evoke target behaviors in most clients. But some clients need additional stimuli. Children and adults in language therapy often need physical stimuli, which are pictures, objects, and demonstrated events (e.g., movements of a toy car). In teaching words and various elements of grammar, such physical stimuli may be necessary to evoke target responses. Physical stimuli may be helpful in articulation treatment as well.

Physical stimuli may be used to evoke speech in the beginning stages of treatment. In the final stages, you should evoke continuous conversational speech from all clients without explicit physical stimuli. Target behaviors must be stabilized in naturalistic conversational speech to promote maintenance. Most adult clients with conversational skills do not need physical stimuli to evoke target responses or to maintain continuous speech. There should be no need for physical stimuli in the advanced stages of treatment when conversational speech is the target. In the initial stages of treatment, children who are reluctant to talk may begin to talk when you show them pictures in storybooks, objects that can be manipulated, and events that can be created to arouse interest. Therefore, when concrete representation of target responses is needed, physical stimuli are unavoidable.

How to Effectively Use Physical Stimuli

1. Prefer objects over pictures. If at all practical, ask the child to bring the relevant stimulus objects from home.

2. Select pictures that are three-dimensional, colorful, and realistic. Find them in popular magazines.

3. Use pictures and objects in the early stages of treatment. In later stages, especially when continuous speech is evoked, do not use pictures or use them sparingly. When the child is capable of continuous speech, do not use pictures. Find other ways of making the child talk. Talk about what interests the child.

4. Use pictures in storybooks. Read the story to the child and ask him or her to retell the story while looking at the pictures.

5. Discontinue the use of pictures as soon as possible. Do not overuse pictures in the later stages of treatment when conversational or more naturalistic speech should be evoked.

Creating New Responses

Many clients with severe physical disabilities resulting in communicative impairments cannot imitate modeled responses. Because of neurological problems, clients may be unable to move their articulators. Children who are nonverbal also are unable to imitate verbal responses. In treating such clients, you cannot just model the target response and expect them to imitate it. A response that is not even imitated is nonexistent in the client's repertoire. You need procedures to create new responses that do not exist.

Shaping, or *successive approximation,* is a highly researched method of creating new responses. The method allows you to shape a nonexistent complex response from simple responses that do exist in the client's repertoire. In each of several successive stages of treatment, you teach a simple response that takes the client one step closer to the final target response.

Breaking a target response into its simpler components is the key to shaping it (Hegde, 1998a, 2008c). Even the most severely involved client may be able to make some movement that is remotely related to the target response. You then start with this movement and shape something more complex out of it by adding other components. The basic idea in shaping is that you teach what the client can learn in each step. But you do not just evoke random responses that the client happens to learn. You teach responses that are systematically related to the final target behavior. Each new response mastered by the client should be a move in the right direction.

Manual guidance is physical assistance in shaping a response. When the client cannot make a physical movement at all, you may have to manually assist that movement and reinforce the client for any success. In manual guidance, you gently but firmly make a movement happen. For example, a boy with a severe articulation disorder may not move his tongue tip for an articulatory position. But the movement is possible, it is only not probable. Therefore, you may take a tongue depressor and move the tongue tip in the desired direction. A woman with aphasia may have great difficulty in moving her hand to point to a message on an electronic display, but the movement can be assisted by taking her hand and pointing to the message. When a boy who is profoundly mentally handicapped does not open his mouth to produce a vowel, you apply a downward pressure on the chin to make the jaw drop so the mouth is opened. A man with a high-pitched voice does not produce or imitate voice of lower pitch, but as you apply a slight finger pressure on the thyroid cartilage when he produces a prolonged vowel, his pitch may drop. These are all techniques of manual guidance that help shape a target response.

Shaping Correct Articulation

To shape target phonemes, analyze them to identify their simpler components. Then find out if the client can perform any of the components that may be used to shape the target phoneme. For example, a boy with a severe articulation problem cannot produce a phoneme in words. But can he produce it in syllables? If not in syllables, can he produce it in isolation? If not in isolation, can he move the tongue tip in the right direction? Can he make an appropriate lip movement? Can he make any kind of movement of the articulators? Can he open his mouth? If not, can you make him open his mouth with manual guidance? Can you make his tongue or lips move with manual guidance? In designing a treatment program for a client like this, you need shaping. In this example, the production of the phoneme (in syllables or words) is the **final shaping target.** The one response the client is capable of that is some-how related to the final target (e.g., movement of tongue or lips, with or without manual guidance) is the **initial response.** All other responses help bridge the gap between the initial and final response and are called the **intermediate responses.**

How to Shape Correct Articulation

1. Define the final or the terminal target sound or syllable production.

2. Find the simplest response that the client can perform and that is related to the final target sound or syllable production.

3. Specify intermediate responses that should be shaped.

4. Shape the simplest response first by modeling and imitation.

5. Add intermediate responses.

6. Continue to shape until the final target sound or syllable production is achieved.

Shaping Language Skills

Children who are nonverbal and those with severe movement problems are excellent candidates for shaping. Simple, single-word utterances are the most likely initial targets for these clients. The most difficult part of treatment will be this initial stage of establishing a set of basic words. The need for shaping is greatest in this stage.

In teaching word productions to children who are nonverbal and thus do not imitate words or syllables, first you should find an articulatory movement that can be made. For example, a girl who is nonverbal may be able to open her mouth with manual guidance. With some gentle, downward pressure exerted on her chin, you may get her to open her mouth. Next, as the mouth opens, you may ask her to expel some air through the mouth. Model this and give some manual assistance; a slight push on the abdomen as the mouth opens will result in some audible expulsion of air. This audible airflow may be a basis to shape an /h/. In the successive stages, you can shape the articulatory movement for /l/ and /o/. You gradually can shape these responses into a "hello."

How to Shape Basic Language Skills

1. Define the final or the terminal language response (such as the production of a word).

2. Find a simple response that the client can perform and that is related to the final target sound or syllable production.

3. Specify intermediate responses that should be shaped.

4. Shape the simplest response first by modeling and imitation.

5. Add intermediate responses.

6. Add additional language elements to shape phrases and sentences.

Shaping Voice Characteristics

Many clients with voice disorders cannot imitate target voice characteristics. Therefore, shaping is a primary technique of voice therapy. In effecting changes in fundamental frequency (pitch), vocal intensity (loudness), oral or nasal resonance, hard glottal attacks, hoarseness, and harshness, you may have to use shaping in the initial stages of treatment.

Clinicians also use manual guidance in voice therapy, which is often described as *digital manipulation* in textbooks on voice disorders (Boone, McFarlane, & Von Berg, 2005; Case, 2002). In this procedure, your application of a slight finger pressure on the thyroid cartilage as the client produces a prolonged vowel tends to lower the pitch. The lower pitch is a result of increased mass of vocal folds due to their shortening as the digital pressure pushes the thyroid in the backward direction. Once the client achieves a lower pitch on a vowel, you must shape the pitch in producing words and phrases. The new pitch must be practiced in successively longer utterances until it is sustained in conversational speech.

In experimenting with different head positions that might facilitate a more normal sounding voice, manual guidance may be necessary. You might manually help the client change the head position to change a certain characteristic of voice. Keeping the head straight, tilting it toward the left or right side, or flexing the neck in a downward direction are all useful in changing vocal characteristics. In some cases, along with instructions and modeling, manual guidance also may be necessary.

A male speaker's high pitch is reduced in small steps. Any reduction in pitch is reinforced initially. In subsequent steps, speaking with progressively lower pitch is reinforced. The process is continued until the most desirable pitch is established. In most cases, the first step might be to produce a slightly lower pitch on single words. In the next step, the new or even lower pitch is practiced while speaking short phrases. Finally, the lower pitch is used in sentences and conversational speech. A sequence similar to this may be effective in shaping other voice targets.

In shaping target voice characteristics, you might use mechanical devices that give automatic feedback to the client. For example, you may use the Visi-Pitch, PM 100 Pitch Analyzer, and Phonatory Function Analyzer to modify the pitch of a client. You may use an instrument called Tonar II to modify nasal resonance (Boone, McFarlane, & Von Berg, 2005). These devices work on the principle of shaping. In each successive step of treatment, the client achieves a progressively higher or lower pitch, decreased or increased nasal resonance, and so forth.

How to Shape Voice Characteristics

1. Define the final or the terminal voice quality or characteristic (such as a specified vocal pitch or loudness).

2. Select a simple response level at which the desired vocal target may be imitated (such as in producing a sound, syllable, or word).

3. Specify intermediate responses that should be shaped (words, phrases, sentences).

4. Shape the simplest response first.

5. Add intermediate responses.

6. Shape the desired vocal target in conversational speech.

Shaping Fluency

As the name of the technique suggests, shaping is a part of the fluency shaping technique. As noted before, shaping is not needed in pause-and-talk, response cost, or fluency reinforcement. As you use fluency shaping in treating stuttering and cluttering, you need to shape skills of fluent speech in sequenced steps. Whether it is management of airflow, gentle phonatory onset, or reduced rate of speech, you must take one skill at a time and shape it. Then you put them together and have the client practice the skills starting at the one- or two-word level. As the client maintains fluency, you introduce more complex responses until the client practices fluent speech in conversational speech outside the clinic. This sequence of treatment also is based on shaping.

To use the fluency shaping effectively, you must teach interrelated skills, each carefully shaped and then integrated. In the beginning, start with inhalation and slight exhalation before phonatory onset. Let the client practice this skill without phonation. Then add gentle phonatory onset. Ask the client to produce a syllable or a word. When the airflow management and gentle onset are established, add rate reduction by syllable stretching. Target single words at this stage. Before saying the word, teach the client to inhale, exhale slightly, achieve smooth onset, and speak with prolonged syllables. Teach the client to especially stretch the initial syllables and vowels.

When single-word utterances are free from stuttering, ask the client to produce two-word phrases. Monitor all the skills taught so far. If the client maintains speech free from stuttering, have the client practice skills of fluent speech while producing sentences and conversational speech.

An important part of most stuttering treatment programs is to shape normal sounding prosody when stutter-free speech is established. Rate reduction through syllable stretching induces a monotonous speech that is unacceptable in the natural environment. The client is unlikely to speak at that slow rate outside the clinic. This means that fluency may not be maintained. To strengthen fluency at a near-normal rate of speech, you should fade the excessively slow rate and shape normal prosody.

By allowing the client to slightly increase the rate, you can ensure that fluency is maintained while shaping normal prosody. In carefully planned steps, allow the rate to increase. Typically, increased rate brings back normal patterns of intonation. In some cases, you may have to shape intonation as well. Shaping pitch variations in conversational speech will usually be effective. Excessively slow speech tends to be too soft. Therefore, shaping louder speech will also help in reducing monotone.

How to Shape Fluency Skills

1. Define the final or the terminal target level of fluency behavior (such as less than 5% dysfluency in conversational speech).

2. Select a simple response level at which the client can practice the skills of fluency (words or phrases).

3. Select the first fluency skill to be shaped (airflow management).

4. Shape the skill at the simplest response level.

5. Specify intermediate skills that should be shaped (rate reduction, gentle phonatory onset, maintaining the airflow throughout an utterance).

6. Shape the intermediate skills.

7. Shape the skills of fluency in conversational speech.

Shaping Swallowing Skills

Treatment of swallowing also requires shaping of various target skills the individual cannot readily exhibit. Although the dysphagia treatment literature is not explicit about many behavioral procedures including shaping, clinicians use the method in treating most clients. Whether it is improved muscle control through various exercises, or indirect or direct treatment of specific swallowing problems, shaping is essential. All clinicians ask their patients to perform some simpler, easier, or less risky tasks related to normal swallowing before demanding more complex, difficult, and riskier tasks; this is shaping. For example, many patients with swallowing disorders cannot effectively hold and manipulate food in their mouths. The food may spill over, leak out of the sides of the mouth, or it may prematurely enter the airway. To treat such problems, the clinician may start with an exercise of grossly manipulating a nonfood item in the mouth (e.g., a rolled 4" × 4" gauze pad). Initially, the patient holds the pad between the tongue and the palate as the clinician holds the outer edge of the pad; next, the patient moves the gauze from one side of the mouth to the other, then slides it back and forth; when this skill is mastered, the patient is asked to move the gauze in a circular fashion; when the patient has learned to make such movements of the gauze, a Life Savers candy tied to a thread held by the clinician may be introduced for oral manipulation. In successive shaping steps, the patient may learn to orally manipulate chewing gum without the clinician controlling it (Logemann, 1998). Such steps in treating swallowing difficulties illustrate shaping.

Because a wide variety of skills, exercises, and direct and indirect treatment strategies are used in treating swallowing disorders, it is not practical to describe all the shaping procedures the clinicians might use. A second example will help illustrate the principle of shaping in treating aspects of swallowing disorders.

How to Shape Swallowing Skills

1. Define the final or the terminal target skill for the specific procedure being implemented (e.g., "holding the lip closure for 2 minutes"; "grossly manipulating a rolled 4" × 4" gauze pad without losing it"; "manipulating a liquid bolus from side-to-side in the mouth without losing it").

2. Select the simple or easier response that is related to the defined terminal response (e.g., "holding the lip closure for 10 seconds"). Have the patient practice it and reinforce it positively (e.g., "grasping the gauze between the tongue and palate"; "manipulating a liquid paste bolus before attempting a liquid bolus").

3. Select the next level of response difficulty (e.g., "holding the lip closure for 20 seconds"). Have the patient practice it, and positively reinforce the correct responses.

4. Select the next level of response difficulty (e.g., "holding the lip closure for 30 seconds"). Reinforce correct responses.

5. Specify additional levels of difficulty as needed (e.g., "holding the lip closure for 1 minute").

6. End the exercises when the patient can hold the lip closure for 2 minutes (the defined target duration).

How to Effectively Use Shaping

As you have seen, carefully planned steps in which progressively more complex communicative or swallowing behaviors are shaped are essential in the treatment of speech, language, voice, fluency, and swallowing problems. Therefore, use the following general guidelines in shaping target behaviors.

1. Select the final target behavior for the client. Make an analysis of this behavior so you know how to simplify it. Remember that the simplification of a target behavior is client specific. That is, the same target phoneme, language feature, voice characteristic, fluency, or swallowing will have to be simplified more or less and in different ways to suit each individual client. But you should know the several ways of simplifying target communicative and swallowing behaviors.

2. Experiment with each client to find out what relevant response the client can imitate. This will be the initial response to be taught. If a more complex response related to the final target can be imitated, do not select a simpler response. Simplify a response only to the extent needed, not to the extent possible. This is because you have to move the client through the simpler to the more complex final response. Generally, the more complex the initial level, the faster the treatment progress.

3. Teach progressively more complex responses, but always make sure the client is moving in the direction of the final target response, or not facing risks in case of patients with dysphagia (e.g., aspiration).

4. Use instructions, modeling, and manual guidance as found necessary or appropriate at each step of training.

5. Reinforce imitated responses. To begin with, accept approximations of modeled responses. Subsequently, reinforce more accurate productions. Do not reinforce the initial and intermediate responses excessively. If you do, you will have difficulty moving the client to higher levels of training. Stabilize only the final target response.

6. Fade modeling and instructions. Also, fade any undesirable aspects of the shaped response. For example, fade the slow rate and the monotone of the speech of a person who has been treated for stuttering with the fluency shaping technique. Fade any unusual postures you may have taught to sustain a certain voice quality.

Increasing the Frequency of Responses

Instructions, modeling, and shaping are useful in creating nonexistent communicative behaviors or swallowing responses. But these procedures will not be effective if the client's responses do not meet certain consequences. A client's response may be a crude approximation of the modeled or described response, a perfectly imitated response, or a correct, unimitated (simple instructed) response. In each case, the response may not last if certain environmental consequences do not follow it.

How to make certain consequences follow a response is the topic of this section. These consequences help increase the frequency of newly established responses. The consequences also help strengthen and sustain responses taught in treatment sessions. In this section, you will learn about procedures to increase the frequency of new responses. In the next section, you will learn about procedures to strengthen and sustain responses.

Positive Reinforcement

Normally, what the listener does when a speaker says something is the consequence for the speaker's speech. One person (a speaker) may say "Hi!" and the other (listener) may either say "Hi!" or ignore the speaker. The child might say "Mommy!" and the mother may pick up the child. Therefore, in everyday conversations, one person's speech is followed by another person's speech or nonspeech behavior. These listener behaviors are the consequences of speech, and they will determine if the speaker will say the same thing next time.

In treatment, especially in the initial stages, the communicative behaviors and what follow them are not as naturalistic as they typically are. For one thing, the communicative behaviors may be either absent or not effective—that is why the client is seeking help from the clinician. A child who is nonverbal, a woman with aphasia, a man with a laryngectomy, and a person who stutters all need to do something different in their attempts at communication. Therefore, clinicians set up target behaviors for them. Normally, you only respond to a speaker's communicative behavior. But, clinically, you also teach your clients what to say or how to say something, and then you react to their communicative attempts in ways that are clinical. These clinical ways of reacting to a client's speech or attempts at speech are the consequences that either increase or decrease the client's speaking behavior.

There are two kinds of consequences. One kind, when it follows a response, makes the response more likely under similar circumstances. The other kind makes the response less likely in the future; these consequences help decrease undesirable behaviors and are described in Chapter 9.

Those consequences that follow a response and increase its frequency are called **positive reinforcers.** The procedure of increasing responses by making positive reinforcers follow them is called **positive reinforcement.** To increase the frequency of new target responses, whether communicative or safe swallowing, you must reinforce them positively.

Because no event will reinforce a response all the time, you should constantly evaluate the effects of any applied consequence to see if it continues to reinforce, keeping in perspective that *to reinforce always means to increase a skill.* Initially, you should select a potential reinforcer, arrange it as an immediate consequence for a response, and watch what happens. Count the number of responses the client produces (e.g., a correct phoneme or morpheme production, a safe swallow) when the consequence is being used. If the response rate increases, then you call that consequence a reinforcer. If the response rate did not increase, your *potential* reinforcer was not an actual reinforcer for that client on that occasion. Note that reinforcers always are defined after they are demonstrated to increase a response rate.

There are many types of potential positive reinforcers (Hegde, 1998a, 2008c). All are known to be effective some of the time with some clients under certain conditions. Most of them will work with clients on certain occasions. However, what worked with a client during one treatment session may not work in another session. What worked with one client may not work with another. Some of the consequences are more powerful than others. No consequence will work with every client every time.

Primary Reinforcers

Events that increase a response rate because of their biological (survival) value are called **primary reinforcers.** Potential primary reinforcers include food and drink, whose survival value is obvious.

In some cases, a communicative response followed by food may be learned faster. It is often pointed out that food is an unnatural reinforcer for communicative behaviors. When a little girl correctly names the family dog the first time, no one puts some applesauce in her mouth. However, some communicative behaviors are reinforced primarily. For these behaviors, only the primary reinforcers will do. For example, your requests for food and drink are reinforced primarily; no other consequence will do. Therefore, it is not correct to say that speech and language behaviors are never primarily reinforced. It is correct to say that *some* speech and language behaviors are reinforced *primarily* and *most* are reinforced *socially.*

In directly treating swallowing disorders and in teaching certain compensatory strategies of swallow, primary reinforcers are essential and are never faded out.

In treating communicative behaviors, clinicians use primary reinforcers for clinical reasons, not because they are natural. Food and drink need to be used when other, more natural events do not have an effect.

How to Use Primary Reinforcers

1. In treating disorders of communication, use food and drink only when other reinforcers do not work; continue to use food and drink as the treatment regimen in swallowing disorders requires. Expect to use primary reinforcers with infants and with persons who are nonverbal and profoundly intellectually disabled who are undergoing communication training.

2. Use primary reinforcers only with parental or guardian permission. Select primary reinforcers only after discussing them with the client or, more likely, with the family members. Consider their objections or recommendations about the kinds of food to use. Select healthy food items. Avoid foods that are not recommended for medical reasons.

3. Ask parents to withhold the reinforcers before the session, but stay within limits and do not overly deprive the client. Better yet, arrange treatment sessions around snack time or lunch time so that the infant or the child is motivated for your primary reinforcer.

4. Use social reinforcers always paired with primary reinforcers. For instance, praise a child for the correct response as you offer a sip of juice.

5. Fade the primary reinforcer eventually, and keep only the social reinforcers. Note the exception in treating swallowing disorders.

Social Reinforcers

Reinforcing effects of some events depend on past experiences. These events reinforce because of their association with other kinds of reinforcers. Events that reinforce because of past experiences are called **social,** or **conditioned, reinforcers.**

Social reinforcers are natural reinforcers for many kinds of verbal responses. In everyday communication, social reinforcers are used frequently. In communication, attention to a speaker, a smile, a nod, a touch, a pat on the shoulder, verbal approval (e.g., "I agree," "I like your viewpoint"), verbal praise (e.g., "You put it nicely"), and other kinds of verbal and nonverbal responses from the listener can be potential reinforcers. Therefore, they are preferable in treatment sessions. Even when you use primary reinforcers, you also should use social reinforcers. This means that social reinforcers are used in all stages of treatment and in the treatment of communication as well as swallowing disorders.

How to Use Social Reinforcers

1. Use smile and touch along with primary reinforcers, especially with infants and clients who are profoundly mentally handicapped. Add praise and other verbal stimuli as they seem to gain reinforcing value for the client.

2. Use social reinforcers naturally. When you say "Good boy!" or "Excellent job!" or "I like that!" smile and show proper emotional expressions that go with such statements. You should sound and look happy when a correct response is produced. Use appropriate patterns of intonation so you do not sound like a robot when praising the client.

3. Keep the social reinforcers as you fade the primary reinforcers, except perhaps in treating swallowing disorders where such primary reinforcers as food and drink are essential elements of most treatment strategies.

Conditioned Generalized Reinforcers

Certain events that have a more pervasive effect on behavior are called **conditioned generalized reinforcers.** These events become reinforcing because of their association with other reinforcers. In that respect, conditioned generalized reinforcers are similar to social reinforcers.

The two are different only in one respect. An ordinary social reinforcer has to effect a change by its own power. However, a conditioned generalized reinforcer can affect a response through several other events or objects that may be gained by it. For example, a token, which is a conditioned generalized reinforcer, may be effective because it can be exchanged for a variety of other reinforcers. A token is not just a token. It can mean anything you say because it can be exchanged for many other reinforcers; therefore, it may be effective on most occasions. But verbal praise is only verbal praise. On a given occasion, either it is effective or it is not.

You can use plastic chips for tokens that may be exchanged for other reinforcers the child chooses in a session. Similarly, check marks entered in a booklet or stars and stickers pasted on a sheet of paper, points accumulated, marbles given, and coins earned may be exchanged for chosen reinforcers. You can use anything as a token, provided it is dispensed easily for correct responses and exchanged later for a reinforcer. This points out one important requirement of such conditioned generalized reinforcers as tokens: You should always have backup reinforcers. If you cannot afford to do that, do not use tokens. A clinician who is simply giving tokens or stickers that are not exchanged for a "real" reinforcer is not to using conditioned generalized reinforcers.

Tokens are the most flexible of the reinforcers. For the child who does not respond to juice, you can offer an opportunity to play if a certain number of tokens are earned. If this does not work, you can offer to read a story for the same tokens. You may offer still other choices for the child: a small toy, a piece of gum, or an inexpensive gift. But tokens may be exchanged for reinforcers that cost little or nothing: a walk through the clinic or the campus with you, a visit to the campus bookstore or library, or a chance to draw on the blackboard.

Although the effects of conditioned generalized reinforcers in treating swallowing disorders have not been studied, it is likely that their use is limited. The reinforcer in swallowing treatment sessions is typically primary: food and drink. Tokens or points may be awarded to patients in muscle exercises and indirect treatment target training when food is not used. Whether such conditioned generalized reinforcers will be effective is unknown.

How to Use Conditioned Generalized Reinforcers

1. Consider the cost of a backup reinforcement system before you design a token system. Your clinic may not have any funds to purchase backup reinforcers. Do not promise a child that the parents will back up your tokens unless the parents previously have agreed to it.

2. Maintain a supply of backup tangible reinforcers or backup activities.

3. Ask the child to choose the reinforcer at the beginning of the session.

4. Tell the child how many tokens are needed to receive the backup reinforcer.

5. Set a realistic number of tokens so that the child will have enough of them to get the chosen backup reinforcer. If not, all the correct responses given in the session may be technically unreinforced. Therefore, set a number the child is likely to achieve.

6. Use various activities that do not cost anything as backup reinforcers. Limiting your backups to toys, food, and other tangibles will cost you. Such activities as reading a story to the child, working on a puzzle, listening to music, working on an art project, or a brief opportunity to play outside may be just as effective.

Feedback

Both adults and children wish to know how well they are doing in therapy. When that information is systematically given to them, their performance tends to improve. The information given back to a person or a mechanical system about how the person or the system has been performing is called **feedback.** In behavioral treatment procedures, feedback is a reinforcer for correct behaviors and corrective stimulus when the response is wrong.

Feedback became a powerful tool in changing behavior with the invention of mechanical feedback devices. These devices are especially helpful in giving information about neurophysiological activities that cannot be readily observed. For example, without the help of a mechanical device, you cannot give feedback to a person about the electrical activity of muscles. Such information given back to a person about his or her neurophysiological activities through a mechanical device is called **biofeedback.**

Biofeedback is used in treating stuttering and voice disorders. Several mechanical devices are available to monitor phonatory onset, continuous phonation, and muscle tension. Several kinds of electronic units help reduce the rate of speech in those who stutter by giving delayed auditory feedback (DAF) of their speech. Newer instruments give feedback on phonatory onset and airflow management. Electromyographic instruments help reduce a speaker's muscle tension.

Biofeedback has been successful especially in treating voice disorders. As mentioned earlier, such instruments as PM 100 Pitch Analyzer, the Phonatory Function Analyzer, and the Visi-Pitch give feedback to clients on their vocal pitch and their attempts at changing it. Nasal resonance problems may be altered by the Nasometer, which displays a ratio of oral and nasal resonance. In gradual steps, the client can increase the ratio in favor of the target resonance.

Increased use of computers in treatment will make mechanical feedback more common in therapy. Yet, feedback given to clients in treatment need not be mechanical. You may tell a man who stutters that his rate of dysfluency in the previous 5 minutes of conversation was 15% compared to 17% in the previous session. You may inform a woman that her hoarseness has been reduced some 50% over the past three sessions. A boy in articulation treatment may learn that his correct production of /s/ has increased from 30% to 90%. Such information about performance levels is feedback, and when used systematically, it can increase the rate of responses.

The effect of positive and corrective feedback in treating disorders of communication is well documented (Hegde, 1998a). Although no experimental data on the effects of feedback on swallowing responses in treatment are available, there is no reason to assume that feedback will not work. Most clinicians positively reinforce any successful attempt at swallow and give corrective feedback when the attempts fail.

How to Use Feedback to Increase Target Skills

1. Give informational feedback in a comparative manner. Say where the client was and how close the performance is to reaching the final target or some intermediate criterion of performance.

(continues)

2. Show progress graphically that most clients, including children, can appreciate. Use colors whenever practical. If available, use computers that provide colorful displays on the progress and movement toward the target.

3. Give feedback throughout the session so you can make it contingent on responses.

4. Combine mechanical feedback with verbal praise.

5. Discontinue negative feedback when the client makes little or no progress. Something is not working right. Perhaps you should change the treatment procedure or further simplify the target response.

High-Probability Behaviors

An interesting fact about behavior is that one action of a person can reinforce (increase) another action of the same person. A behavior that reinforces another behavior is of *high probability*. That is, it is exhibited frequently. The behavior that is reinforced (increased) is of *low probability*. It is exhibited infrequently. The unique aspect of **high-probability behaviors** as reinforcers is that both the reinforcer and the reinforced are the behaviors of the same person. Typically, clinician's actions reinforce the client behaviors. In this special case, the client's more frequently exhibited behavior reinforces his or her less frequently exhibited behavior.

In using high-probability behaviors to reinforce low-probability behaviors, the clinician does not give anything except an opportunity to perform that highly desired behavior. But that opportunity is given only when the client performs what he or she is not likely to perform. Thus, the clinician increases the frequency of an unlikely behavior.

Target communicative behaviors are of low probability. The goal of treatment is to increase their frequency. To do this, first you must find a behavior that the client exhibits frequently. Does the client frequently paint, sing, read, listen to music, ski, go to movies, or talk to friends on the phone? Can any of these actions be used to reinforce target communicative behaviors under treatment?

Some high-probability activities can be allowed in the treatment session itself. For instance, every time the child gives a certain number of correct responses, you may read aloud a brief story or part of a longer story that the child has selected. Opportunities to draw or paint, put puzzles together, and listen to a song played on a tape recorder are among other activities that can be used to reinforce target responses in the clinic.

Opportunities for other behaviors cannot be provided in the clinic. The child or an adult client cannot ski or see a movie in the treatment room. Often, these are the behaviors of highest probability with the greatest reinforcement potential. These behaviors may occur days or weeks after treatment sessions in which the target responses are produced. High-probability behaviors in such cases are at best delayed reinforcers.

To bridge the gap between the eventual high-probability behavior and the target responses, use a token system. Reinforce each correct response with a token.

Require a certain number of tokens to engage in that cherished behavior. Obviously, in the case of children, you should have the approval of parents who will make such opportunities available. For example, the parents of an adolescent boy receiving language treatment may take him to a ski resort after accumulating a certain number of tokens in the treatment sessions. In the case of adults, you should have some system to verify the client's compliance with the arrangement.

The use of some high probability behaviors in reinforcing low probability safe swallowing has not been investigated. Whether this can be done is an interesting research question.

How to Use High-Probability Behaviors as Reinforcers

1. Find potential high-probability behaviors while talking with parents and clients.

2. Control unauthorized opportunities for the selected high-probability behavior. You do not have a reinforcer if the client gets to ski every weekend regardless of the number of tokens earned.

3. Require a number of tokens that will ensure the opportunity for the high-probability behavior, especially in the beginning. Increase the required number of tokens in gradual steps.

4. Give brief but frequent breaks for the high-probability behaviors, especially with young children.

5. Select behaviors that take a relatively longer time to complete. A longer story may be read in chunks. A complex puzzle may be completed in stages. Require a small number of tokens to read a few paragraphs or to fit a few pieces of the puzzle.

Instructions, modeling, shaping, and reinforcing consequences discussed so far help you create new responses and increase the frequency of new and existing responses. But to strengthen and sustain those responses, you need to use reinforcers in certain ways. Those procedures are discussed next.

Strengthening and Sustaining Target Behaviors

Target communication skills you teach your clients may not be strong enough to last. To strengthen and sustain responses you shape or increase, you must use reinforcers differently in different stages of treatment. A pattern of reinforcement arranged for a pattern of responses is called a **schedule of reinforcement.** One kind of schedule must be used to create and increase responses and another kind to *sustain and strengthen* them.

In a **continuous schedule,** every response is reinforced. This schedule is necessary in the early stage of treatment when the response needs to be shaped or increased to a higher frequency. A continuous schedule is helpful in establishing a behavior but not in sustaining it. A continuously reinforced response is susceptible to extinction when reinforcement is stopped. After dismissal, the client may not maintain the target responses because of infrequent reinforcement or lack of it in the natural environment.

A paradoxical effect of reinforcement schedule is that responses are strengthened more when they are reinforced intermittently, rather than continuously. On an intermittent schedule, some responses are reinforced and others are not. There are many patterns of reinforcement and nonreinforcement resulting in many intermittent schedules.

In a **fixed–ratio schedule,** a response is reinforced after a fixed number of unreinforced responses have been made. For example, a fixed ratio of 10, abbreviated FR10, means that you reinforce every 10th response. This schedule creates a pattern of 9 unreinforced responses and a 10th reinforced response. An FR1 means that every correct response is reinforced.

A fixed-ratio schedule is easy to arrange and is used frequently in clinical and educational work. After a period of continuous reinforcement (FR1) to establish a target response, you should gradually stretch the ratio. For example, you may initially reinforce a child continuously for naming a set of pictured stimuli. When the child's correct response rate increases substantially, say from 10% to more than 50%, you may shift to an intermittent schedule. Your first intermittent schedule may be an FR2 (every second response is reinforced). When the response rate shows a further, significant increase, you may switch the schedule again, perhaps to an FR5. A fixed ratio allows you to make a progressive reduction in the amount of reinforcement delivered for correct responses.

In a **variable–ratio (VR) schedule,** the number of responses required before giving a reinforcer varies around an average. Compared to a fixed ratio of 5, in which every fifth response is reinforced, in a variable ratio of 5 (VR5), an average of 5 responses are required before a reinforcer is given. Because the schedule is based on an average, the actual number of responses required on any given occasion will vary. You may reinforce the 7th response on one occasion and the 3rd on the next. The variable ratio is not a random method of reinforcement. The variable ratio is determined beforehand and reinforcers are given so as to conform to an average number of unreinforced responses.

Variable ratio produces a strong response rate. Whenever possible, use this schedule in the latter stages of treatment. Use a variable ratio schedule especially when you monitor the target behaviors in conversational speech.

Typically, a schedule specifies which behavior will be reinforced and how frequently. But there is an unusual schedule that specifies which behavior *will not be reinforced.* This schedule is called the **differential reinforcement of other**

behavior (DRO). Sometimes, what matters most is that a client *not* exhibit a certain behavior. In such cases, there can be one or a few unacceptable behaviors, with many other acceptable behaviors that could be produced instead. So your schedule specifies what behavior or behaviors will not be reinforced. This means that many other alternative behaviors can be reinforced.

Suppose you are working with a small group of children and a boy in the group refuses to sit in his chair. He moves around and disturbs other children working on their assignments. In this case, not sitting in the chair is the troublesome behavior; instead, the child could be reading, sitting quietly, working on his arithmetic, coloring, and so forth. Therefore, you tell the child that he will be reinforced provided that he does not leave the chair. You reinforce any of the desirable behaviors, including just sitting in the chair.

Two other frequently discussed schedules are the fixed interval and the variable interval. Whereas the ratio schedules are based on the number of responses that go unreinforced between reinforcers, the *interval schedules* are based on the time that lapses between reinforced responses. In a **fixed interval (FI) schedule,** an invariable period of time lapses between any two opportunities for presenting a reinforcer. In a **variable interval (VI) schedule,** the amount of time that lapses between two such opportunities is varied around an average.

An important thing to remember about the interval schedules is that the reinforcer is not automatically given after the specified fixed or variable time interval passes. The lapse of the interval creates an *opportunity* to earn a reinforcer. The first response made *after* the interval is over is reinforced. That first response may or may not be made precisely at the end of the interval. Always remember that a reinforcer must be given immediately after a response is made.

Interval schedules have not been used frequently in treating communicative disorders, although they have some potential. In treating voice and fluency disorders, you can use interval schedules. For example, a stuttering speaker's fluent speech may be reinforced on a VI10 s (variable interval of 10 seconds). In this schedule, you reinforce if the speaker maintains fluency during 10-second intervals *on the average*. Similarly, a speaker with hoarseness may be reinforced for clear voice on a fixed or variable time schedule.

Reinforcement schedules and their differential application apply to swallowing disorders as well. In the initial stages of training, whether it is a compensatory action, a muscle exercise, or a direct treatment target, the clinician will reinforce all successful attempts. Gradually, the clinician will thin out reinforcement as the patient becomes more proficient in swallowing.

Clinical Use of Reinforcement Schedules

Generally, variable ratio and variable interval schedules produce stronger responses than fixed-ratio or fixed-interval schedules. But all intermittent schedules produce stronger response rates than the continuous schedule. There are several other reinforcement schedules that may be helpful in treating various disorders of communication. See Hegde (1998b) for details.

How to Effectively Use Different Reinforcement Schedules

1. Begin with continuous reinforcement. During response shaping and modeling, reinforce every correct response.

2. Switch to a fixed-ratio schedule when nonimitated (spontaneous) response rates show a substantial increase over baselines.

3. Start with a small ratio, perhaps an FR2.

4. Increase the ratio in small steps as the correct response rates continue to increase.

5. Use a large ratio during conversational speech. An FR10 or larger should work. If possible, use a variable interval ratio.

6. Lower the schedule if a switch to a thinner schedule of reinforcement causes a decline in the correct response rate.

7. Use DRO when many desirable behaviors are incompatible with one or a few undesirable behaviors.

Sequence of Treatment

Treatment is started after you have assessed the client's communicative behaviors and selected the target behaviors. However, before you begin treatment, you must establish baselines of target behaviors.

Baselines of Target Behaviors

Baselines are a client's pretreatment response rates. Baselines are necessary to assess the client's improvement with treatment. The client's progress may be judged continuously against the baselines.

The assessment data are not enough to evaluate the client improvement in treatment because the data may be dated by the time you start treatment. More importantly, measures of communicative behaviors taken during assessment are limited, not repeated and, hence, are of questionable reliability. Therefore, you need to establish baselines just before starting treatment to get current, reliable, and comprehensive data on a client's status before treatment.

In baserating behaviors, take *repeated measures* to establish reliability. For example, instead of taking one conversational speech sample to assess articulation, language features, or stuttering, take two or more samples to find a somewhat stable rate of those behaviors. Because you can concentrate only on the immediate target responses, you can afford to take more extensive measures than is possible during assessment. For example, during assessment, you may get a rough idea of most if not all phonemes in error. In establishing in-depth baserates before starting treatment, you select only a few phonemes on which the treatment will be started soon. You baserate new phonemes when you are ready to teach them. This method always gives you both reliable and current pretreatment response rates.

To obtain comprehensive baselines, *sample responses adequately*. For example, it is not sufficient to give one or two opportunities to produce a phoneme or a grammatical morpheme. Typically, this is all a standardized test can do. Therefore, you must prepare an adequate number of stimulus materials to evoke the target responses on repeated trials. For baserating speech and language targets, roughly 20 stimulus items are needed to measure the production of each target response. When combined with repeated speech and language samples, such measures reflect pretreatment response rates more accurately than standardized test results. However, read the cautionary note on baserating swallowing disorders in "How to Baserate Target Behaviors."

How to Baserate Target Behaviors

1. Baserate only those behaviors that you plan to teach immediately. Repeat a baseline before teaching any behavior, even if it was baserated a few weeks earlier. Because behaviors tend to change, only a baseline taken just prior to treatment is valid.

2. Write instructions to the client. Also, write questions to evoke the target responses. You need questions to evoke responses to pictured stimuli. Select physical stimuli (pictures or objects).

3. Plan how you might take conversational speech samples. To sample language structures adequately, you should direct conversation so that opportunities for producing infrequently used language structures are presented. See Appendix G for guidelines on taking and analyzing speech samples.

4. Write at least 20 articulation and language response exemplars for each target behavior. An exemplar may be a word, phrase, or sentence that contains a target response. For instance, the word *soup* or the phrase *hot soup* or the sentence *I like soup* contains the /s/, a potential target response for a child who misarticulates it. Each of those three is an exemplar. Similarly, in teaching the present progressive *ing*, you might have such exemplars as *walking, boy walking, boy is walking*, and so forth. Your exemplars may be of one kind only. You may have 20 words, phrases, or sentences

(continues)

depending on the initial level of training. They are likely to be words or phrases. See Hegde (1998c) for a variety of target behavior exemplars that you can use to baserate as well as treat speech and language targets.

5. Present the 20 stimulus items on discrete trials. A discrete trial gives the client one opportunity to produce the target response. Typically, you show the picture or object, ask a question, and wait for the response. Also, baserate imitative responses on a set of trials in which you model the responses after asking the question.

6. Take an adequate conversational speech sample. Ask the client or parents to supply taped conversational speech samples from home to assess the target behavior rate in extraclinical situations.

7. Record each response on a recording sheet. See Appendix Q for a sample discrete trial baseline recording sheet.

8. Calculate the percentage correct speech (articulation, fluency) and language response rate separately for discrete trials and for the conversational speech samples. Also, calculate the response rates separately for clinical speech samples and home samples. For fluency clients, calculate the percentage dysfluency rates based on the number of words spoken. For voice clients, you may calculate durations of conversational speech that are free of problems and those durations that are characterized by such problems as hoarseness or nasality.

9. Repeat the measures if any two measures for the same response mode and situation are not comparable. For instance, if two clinic speech samples show different baselines, then you need to repeat them. Similarly, if two home samples disagree widely, you need additional home samples. Home and clinic samples may vary in the case of stuttering and voice characteristics. But the response rates should not vary much in case of articulation and language.

10. Write objective statements to summarize the baseline data. Such objective statements help evaluate the effects of subsequent treatment by giving a quantitative specification of a client's status before treatment.

11. The treatment literature on swallowing disorders does not offer guidelines on baserating specific problems the patients may exhibit (Groher, 1997; Logemann, 1998). The Modified Barium Swallow Study, a procedure in which the swallowing problems are studied, may be considered a baseline procedure, provided the clinician offers multiple trial swallows. Just before the treatment is begun, the clinicians may baserate by trial swallows; however, extended baserates of the kind suggested for speech and language skills may expose the individual to unnecessary risks of aspiration.

Take note of the following examples of objective statements summarizing baseline data:

- The child's correct articulation of /s/ in conversational speech, measured across three samples, was 20%. Each sample contained at least 10 opportunities to produce the phoneme.

- The client's rate of dysfluency on two home samples of at least 2,000 words each was 13% and 15%, respectively.

- The client's longest fluent utterances, measured over two conversational speech samples of 800 words each, typically lasted 10 seconds. (Note: This is a durational baserate of fluency. The measure is a statistical mode—which is the most frequently occurring event—not an average.)

- The client's voice was judged hypernasal on 90% of utterances that did not contain nasal speech.

- The client was hoarse 90% of the time she spoke during two base-rate sessions. She spoke at least 500 words or more in each session. (Note: another durational baserate measure.)

- The patient did not recall the names of five of his close relatives, including his wife. The patient was asked to name them on three occasions—each separated by 24 hours.

- Ten percent of the words spoken by the patient were jargon.

Initial Treatment Sequence

Number of Target Behaviors

After establishing baselines, you begin teaching the target behaviors. The first question you face is: How many behaviors can I teach in individual sessions? There is no single rule that you can follow in all cases. Much depends on the disorder of the client, severity of the disorder, the rate at which the person learns, age, education, intellectual capacity, and other client characteristics. But equally important are the clinician's expertise, the duration of sessions, and whether the client is treated individually or in a group.

To begin with, try the following recommendations; if they do not work, analyze the data to find out what went wrong.

1. Be ready to initiate training on three to five phonemes in syllables or words.

2. Plan on initiating training on two to four grammatical morphemes, syntactic structures, and other language features while working with a child who has language disabilities.

3. Be prepared to instruct and model all the basic skills of fluency (e.g., air-flow management, syllable prolongation, and gentle phonatory onset) in

the first full session of treatment. In a 30-minute session, you should have sufficient time to instruct and initiate practice on all of them. In the case of persons who learn fast, you can move from the single-word level to two-word phrases or even to short sentences in one or two sessions.

4. Expect to instruct and model the target behaviors and initiate training on voice targets in the first treatment session. If you use a feedback instrument, be ready to fully demonstrate it and start training the client on it. Depending on the client's learning rate, the treatment should move from words to phrases and sentences in the first session or two.

5. Experiment with two to four target behaviors while treating clients with neurogenic speech or language disorders. The rate of learning in these clients may depend on their general health status; therefore, you may need to probe with a slightly different number of target behaviors to judge, on an individual basis, the best course of action.

6. In treating swallowing disorders, always consider the patient's safety as the primary criterion to determine the number of specific targets to be treated in a single session; start with a single target (e.g., a specific food consistency or a particular posture) and add multiple targets as the patient's pattern of swallowing disorder and the underlying neuroanatomic deficits warrant.

Structure of Treatment Sessions

Treatment sessions may be highly structured or loosely structured. Tightly structured sessions are more formal and loosely structures sessions are more naturalistic. When you use discrete trials, you are more structured than when you use conversational speech to train target behaviors. In treating swallowing disorders, selected boluses or exercises may be presented on discrete trials, but eventually the patient may be asked to eat in the typical manner.

The argument you often hear about tight versus loose structure of treatment sessions is not that important. Two factors dictate the structure of treatment sessions: the client and the stage of treatment. First, a client who is minimally verbal or nonverbal or has multiple misarticulations often responds better under a structured format. Many neurologically involved patients also perform better with a structured format. Children with attention deficits need structured formats. Patients with dysphagia also respond better when the treatment is carefully structured.

Second, during the early stages of treatment, most clients benefit from structured format. They can better focus on target behaviors and get used to the clinical process sooner if it is structured and somewhat simplified. However, during the latter stages of treatment, all clients need the loose format. During these stages, the target behavior is more likely to be conversational speech, which cannot be implemented within a structured, discrete trial format.

In essence, use the tight structure if the client needs it, but use the loose structure if the client can handle it. In the latter stages of treatment, always use the loose structure, so the treatment resembles communication in natural settings.

Discrete Trial Procedure

The initial training is better started with some structure, especially when the targets are narrowly defined articulation and language skills. Therefore, in most cases, use the structured discrete trial procedure to establish the target speech and language responses. The discrete trials are less useful or not needed in treating fluency and voice problems.

Discrete trials also may be useful in several stages of swallowing treatment. An exercise to strengthen the tongue muscles may be practiced on discrete trials, with a brief break between trials. Each bolus of food may be presented on discrete trials. These discrete trials may be faded into more natural and continuous eating.

See Appendix L for steps in administering discrete treatment trials. In the treatment of articulation and language disorders, a discrete trial consists of (1) stimulus presentation; (2) asking a question that normally evokes the target response; (3) modeling; (4) giving a few seconds for the client to respond; (5) consequating the response; (6) recording the response; (7) marking the end of the trial by pulling the stimulus away; and (8) starting the next trial after a few seconds.

Practice the stimulus presentation so that you can administer each trial quickly, smoothly, and efficiently. Instruct, ask questions, and model responses as described earlier. In evaluating consequences, make a quick judgment about the accuracy of the client responses. If the response is correct, immediately reinforce it. If it is wrong, use one of the response reduction procedures described in Chapter 9. Record every response of the client on a recording sheet (see Appendix L for a sample).

Movement through the Treatment Sequence

When the treatment is working, you will see systematic increase in a client's target behaviors. As this happens, you begin to make important clinical decisions. To take a client from the initial imitation of a narrowly defined target response to the final stage of conversational speech in natural settings, you must move from one stage of treatment to the next. Similarly, in treating swallowing disorders, the clinician takes a client from certain initial, simpler, or easier swallow targets to more complex targets. For example, the bolus size may be gradually increased; food viscosity may be gradually changed until more typical foods are presented.

Each movement is progress. But each movement requires a clinical decision. A wrong decision made at a juncture might retard the client's progress. For example, if you spent too much time reinforcing the isolated production of a phoneme, it may be difficult for you to move the client on to the word level of training. The following general guidelines should help you make decisions to move to a different level of training. The guidelines are also clinical criteria of movement through stages of treatment.

Criteria for Clinical Decisions

When Do I Stop or Reinstate Modeling?

1. Stop modeling when the client imitates the initial target response on at least five consecutive trials.

2. Reinstate modeling when you observe incorrect responses on three to four trials with no modeling. Again, stop modeling after five correctly imitated responses. If you have to stop and reinstate modeling repeatedly, continue modeling until the client gives 10 or more imitated responses. Alternatively, see if the client can give correct responses if you continued a little longer without modeling.

Training Criteria for Target Response vs. Behaviors

To understand some of the subsequent criteria, you should make a distinction between a target response and a target behavior. As you know, you use some 20 words in teaching a phoneme. The production of each word that contains the target phoneme is a target response; the correct production of the phoneme in varied contexts and in conversational speech is the target behavior. Likewise, in teaching a grammatical morpheme, you may have some 20 or so sentences that contain that target morpheme. The production of each sentence is a target response; the production of the morpheme in varied contexts and in conversational speech is the target behavior.

Each specific response is an exemplar of the target behavior. On the one hand, the word *soup* is an *exemplar* of /s/ (or another phoneme in it). The word *walking* is an exemplar of the present progressive. On the other hand, the production of the phoneme /s/ and the present progressive in varied linguistic contexts (e.g., different words, phrases, sentences) and in varied natural settings (e.g., home, classroom, occupational setting) are target *behaviors*. In the treatment of swallowing disorders, presentation of a single bolus is an exemplar; if the single bolus is swallowed safely, the exemplar training has been successful. However, to say that the swallowing behavior has been trained, the patient has to master a *class of swallowing acts*, to be exhibited in varied contexts (e.g., healthcare facility, restaurant, home), not just a single swallowing act.

When we say that a client has multiple articulation targets to learn, we do not mean the 20 or so sentences for each phoneme; we mean the number of phonemes to be taught. Similarly, when we say the child has multiple grammatic morphemes to learn, we do not mean any particular word or sentence that contains a morpheme; we mean such classes of responses as the regular plural, present progressive, an article, a preposition, and so forth (Hegde, 1998a, 2008c).

You also can think of a target behavior as a group of similar responses and a target response as any one of those responses. We teach the more concrete individual responses to have the client master the more abstract target behavior.

When Is a Target Response Tentatively Trained?

A target response is tentatively trained when the client gives at least 10 consecutively correct, nonimitated (spontaneous) responses. Suppose you were teaching a child the present progressive *ing* in words. Perhaps you were teaching four words with the target feature in it. When the child correctly produces the word *walking* 10 times in a row, you could consider that response (not the behavior) to have been tentatively learned.

Extend this logic to (1) a child under articulation training; (2) a man under voice therapy who is being trained to say individual words without nasal resonance; and (3) a woman who is aphasic and is receiving treatment for naming problems.

Such specific quantitative criteria often are not specified for treating swallowing disorders; clinical judgment may replace quantitative criteria. However, one may adopt somewhat flexible quantitative criterion in individual cases. For example, a particular target such as the head tilt posture during swallow may be considered successfully trained if the patient safely swallows on 5 or 10 consecutive swallow trials when boluses of certain size and consistency are presented.

Explanation of the Criterion This is a highly tentative criterion. Much work needs to be done to complete the teaching of the target behavior, but the client has met a tentative training criterion on one exemplar (response). You should stop training an exemplar at some point, and this is a suggested point. You can redefine this criterion just as appropriately as 15 or 20 consecutively correct responses.

When Is a Target Behavior Tentatively Trained?

A target behavior is tentatively trained when the client meets a tentative probe criterion of at least 90% correct response rate on probe trials.

The tentative training criterion for a target behavior is based on an external procedure. That is, you cannot decide that a behavior (e.g., the /s/, the present progressive, oral resonance, normal voice quality, naming) is tentatively trained because the responses on selected training words or phrases during treatment have been correct. Instead, you conduct a *probe* to decide whether a target behavior has been tentatively trained. The procedure applies to both communicative and swallowing treatment targets.

Probe Procedure

To find out if the target behavior under training meets the probe criterion, conduct probes. A **probe** is a procedure to find out if a trained response is produced (a) when the treatment variables (e.g., modeling, positive reinforcement, corrective feedback) are withheld or (b) the response is produced on the basis of generalization, also when the treatment variables are withheld. For example, a phoneme trained in a few words may be correctly produced in other, untrained words. A grammatical morpheme trained in a few sentences may be produced in other, untrained, and varied sentences. Hold a probe when you have trained four to six target responses (e.g., four words or phrases). You may probe through discrete trials or speech samples. On *discrete trial probes*, you alternate the trained and the untrained stimuli. For example, of the 20 words you had baserated for teaching /s/ in words, assume that you have used 4 words in training. The client has met the tentative training criterion on each of those words. Now you probe to see if /s/ is tentatively trained. To do this, prepare a probe list on which the first word is the one already trained. The second should be one of the words not used in training. The third is again a trained word, followed by an untrained word. Reuse the trained words until all the untrained words have been alternated with them.

Do not model any words on probe trials. Show pictures to have the child name them or ask the child to read the printed words on the probe list. Reinforce the correct production of the trained words as you will have done on training trials; do not offer consequences (reinforcers or corrective feedback) for right or wrong productions of the probe words.

Count the number of correct productions of untrained words only; ignore productions of trained words. Calculate the percentage of correct untrained word productions. This is your probe response rate. If this is at least 90%, you may assume that the target behavior has been tentatively trained.

Tape record a brief conversational speech sample, making sure that at least 20 opportunities were available for producing the target behavior. Count how many were correctly produced. Calculate the percentage correct probe rate for the conversational speech to see if it meets the criterion.

Use the same probe criterion at the level of words, phrases, or sentences. When you have completed training in sentences, use only the conversational speech probe to calculate the percent correct probe response rate.

Note that a behavior is trained only when some untrained exemplars of that behavior are produced correctly. You can use the same procedure to probe various language targets. For clients who stutter or for those who have voice problems, probes should be conducted at the level of response topography on which the training was just completed (phrases, sentences, conversational speech). Record the responses without offering consequences to any of the behaviors. Measure the target behaviors of interest in the same way you did during baserate sessions. Calculate the percentage of probe response rates (e.g., percentage dysfluency rate or the percentage of utterances without hoarseness) and compare them against the percentages recorded during baserate sessions. Appendix H shows a sample probe recording sheet.

In treating swallowing disorders, probes may be presented as well. A *probe* in swallowing may be a liquid or solid bolus that has been presented for a duration of training for swallow while withholding positive reinforcement or corrective feedback. If the patient can swallow without these and other treatment variables, then the minimal probe criterion is met. If the client is presented food that is slightly different from that presented during training trials and the patient swallows without aspiration, then somewhat generalized swallowing response is documented. For instance, when the client begins to safely swallow thickened liquid, the clinician may probe to see if thinner liquids may be equally safely swallowed in the absence of treatment variables.

When Do I Make Topographical Shifts in Training?

Make the first topographic shift when a behavior meets the tentative probe criterion at the initial response level. For example, when the initial probe shows 90% correct production of /s/ in untrained words, shift training to phrase level. When the phoneme production is 90% on probe phrases, shift to sentences. When the probe for sentences shows 90% correct, move to more natural conversational speech. Move again to more natural settings when, within the clinic, the target phoneme is produced at 90% accuracy on conversational probes.

As you can see, topographical shifts involve movement through a hierarchy of response complexity. Such shifts occur when you move to words from syllables, to phrases from words, and to sentences from phrases. Topographical shifts are necessary in the treatment of most disorders of communication and swallowing.

It is likely that in most cases, you will have started training on three or four behaviors. The initial topographical level of training on most if not all of these behaviors may be syllables or words. The level is rarely conversational speech. But the final topographical level is always conversational speech.

The progress on multiple target behaviors under training is likely to vary. Each behavior is shaped through its own topographic sequence. One behavior may move through fewer sequences than the other. Some behaviors will meet the tentative training criterion sooner than others.

When one of the target behaviors meets the final criterion or any time you have extra treatment time, select another behavior for training. Start with a simple topography and move through a sequence.

Design a similar or modified sequence to training language, fluency, and voice characteristics. Note that the probe criterion may be higher for fluency. Generally, 90% fluency is too low, as most people who stutter do so only on 10% of the words they speak. A probe criterion of 98% or better is desirable.

Be flexible in applying the suggested guidelines on topographical shifts. Do not always assume that all clients need to be started at the syllable or the word level—the two lowest levels of oral communication training. In teaching fluency skills to a person who stutters, for example, try the phrase or even simple sentence level. If the client can sustain airflow, gentle onset, and syllable prolongation at the word or simple sentence level right away, the treatment has topographically progressed so much. If the client cannot manage the skills at the selected (more complex) level, you will find out in a matter of minutes. No harm is done. You just quickly drop to a lower level of training. Therefore, always starting at the lowest level of response topography is inefficient. Persisting at the lowest level is worse; the client may perseverate at that level when you move on to a higher level. In such cases, *you* will have taught the client to perseverate.

In treating swallowing disorders, different kinds of complexities may be gradually increased across training trials or sessions. For some patients, a postural adjustment may be the initial target; soon, more direct swallowing procedures may be implemented. Some patients may swallow better thickened liquids before they can manage to swallow thinner liquids. Such shifts in training strategies depend on the nature of the swallowing disorder in a client and his or her response to treatment strategies.

What Do I Do When Probe Criteria Are Not Met?

Provide additional training when clients fails to meet a probe criterion. A client may fail the probe criterion at any level of training. When this happens, give additional training at the same level. For example, the child who fails the tentative probe criterion at the word level of phoneme training should be trained on new exemplars. Teach two to four new exemplars before you probe again. In some cases, especially when you already have trained 8 to 10 exemplars, a few additional training trials on all of the trained exemplars may be sufficient to have the client meet the probe criterion.

In treating swallowing disorders, too, frequent probes may suggest the need for additional training trials. For example, if a certain postural adjustment, such as a head tilt toward to stronger side of the mouth, is practiced on 10 trials with positive reinforcement and corrective feedback, the clinician may probe two or three times to see if the client can swallow safely without the feedback. If he or she cannot, additional training trials on the postural adjustment may be offered. Nonetheless, the clinician should be ready to abandon the training on a failed strategy and apply a more promising strategy.

When Is a Target Behavior Finally Trained?

A target behavior finally is trained when its production in conversational speech in natural settings is acceptable. Note that different criteria may apply to different communicative behaviors. Phonemes and language structures may be considered finally trained when they are produced in conversational speech at a minimum of 90% accuracy. Fluency may be considered trained when the client's rate of dysfluencies in conversational speech in extraclinical situations does not exceed 3% or 4%. Normal voice characteristics may be considered trained when they are sustained at least 90% or 95% of utterances or of speaking time. A swallowing problem may be considered effectively treated when the patient can swallow liquid, solid, or semisolid food without aspiration at a rate that is essential to maintain the physical health of the individual.

The target behavior is finally trained when the client is ready for dismissal. You dismiss the client from services only when the communicative behaviors are produced under natural conditions or safe swallowing skills are established.

The various criteria described so far are suggested guidelines for making clinical decisions. They have worked in clinical research. But always remember that no criterion is a rule you cannot violate and that all criteria depend on client performance. Design your criteria that are supported by clinical data. Each client's response rates you record are your clinical data. These data are your ultimate guiding principles.

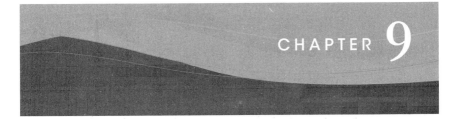

CHAPTER 9

Controlling Undesirable Behaviors

Chapter Outline

- Behaviors to Be Reduced
- Assessment of the Maintaining Causes of Undesirable Behaviors
- General Strategies for Decreasing Undesirable Behaviors
- Direct Strategy for Decreasing Behaviors
- Indirect Strategy for Decreasing Behaviors
- General Guidelines for Reducing Undesirable Behaviors
- Aversive Nature of Response-Reduction Procedures

In Chapter 8, we suggested that reducing the frequency of undesirable behaviors is an important clinical task. While implementing procedures to increase desirable communicative behaviors, you may use procedures that reduce undesirable communicative responses. In many cases, you also must reduce undesirable general behaviors (e.g., crying during treatment sessions, crawling under the table) that interfere with treatment.

Often, undesirable communicative behaviors are the ones the client or the parents complain about. Parents are more likely to complain that their child does not speak well or that he or she stutters. They are the behaviors that need to be replaced by appropriate communicative behaviors (Hegde, 1998a, 2008c).

Behaviors to Be Reduced

Among others, reduce the following *undesirable* or *inappropriate communicative behaviors* while working with your clients.

1. **Language disorders.** Undesirable communicative behaviors to be reduced in clients with language disorders include, among others, the following: gesturing; crying or fussing when something is wanted; using inappropriate words; inappropriate production of semantic, syntactic, and morphologic features or a combination of these; and inappropriate use of language in social situations.

2. **Articulation and phonological disorders.** Misarticulation of isolated speech sounds or patterns of misarticulations are the behaviors to be reduced.

3. **Voice disorders.** The behaviors to be reduced include breathiness, hoarseness, harshness, inappropriate pitch or loudness, hyper- or hyponasality, hard glottal attacks, and vocally abusive behaviors.

4. **Fluency disorders.** In stuttering treatment, behaviors to be reduced include dysfluencies, speech rate, abrupt initiation of sound, inappropriate management of airflow, muscular tension associated with speech production, and avoidance of words and speaking situations. In the latter stages of fluency shaping treatment, you need to reduce monotonous and excessively slow speech that was targeted in the initial stages. In treating persons with cluttering, you need to reduce dysfluencies, imprecise articulation, excessively fast rate of speech, and poor organization or formulation of sentences.

5. **Swallowing disorders.** In treating swallowing disorders, clinicians try to reduce or eliminate a variety of problems including failure to prepare a bolus by not chewing; difficulty holding the bolus or abnormal holding in the mouth; spilling food from the mouth; premature swallowing resulting in aspiration; absent, delayed, searching, thrusting, or disorganized tongue movements; food residue in various parts of the mouth and the valleculae; piecemeal swallow; inadequate velopharyngeal closure during swallow; food coating on the pharyngeal wall; aspiration due to various deficiencies; laryngeal penetration of food; and so forth.

Among others, reduce the following *undesirable general behaviors* that interfere with treatment.

1. **Inattention.** Especially a problem with children, inattention and distractibility interfere with treatment. Unless you reduce these behaviors, you cannot concentrate on fostering the desirable target behaviors.

2. **Crying, fussing, and other emotionally laden conduct.** These are among the strong disrupters of the treatment process. Such client behaviors emotionally upset the clinician who does not know how to handle them.

3. **Out-of-seat and other uncooperative behaviors.** Children who begin to move around in the therapy room, crawl under the table, constantly grab things on the table, kick the table leg, make faces at the observation mirror, or simply wiggle around in their seats cannot focus on treatment targets.

4. **Absenteeism.** A larger problem is a no-show or frequent cancellation of treatment sessions. Obviously, clients who do not attend treatment sessions cannot be helped.

5. **General unresponsivity.** Many clients show a generalized unresponsivity to treatment. Stimuli and treatment processes do not interest them. In such cases, lack of motivation for responding and working with the clinician seem to be the main problems that interfere with the treatment process.

6. **Distracting verbal behaviors.** Children who constantly ask "Are we done yet?" and "You know what?" are trying to distract you from treatment they do not enjoy. Such distracting verbal behaviors, too, need to be reduced or eliminated.

Many clients interweave undesirable behaviors with appropriate responses. The undesirable communicative behaviors, such as the undifferentiated gestures of the nonverbal and the speech sound errors of a child with misarticulations, may be more frequent in the beginning but decline as treatment proceeds. The best way of reducing undesirable communicative behaviors is to increase the desirable counterparts. For instance, the most effective way to reduce misarticulations is to increase correct productions of speech sounds.

Undesirable general behaviors that interfere with treatment often need some special procedures. An occasional interfering behavior is not a serious problem. At times, children wiggle in their chairs and fail to pay attention to the stimuli presented. These may be controlled easily by instructions and reinforcement. But when the client consistently exhibits interfering behaviors, you must take special steps. To reduce persistent undesirable behaviors, you need to make a functional analysis, which is an assessment of the causes of those behaviors.

Assessment of the Maintaining Causes of Undesirable Behaviors

If you can assess the potential maintaining causes of an undesirable behavior, you can reduce or eliminate them more efficiently. It may not always be possible to find out what maintains undesirable (or desirable) behaviors. It is difficult to say how stuttering, misarticulations, inappropriate or inadequate language, and voice quality deviations are maintained. Similarly, it is often not clear why a child is crying, wiggling in the chair, or exhibiting other interfering behaviors. A clinician's commonsense reason for such behaviors may or may not be valid.

You can take some steps prior to starting treatment to find out potential maintaining variables. While establishing baselines, you may introduce the variable you suspect is maintaining an undesirable behavior to see what happens. For example, a child may begin to leave the chair when a difficult task is presented; if this is your observation, periodically present difficult tasks and note the response. If easier tasks kept the child in the chair and difficult tasks drove the child to wander, you will have assessed the potential cause of the child's interfering behavior. Baselines that also are used to find out the maintaining causes of behaviors being measured are called functional analysis baselines (Mason & Iwata, 1990). A functional analysis helps you determine causes of behaviors.

In hindsight, successful treatment sometimes tells you what maintained an undesirable behavior. For example, you may find out that a nonverbal child's undifferentiated gestural or vocal attempts at communication have decreased after learning useful and effective verbal communication. A child who can request something in words is less likely to cry, fuss, or point to things wanted. In such a case, you might think that parental reinforcement maintained the undifferentiated attempts at communication.

In applied behavioral analysis, scientists have made systematic attempts at finding maintaining causes of some interfering behaviors. For example, studies of experimental analysis of self-injurious or self-stimulatory behaviors have suggested that these and possibly other undesirable behaviors may be maintained by *positive reinforcement, negative reinforcement,* or *automatic reinforcement* (Cooper, 2007; Hegde, 1998a, 2008c; Malott & Trojan, 2008).

Most often, attention is the positive reinforcer that maintains undesirable behaviors. A teacher who otherwise ignored a child may promptly attend to a child's misbehavior, thus inadvertently reinforcing the troublesome behavior. These behaviors are most effectively reduced by **extinction** (withholding attention).

To find out if an undesirable behavior is maintained by positive reinforcement in the form of attention, first measure the frequency of the behavior prior to treatment. Then, pay attention to that behavior to see if its frequency increases. You then withdraw attention to see if the frequency of the behavior decreases. If the behavior increases as you pay attention and decreases as you ignore it, then the undesirable behavior is most likely maintained by positive reinforcement.

Negative reinforcement maintains an undesirable behavior when that behavior terminates an aversive event. As in the example given earlier, a child, faced with a difficult task the clinician demands (an aversive event), may exhibit an undesirable behavior (Hegde, 1998a, 2008c). Observing this behavior, the clinician may stop making those demands. In this case, the child escaped from the difficult task by exhibiting undesirable behavior. This is negative reinforcement; the undesirable behavior is strengthened and is more likely to be exhibited in the future because it helped reduce or eliminate the aversive event. One way of reducing such negatively reinforced undesirable behaviors is to prevent escape by not terminating the task demand. The clinician should continue to make the demands and reinforce compliance.

As noted earlier, you may find out if an undesirable behavior is maintained by negative reinforcement by presenting some difficult tasks and see if the behavior increases in frequency. If it does, the behavior most likely is maintained by negative reinforcement. For example, you might present a series of trials on which a non-verbal child who frequently exhibits undesirable behaviors is asked to imitate relatively long and unusual words, a difficult task for the child. Having failed to give correct responses on repeated trials, the child may begin to exhibit the undesirable behavior (e.g., crying or reticence). These behaviors are the child's way of escaping from a difficult (hence aversive) task demand. The escape negatively reinforces the undesirable behaviors.

Automatic reinforcement is presumed when behaviors do not seem to have environmentally generated maintaining causes. Neither externally delivered positive reinforcement nor negative reinforcement seems to account for the frequency of the behavior under observation. Therefore, undesirable behaviors are presumed to generate *neural* or *sensory consequences* that reinforce those behaviors. Lack of stimulation and activity frequently are cited reasons for undesirable behaviors that are maintained by automatic reinforcement. In these children, providing opportunities for play and other kinds of activities and for manipulation and exploration of toys and other materials tend to reduce their undesirable behaviors.

To find out if automatic reinforcement maintains undesirable behaviors, you need to leave the child alone in a room and see if the behaviors occur. Automatic reinforcement is most often presumed in case of stereotypic or self-stimulatory behaviors. A boy with autism may rock himself endlessly when left alone. It is difficult to point out positive or negative reinforcement for such behaviors. A reasonable assumption is that such self-stimulatory behaviors generate their own neural or sensory consequences that are reinforcing.

General Strategies for Decreasing Undesirable Behaviors

Procedures that reduce behaviors make no distinction between desirable versus undesirable or good versus bad behaviors. Behaviors are described in such evaluative terms from a personal and social viewpoint. Procedures that decrease behaviors may decrease any behavior: desirable, undesirable, good, or bad. Therefore, the prudent clinician's job is to apply response reduction procedures to only the undesirable behaviors. Similarly, reinforcement also will increase good or bad behavior. The same prudent clinician's job is to apply response reinforcing consequences only to desirable behaviors.

Extinction and *punishment* are two main behavioral procedures to reduce undesirable behaviors. Several procedures typically described under extinction and various forms of punishment are included here and are considered appropriate for therapeutic use. It should be noted that the scientific and therapeutic meaning of punishment does not share the negative connotations of *punishment* in everyday language. Nonetheless, we wish to minimize the use of the term *punishment* because its scientific meaning constantly is confused with its everyday meaning of a collection of many painful, exploitative, and vain procedures that most societies and governmental agencies employ. We prefer the term **corrective feedback** to *punishment* (Hegde, 1998a, 2008c). Also, the response reduction procedures recommended here do not include all of the punishment procedures researched in behavioral analysis. Therefore, we have taken a more descriptive approach in classifying response reduction procedures that you may use in clinical treatment.

Direct and Indirect Response Reduction Strategies

We classify the response reduction strategies as either direct or indirect. This classification depends on whether a treatment contingency is placed on the behavior to be reduced or on another behavior. In the **direct response reduction strategy,** you place a contingency on the behavior to be reduced. *Placing a contingency on a behavior* means that you take an immediate action (e.g., saying "No") followed by a behavior that needs to be decreased.

In the **indirect response reduction strategy,** you place a contingency on a *desirable* behavior whose increase will have an indirect effect of decreasing an undesirable behavior. Note that the behavior to be reduced is not directly manipulated. An important point to remember is that an *undesirable behavior may be reduced by increasing a desirable behavior* that replaces the undesirable behavior.

Another important point to remember is that only direct response reduction procedures may be defined as punishment or corrective feedback. Although indirect procedures also help us reduce behaviors, they are not response reduction procedures. The indirect procedures increase desirable responses; they are reinforcement procedures. You should not say that we use reinforcement procedures to decrease behaviors. By definition, reinforcement procedures increase behaviors. When used in a program of response reduction, the *reinforcement procedures increase desirable behaviors.* Presumably, this makes the undesirable behavior unnecessary. This is an important reason for classifying some response reduction strategies as indirect.

In the following sections, we return to this distinction to make it clearer to you. Specific procedures and examples show how a contingency is placed either on the behavior to be reduced or on a different behavior to be increased. Always, the behavior to be increased is productive and desirable.

Direct Strategy for Decreasing Behaviors

In the direct strategy, you concentrate on an undesirable behavior and place a contingency on it (do something immediately). The effect of this contingency (your immediate action) is to directly reduce that behavior (Hegde, 1998a, 2008c).

There are several procedures in which the behavior is directly reduced. These procedures fall into two major categories: stimulus presentation and stimulus withdrawal. We describe specific procedures under these categories.

Stimulus Presentation

Responses may be reduced by *presenting a stimulus immediately after a response is made.* Research has shown that several response-contingent stimuli (stimuli delivered soon after a response is made) can reduce behaviors. Stimuli that reduce behaviors are *corrective.*

Most frequently used corrective stimuli are verbal. Such verbal stimuli as "No," "Wrong," and "Not correct" can reduce behaviors if presented immediately after the production of an incorrect response. Most clinicians indicate to the client in some way that a given attempt to produce the target response was not acceptable. The indication may be more or less subtle. The clinician may shake his or her head in a disapproving manner, show other facial or hand gestures of disapproval, or use explicit verbal stimuli. In all cases, the clinician will have used stimulus presentation as the method of reducing the undesirable response.

Verbal corrective stimuli (such as "No" or "Wrong") by themselves may not be effective in reducing a behavior. They may be especially ineffective in reducing generally disruptive behaviors (e.g., crying, leaving the chair, or paying no attention). However, when combined with strong reinforcers for desirable behaviors that are shaped in carefully designed incremental steps, verbal stimuli may be sufficient to reduce undesirable behaviors. For instance, clinicians who say "Not correct" for incorrect productions of phonemes also say "Good job!" for correct productions that they shape in small incremental steps. Clinicians who fail to give any kind of corrective feedback for incorrect responses will find the client's errors persisting.

How to Use Stimulus Presentation to Reduce Behaviors

1. *Present the verbal stimulus soon after the response is made.* To do this, you must make quick evaluations of the correctness of client responses.

2. *Present the verbal stimulus in a firm and objective manner.* Say "no" in such a manner to reinforce that you mean it. You should not sound unsure. The message, not necessarily the voice, must be clear and loud.

3. *Use an objective tone devoid of emotionality.* Do not use an angry or otherwise emotionally laden tone. Being a professional, you should not give an emotional reaction to incorrect response.

4. *Vary the words you use.* Do not use the same "No" or "Wrong" throughout an entire session.

Stimulus Withdrawal

Immediately after a response is made, *you may withdraw a stimulus that presumably maintains or increases that response.* While you present stimuli that weaken a response (e.g., saying "No" to a wrong response), you *withdraw* stimuli that reinforce it (e.g., taking a token away when a wrong response is made). In reducing undesirable responses, stimulus withdrawal may be more effective than stimulus presentation.

There are three specific procedures of stimulus withdrawal: time-out, response cost, and extinction. In all three, reinforcing events or consequences are withdrawn or made unavailable immediately following a wrong response or at the earliest sign of that response.

Time-Out

A frequently used method of behavior reduction is time-out from reinforcement. **Time-out** is a period of time during which all reinforcing events are suspended contingent on response and, as a result, there typically is a decrease in the rate of that response.

The clinically useful forms of time-out include exclusion and nonexclusion time-out. In **exclusion time-out,** the child is excluded from the current setting and the stream of activities. For example, you might ask a child to sit in the corner the instant he or she exhibits an undesirable behavior. All activities are terminated; the child is told to sit quietly. In this case, the setting is changed from the regular seating place to the corner. This is exclusion time-out.

In **nonexclusion time-out,** an undesirable behavior is followed immediately by cessation of all activity, but there is no physical movement and there is no change in the setting. For example, in stuttering treatment, you signal the client to stop talking for 5 seconds as soon as you observe a dysfluency or stutter. You avoid eye contact for the duration. At the end of the duration, you signal the person to resume talking. In this case, it is presumed that talking is reinforcing and interruption and silence are aversive. This aversive consequence presumably reduces the behavior on which it is made contingent. As you can see, nonexclusion time-out is time-out from the ongoing activity only; the person is not removed from the immediate setting and the activity is the presumed reinforcer.

Many research studies have shown that time-out can reduce several forms of undesirable behavior. Unfortunately, time-out is also most often misused. Careless use of time-out may have a paradoxical effect on behavior: The behavior might increase in frequency. This is likely to happen when the time-in period and setting are not reinforcing and the time-out duration and setting are. *Avoid the following conditions under which time-out may increase the undesirable behavior.*

1. *Time-out provides unintended negative reinforcement.* An uncooperative behavior may bring relief from aversive treatment trials. For instance, as soon as fussing begins, you send the child to the corner. But this action terminated difficult treatment trials, which were the cause of fussing (just what the child ordered, one might say). Consequently, the child's fussing behavior is negatively reinforced. When you resume treatment, the child may exhibit the undesirable behavior with added strength, because this is how he or she can terminate treatment trials. Often, treatment is aversive because the selected target behavior is too difficult for the child. The desirable behaviors do not increase and you say "No" to the child all too frequently because of wrong responses.

2. *Time-out provides unintended positive reinforcement.* During time-out, the child may pull a small toy from his or her pocket and begin to play. A picture on the wall may provide positive reinforcement when you send the child to a corner. When asked to sit outside a classroom or treatment room, the child may enjoy watching people walking by or some activity going on outside. These events may positively reinforce the child's undesirable behavior because it is only through those behaviors that the child gets to watch reinforcing stimuli or outside activities. As soon as treatment is resumed, you may see an especially strong display of the undesirable behavior. Obviously, this troublesome behavior is the ticket to outside fun.

Advantages of Time-out Prudently and sparingly used, time-out has many advantages. Compared to several other response reduction procedures, time-out is only mildly aversive. It is not a difficult procedure to learn and use. Brief time-out periods do not waste much teaching time. Therefore, consider using time-out to reduce undesirable behaviors in your client.

How to Use Time-out

1. *Avoid too brief or too long durations of time-out.* Durations that are too long may be ineffective, because they may allow opportunities for other behaviors and take valuable time away from treatment. An appropriate duration depends on the nature of the behavior to be reduced. In reducing stuttering, for example, 5- to 10-second durations may be effective; longer durations are unnecessary. In controlling more global uncooperative, destructive, or inattentive behaviors, longer durations may be necessary. In most speech and language treatment sessions, the duration would not exceed 5 minutes.

2. *Avoid exclusion time-out, as it is the least desirable procedure.* Do not use it unless you have tried nonexclusion time-out, extinction, response cost, and other procedures first and have found them ineffective.

3. *Signal the beginning of the nonexclusion time-out with a stimulus.* For example, you may raise your index finger to signal to a stuttering person that a 5-second time-out has begun and that speech must be terminated. In exclusion time-out, a young child may be guided physically to a time-out area without any signal. But in all cases, either a verbal statement or a nonhuman sound such as a buzzer should announce the end of the time-out period.

4. *Avoid physical contact in administering exclusion time-out.* If the child complies with your instruction to go to the time-out area, do not use

(continues)

physical contact. Ask the child to go to the designated area and stay there until the end of the time-out period. Physically guide the child to the area only when the child does not comply.

5. *Use time-out on a continuous schedule.* Impose time-out on every instance of an undesirable behavior. Do not use an intermittent schedule, especially in the beginning of the response-reduction program. Intermittent scheduling may be useful in later stages of training when the undesirable behavior is of low frequency and you wish to keep it that way.

6. *Remove all reinforcers from the time-out area.* When you use exclusion time-out, the area to which you send the child to spend the time-out should not contain reinforcing objects, people, or events. For instance, do not ask the child to sit in a hallway full of people and events. Failure to follow this rule is the main reason why sending a child to his or her own room for misbehaving usually is ineffective. Typically, a child's room is full of reinforcers.

7. *Release the client from time-out only when the undesirable behavior has been stopped.* If the child continues to fuss in the corner, extend the time-out until the child becomes calm.

8. *Enrich the treatment situation with powerful and varied reinforcers.* Time-out is more effective when the return to the teaching situation is highly reinforcing and the time-out situation is dreary and unreinforcing. You will be in serious trouble if the situations are reversed.

Note that time-out will not reduce all behaviors in all clients. Besides, you should constantly watch for paradoxical effects. When you observe even a slight increase in the undesirable behavior being subjected to time-out, you should find an alternative procedure to reduce that behavior.

Response Cost

A procedure of reducing behaviors through response-contingent withdrawal of tangible reinforcers is called **response cost.** The client must give up a reinforcer every time an undesirable response is made.

Time-out and response cost are similar in that both deprive the client of some reinforcers. But their procedures are different. In time-out, you arrange a brief duration of no reinforcement of any kind; during this time, there is no responding; the person may even be moved to another scene that lacks reinforcers. In response cost, you take away a specific, tangible, reinforcer the client has earned or has been given; there is no particular interruption of responses; the client does not move physically; and it is not a duration of time devoid of reinforcers.

Response cost is implemented most effectively and efficiently in a *token system.* **Tokens** are presented and withdrawn depending on the behavior. At the end of a treatment session, the remaining tokens are exchanged for a **backup reinforcer,** usually a small gift in the case of children.

Response cost may be either the lose-only type or earn-and-lose type. In the **lose-only type,** you give the client a certain number of tokens at the beginning of a session. These tokens are not contingent on desirable behaviors; therefore, the client does not earn them. During the treatment sessions, you withdraw a token for every undesirable response. You also may reinforce the desirable responses with verbal praise and other such social reinforcers that you cannot take back.

In the earn-and-lose type of response cost, all tokens are contingent on desirable behaviors. That is, the client must earn them by exhibiting desirable behaviors. While earning them, the client also loses a token for every instance of an undesirable behavior. In this case, both the desirable and the undesirable behaviors evoke the token contingency.

Either the lose-only or the earn-and-lose method may be used individually or in small groups. When used with groups, any individual's undesirable behavior will cost the group a token. The group earns tokens only when all members exhibit the desirable behavior.

Like all other response-reduction procedures, response cost may be ineffective or may increase the rate of undesirable response under certain conditions. *Avoid the following problems in designing a response-cost system.*

1. *Low token loss preceded by high loss may be ineffective.* Typically, you withdraw one token per undesirable response. But in some cases, to make it work, you may have to withdraw multiple tokens per response. If you do this, you should not start with a high number and then go down. For instance, you should not first take away five tokens per undesirable response and then only two. The reduced token loss condition may be ineffective.

2. *The client may run out of tokens.* If that happens, there is nothing to lose and you do not have response cost to reduce the behavior.

3. *Loss of tokens may cause emotional responses.* If such responses do not subside quickly, use another method of response reduction. You should not carry the method to a point where you struggle with the client to take tokens away or that the child is in tears.

4. *The undesirable behavior may increase because of attention.* When you take a token away, you also pay immediate, contingent attention to the undesirable response. If the response increases, use another procedure.

Advantages of Response Cost Along with time-out, response cost is a widely researched method of reducing undesirable behaviors. It is known to be very effective, socially acceptable, and less aversive than some of the other methods of behavior reduction.

How to Use Response Cost

1. *Prefer the earn-and-lose method to lose-only method.* This method allows you to systematically reinforce correct and cooperative behaviors through tokens earned, while reducing undesirable behaviors through tokens lost.

2. *Give more tokens than you take back.* To this end, simplify the target response and shape it, if necessary. The child should experience more success (reinforcers) than failures (token loss). At the end of the session, the child should be left with some tokens to be exchanged for backup reinforcers.

3. *Withdraw tokens promptly.* There should be no delay between the undesirable response and token withdrawal.

4. *Increase the number of tokens withdrawn per response only if necessary.* Do this when a single or fewer token withdrawals are not effective. But do not decrease the number of tokens withdrawn.

5. *Avoid client indebtedness.* If you find yourself withdrawing enough tokens to result in client debt, switch to another response reduction method.

6. *Control potential emotional problems.* Any emotional response will be evident on the first token withdrawal. If this happens, reverse the roles for a few minutes. Let the child be the clinician who withdraws tokens for your wrong responses. For example, assume that the child who stutters gets suddenly upset when you withdraw the first token contingent on stuttering. You can then say, "Hey, you know what? I too have bumpy speech sometimes! You want to take a token away from me?" The child is usually delighted to do this. Keep a few tokens for yourself, exhibit a few dysfluencies, and ask the child to withdraw one for each of your dysfluencies. This strategy is effective in controlling emotional responses. When you return to the procedure, the child is likely to accept it.

As with any response-reduction procedure, watch for excessive and uncontrollable emotional responses and paradoxical increase in undesirable behaviors. Always be prepared to use another response-reduction procedure.

Extinction

The procedure of simply withholding the consequences that reinforce a behavior is called **extinction.** Note that extinction is not a punishment procedure, yet response cost and time-out are. But all three procedures have the same effect on the behavior: reduced frequency. We have grouped extinction along with response cost and time-out to point out that in all three, the locus of contingency management is the undesirable behavior. Though the three procedures are direct compared to procedures that reduce undesirable behaviors by increasing desirable ones, extinction of *positively reinforced behaviors* is less direct than response cost and time-out. But the extinction of *negatively reinforced behavior*, as you will find out shortly, is a direct procedure.

Extinction is a *do-nothing-procedure*. When nobody does anything to sustain a behavior, it will weaken and eventually disappear. It weakens a response by removing reinforcing consequences. Therefore, you can use this procedure only when the behavior to be reduced is either positively or negatively reinforced. Your functional analysis baselines might suggest that the behavior is indeed maintained by these kinds of reinforcement.

Children's *uncooperative behaviors* are prime targets for extinction. Such interfering behaviors as crying, fussing, frequent verbal requests to go to the bathroom or see the parent waiting outside, irrelevant talking (the "You know what?" type of interruptions), and many other similar behaviors are maintained by clinician's unintended reinforcement. The reinforcement may be positive or negative. The clinician may positively reinforce repeated verbal requests to go to the bathroom by paying attention. But leaving the treatment room for the bathroom is a negatively reinforced behavior. The child who leaves the treatment room terminates unwanted treatment. This is negative reinforcement. Note that if the child begins to leave the treatment room, you cannot just ignore the behavior. You need to prevent escape, thus depriving the child of negative reinforcement. *Prevention of escape* is sometimes described as **escape extinction** (Iwata et al., 1990). This procedure implies that extinction is not always a passive or indirect procedure.

Advantages of Extinction Used correctly, extinction is an effective method of reducing undesirable behaviors. Consider it for reducing crying, undesirable interruptions, and similar problem behaviors.

How to Use Extinction

1. *Discuss the problem and the extinction procedure with the parents.* Some parents may be alarmed to see you sitting still when their 3-year-old child is loudly and tearfully crying "Mommy!" If they understand what you are doing and why, they may tolerate the procedure. Extinction is slow and unpleasant for both the child and for those who administer it or watch it.

(continues)

2. *Find out what reinforces the undesirable behavior.* Try to find out if the behavior is reinforced positively, negatively, or with a combination of the two. Also, find out if the behavior is reinforced independent of what you do. For example, a child who leaves the chair and goes to the chalkboard to scribble may be reinforced independently of your actions. Also, the child is reinforced negatively (escaping from your teaching) and positively (scribbling on the chalkboard). In this case, even if you avoid all interactions with the child to eliminate reinforcement, the behavior still may persist because of negative and positive reinforcement.

3. *Remove positive reinforcers inherent to your actions promptly and fully.* Withdraw all attention from undesirable behavior. Avoid eye contact; sit motionless. Be firm, wait it out; do not change anything. For example, once you initiate extinction for crying behavior, do not lecture, do not admonish, do not cajole, do not try to charm the child, do not try to talk the child out of crying, do not reorganize the materials on the table.

4. *Remove positive reinforcers that are unrelated to your actions.* If the child on the floor begins to play with a toy, look at pictures, examine your bag, and so forth, remove the objects promptly and then sit motionless.

5. *Remove negative reinforcers as promptly and fully as possible.* Prevent the child from leaving the seat, walking around, or walking out of the treatment room. Do not stop treatment because the child asks interrupting questions. Do not answer such questions as "Do you know what?" If you answer such questions, you will have positively reinforced such interruptive questioning and negatively reinforced the escape behavior that terminates your teaching.

6. *Do not terminate the extinction procedure when you see an extinction burst,* which is a temporary increase in the rate of a response when extinction is initiated. It often scares the clinician, who quickly turns attention to the client. Do not do this. Continue to withhold reinforcers by sitting motionless and the behavior will eventually subside.

7. *Reinforce desirable behaviors promptly and lavishly.* For example, the instant the child stops crying or fussing, you should smile, hug the child, wipe the tears, praise, give a token, and reinforce the child in other ways. Make the desirable behavior pay off better for the child than the undesirable behavior.

A Word of Caution *Behaviors that are reinforced automatically and those that are destructive or aggressive are not candidates for extinction.* You cannot ignore a self-stimulatory behavior (e.g., rocking by a child with autism), self-injurious behavior (e.g., self-biting by a child with autism), or an aggressive or destructive behavior (e.g., hitting others or destroying property) and expect the behavior to diminish. Such behaviors are automatically reinforced by their sensory consequences. Aggressive and destructive behaviors carry their own reinforcers: Injury to others and destruction of property will reinforce the troublesome behaviors. Therefore, extinction will be ineffective. Do not use extinction to reduce these behaviors.

Indirect Strategy for Decreasing Behaviors

In the direct strategies of stimulus presentation and stimulus withdrawal (extinction, time-out, and response cost), the clinician places the treatment contingency directly on the undesirable behavior to reduce its frequency. To the contrary, in the *indirect strategy, desirable behaviors replace the undesirable behaviors.* You do not place a treatment contingency on the undesirable behavior at all. This approach is so indirect that you do nothing specific to the behavior to be reduced.

The main feature of the indirect strategy is that you reinforce desirable behaviors, increase them, and, as a consequence, decrease the undesirable behaviors. In a sense, you use reinforcement to control undesirable behaviors; by reinforcing desirable behaviors, you weaken undesirable behaviors. But as noted before, you should never make the mistake of saying that "I use reinforcement to decrease undesirable behaviors." Reinforcement only can increase behaviors. *When you use reinforcing procedures, the behavioral reduction is a by-product.* Undesirable behaviors decrease only because other behaviors increase. Therefore, you might say that "I use reinforcement to increase some behaviors so that other behaviors are decreased."

The use of reinforcement to increase some behaviors while other behaviors decrease as a result is known as **differential reinforcement** (Cooper, 2007; Hegde, 1998a, 2008b; Malott & Trojan, 2008). The term *differential* suggests that it is not the straightforward reinforcement of some behavior. There is a *differential* effect of the reinforcement procedure. Although some behaviors increase because of the reinforcement, others decrease as a by-product. This is the meaning of differential reinforcement.

There are several differential reinforcement procedures to help you increase some behaviors that can have a concurrent effect of reducing other behaviors. The difference between some of them is subtle and probably not crucial. But if you understand the difference, you will be a sophisticated user of response reduction procedures. The following four differential reinforcement procedures are important: **differential reinforcement of other behavior (DRO), differential reinforcement of incompatible behavior (DRI), differential reinforcement of alternative behavior (DRA),** and **differential reinforcement of low rates of responding (DRL).** All of these increase certain behaviors and thereby decrease certain other behaviors.

Differential Reinforcement of Other Behavior (DRO)

In this procedure, you *reinforce a child for not exhibiting a specified undesirable behavior for a particular duration.* For example, you may reinforce a child for not wiggling in the chair for 2 minutes. If the child desists in the behavior for that entire duration, you may give the child a token. Gradually, you can increase the duration for which the child should refrain from the undesirable behavior. A child who frequently interrupts you during treatment may be asked not to do it for a period of several minutes. The child is then reinforced for compliance. A verbally or physically aggressive child may be told that he or she will receive a token if aggressive behaviors stop for a certain duration.

The examples of DRO show that what is reinforced is *left open*. The procedure does not require a particular desirable behavior to earn reinforcers. The child need not do anything in particular to get reinforcement; he or she must simply refrain from doing something (the specified undesirable behavior). To earn a reinforcer, a child simply should avoid the troublesome behavior. An aggressive or hyperactive child, for example, may sit quietly for the specified duration to earn reinforcers. But the child may also read, color, work on mathematical problems, or put puzzles together to earn the reinforcer. You look for these and many other forms of acceptable behaviors, none specified ahead of time, to reinforce. Any one of several desirable behaviors and the omission of the specified undesirable behavior results in reinforcement.

Differential Reinforcement of Incompatible Behavior (DRI)

In this procedure, you *reinforce behaviors that are incompatible with the undesirable behavior*. Unlike the DRO, in which no specific desirable behavior is required, a behavior that is topographically incompatible with the undesirable behavior is required in DRI and reinforced when it occurs. A child who is verbally abusive may be reinforced for nonabusive, socially acceptable verbal expressions. A child who snatches toys from other children may be reinforced for giving his or her toy to playmates.

Note that the described abusive actions are *incompatible* with socially acceptable actions in that both cannot be produced at the same time. Snatching and sharing or wandering around or sitting quietly cannot occur simultaneously. Therefore, when the desirable behavior is increased with reinforcement, the incompatible undesirable behavior should decrease. To use DRI, you must find a response that cannot coexist with the undesirable behavior and target that for reinforcement.

Differential Reinforcement of Alternative Behavior (DRA)

In this procedure, you *specify and reinforce a behavior that is an alternative to the undesirable behavior*. Note that an alternative desirable behavior is not necessarily incompatible with the undesirable behavior to be reduced. In DRA, the desirable behavior is just an alternative to, but not incompatible with, the undesirable behavior. For example, you may find out that a child often is disruptive because of lack of academic or social skills. In this case, you may target specific reading or writing skills and adaptive social skills that the child will enjoy more than the disruptive behaviors.

One drawback with the DRA procedure is that because the desirable behavior is not incompatible with the undesirable behavior, both may be exhibited.

While learning better academic and social skills, the child may continue to disrupt. In such cases, it is necessary to teach behaviors that are incompatible with the undesirable behavior. For instance, reinforcing the child to sit quietly for periods of time would be incompatible with disruptive behavior.

Differential Reinforcement of Low Rates of Responding (DRL)

In this procedure, you *reinforce the child when the frequency of undesirable behavior is below the baseline level*. In DRL, you shape the undesirable response down until it is eliminated or reduced to a manageable level. The procedure gradually reduces the behavior. For example, you find out that during treatment sessions, a child asks, "Are we done yet?" once every 2 to 3 minutes. You can then set a criterion of no more than two interruptions in a 10-minute interval. Normally, the child would have interrupted some three to five times during this interval. You can reinforce the child if during the previous 10 minutes the child had interrupted you only two times or less. In using this procedure, you must make sure that you do not reinforce the child soon after an interruption.

Differential reinforcement, especially the DRO, DRI, and the DRA, are procedures that help you replace undesirable behavior with desirable behaviors. In these procedures, while reinforcing desirable behaviors, you make sure that you do not reinforce undesirable behaviors. Therefore, a common theme of these procedures is that (a) the client gains access to reinforcing affairs through desirable behaviors; (b) the undesirable behaviors do not get reinforced anymore; (c) consequently, the undesirable behaviors do not serve the client as they did before; and, therefore, (d) the desirable behaviors replace the undesirable behaviors.

Other Indirect Procedures

Two other indirect procedures that may be used include behavioral momentum and the presentation of a sudden, surprising stimulus. These newer techniques can be effective with many children who exhibit undesirable behaviors or who are unlikely to produce the target behaviors with modeling and shaping.

Behavioral momentum is a procedure in which the *force* of a behavior in progress causes another behavior that may not otherwise be exhibited. In using behavior momentum, you first ask the client to do what he or she is likely to do; as soon as this behavior occurs and it is reinforced, you ask the client to repeatedly and rapidly perform an action that he or she is not likely to perform. The unlikely behavior may be performed because of the force (momentum) of the previous, readily exhibited behavior.

This method has been used to reduce noncompliant behaviors (Mace et al., 1988). For example, assume that a girl does not comply with your request to look at the stimulus picture used in training words. Also assume that she readily will clap her hands when asked to. Then, you could ask her to clap two or three times in succession and immediately ask her to look at the picture. She may then immediately look at the picture. Note that when picture-attending behavior increases, the noncompliance behavior will have decreased. You decreased noncompliance behavior by behavior momentum.

Surprising stimulus presentation also can terminate or prevent an undesirable behavior. A study has shown that sudden loud noise can terminate undesirable behaviors (Charlop, Burgio, Iwata, & Ivancic, 1988). But you may prevent undesirable behaviors by anticipating them and then presenting a sudden and surprising stimulus. For example, a child's imminent crying may be prevented if you suddenly and dramatically pull out a clown or an animated toy just before the crying is about to erupt. You suddenly may turn on the radio, get up from the chair, pull something from a box, or behave in some dramatic fashion. Stimuli that appear so suddenly and dramatically tend to inhibit certain undesirable behaviors.

To prevent undesirable behaviors by sudden stimulus presentation, you must watch the client closely to detect early signs of trouble. The surprising stimulus or action must be presented *before* the response onset; if not, you may reinforce the undesirable response.

Stimuli that terminate undesirable behaviors are aversives; but those that prevent such behaviors are positive reinforcers. For instance, you say "no" to an undesirable behavior that is promptly terminated. The verbal "no" is an aversive stimulus. To the contrary, when you prevent an imminent crying response by suddenly pulling out a clown from your bag, you provoke an incompatible response of surprise, curiosity, and so forth. The sudden appearance of the clown is a positive reinforcer. Be clear about this distinction.

General Guidelines for Reducing Undesirable Behaviors

We have described several procedures of response reduction. Although each of them may reduce responses, you should not think of using an isolated procedure in reducing or increasing behaviors. You must design a comprehensive program of contingency management involving reinforcement for the desirable responses, withdrawal of reinforcers for the undesirable responses, presentation of response reduction consequences for the undesirable behaviors, and others. A combined procedure that simultaneously shapes and reinforces a desirable behavior while withdrawing reinforcers from the undesirable behaviors and presenting them with other response reduction consequences will be the most effective (Hegde, 1998a, 2008c).

Designing an Effective Response Reduction Strategy

Take the following steps in designing an effective response reduction strategy involving multiple contingencies or procedures.

1. *Use only extinction to avoid the use of all other response reduction procedures.* If the undesirable behavior is not frequent enough to disrupt the treatment process, continue to reinforce the desirable behavior and ignore the undesirable behavior. Use one of the response reduction procedures only when this strategy fails to bring the undesirable behavior under a manageable

level. For example, if reinforcement of correct articulation is doing the job, ignore the incorrect productions. However, if the incorrect productions persist, introduce a more active response reduction procedure (verbal "No," response cost, or time-out).

2. *Use procedures that help prevent undesirable responses.* Model the correct response until the client's productions stabilize. You then would not have to use the response reduction procedures, because the client is successful. Prompt the correct response when the client hesitates; such hesitations may signal an imminent wrong response, and you can prevent this by prompting the correct response.

3. *Define clearly and narrowly both the undesirable behavior to be reduced and the desirable behavior to be increased.* For instance, *distorted productions of /s/* is a more clearly and narrowly defined response than *problems of articulation.* Conversely, *production of correct /s/* is a better definition than *improved articulatory skills.* Similarly, *production of part-word repetitions* (and other specific types of dysfluency types) is a more clearly and narrowly defined behavior than *stuttering moment.* Also, *reduced speech rate through syllable prolongation* is a better definition than *controlled rate of speech.* Use response reduction procedures only when you have such clearly defined behaviors on which you can place response contingencies.

4. *Differentially reinforce a desirable behavior that is incompatible with the undesirable behavior (DRI).* For instance, in-seat behavior is incompatible with out-of-seat behavior; any form of cooperative behavior does not coexist with uncooperative behavior; attention replaces inattention; smiling and crying are opposite behaviors. To make the response reduction procedure less aversive, reinforce the incompatible desirable response. When you do this, you will simultaneously increase a desirable behavior and decrease an undesirable behavior. This action will help limit the use of aversive response reduction procedures and minimize the aversiveness of the procedure used.

5. *Differentially reinforce a desirable behavior that will secure for the client what the undesirable behavior seems to secure (DRA).* Technically, this means that you teach a desirable behavior that is *functionally equivalent* to the behavior to be reduced (Carr & Durand, 1985). If it looks like the child is crawling under the table to get your attention, then provide lavish attention to quiet sitting in the chair. Children who are minimally verbal or those who are nonverbal may fuss often because that is the only way they can get their wants satisfied. Teaching mands (requests, demands) may reduce such inappropriate behaviors.

6. *Differentially reinforce the client for reducing the rate of the undesirable behavior (DRL).* If you see systematic reduction in the undesirable behavior, reinforce the child while that behavior is not being exhibited. For example, you might tell a child that he wiggled only once during the last 5 minutes and reinforce when he sits without wiggling.

7. *Differentially reinforce the client for simply omitting the undesirable behavior and for producing any of the many acceptable behaviors (DRO).* For example, in a group, praise a disruptive child for not being disruptive; such praise and other reinforcers may be made contingent on many and unspecified desirable behaviors.

8. *Use varied consequences to reduce a response* (Charlop et al., 1988). Do not use one type of response consequence constantly. For example, in the same treatment sessions, alternate the use of verbal "no," response cost, time-out, and other consequences that reduce the response rate. Similarly, use varied reinforcers to increase the desirable behavior that will replace the undesirable behavior (Egel, 1981). Verbal praise, tokens backed with many reinforcers, frequent feedback on response accuracy, and opportunities for exhibiting high probability behaviors all may be used in a single session.

9. *Use an interfering response to reinforce correct responses* (Charlop, Kurtz, Casey, & Greenberg, 1990). For example, a child frequently may leave the seat to go to the chalkboard and scribble on it. Instead of trying to suppress this interfering behavior with a verbal "no"and such other means, you can make short durations of drawing or writing on the chalkboard contingent on sitting for a few minutes and giving correct responses. You will then have turned an annoying, interfering behavior into a reinforcer of desirable target behaviors.

10. *Use behavioral momentum to decrease certain undesirable behaviors.* Repeatedly and rapidly evoke a likely behavior, reinforce it, and immediately demand the production of the unlikely target behavior. Reinforce its occurrence as well.

11. *Simplify the target skills to eliminate escape from therapeutic work you demand of the client.* Some children crawl under a table, leave their seat, or look away from you because they find the treatment aversive. By their undesirable behaviors, children escape from therapy or instruction (Carr & Durand, 1985; Iwata, 1987; Iwata et al., 1990). Treatment may be aversive to clients for many reasons, but the most frequent reason is that the task is too difficult and the child receives too much corrective feedback and too little reinforcement. Then simplify the task. Shape the target behavior in small steps so that the child is more successful and, hence, receives reinforcement more often than corrective feedback.

12. *Use a strong, sudden, and surprising stimulus to terminate or prevent an undesirable behavior.* Try to terminate an undesirable behavior by presenting a surprising stimulus. Try to prevent the occurrence of an undesirable response by presenting the surprising stimulus as soon as you anticipate its occurrence.

13. *Use a continuous schedule.* Make sure every instance of an undesirable behavior is followed by the response reduction procedure you have selected. Whether it is response cost, time-out, or verbal stimuli, apply it continuously.

14. *Present or withdraw consequences immediately.* Do not hesitate, wait, or be slow in responding to the undesirable response.

15. *Do not allow escape from the response-reduction procedure.* A crying child being purposely ignored should not get out of the treatment room only to be consoled by the parent waiting outside. This will positively reinforce the crying behavior. Similarly, clients under other response-reduction procedures should not be allowed to leave the treatment scene. If they are, the clients will escape from treatment and get negative reinforcement. (Contrast this with #9; these two are different concepts.)

16. *Apply the response-reduction procedure at the earliest sign of the undesirable response.* Do not wait until the undesirable response is completed to apply the procedure. Suppose you wish to reduce a child's behavior of leaving the chair. You should not wait to say "no" until after the child has left the chair and is on the floor. The best time to say "no" (assuming it will be effective) is when you see the slightest movement of the child that suggests an imminent response. In using time-out for stuttering, you should not wait until an instance of stuttering has been completed. Instead, you must watch for the earliest signs of stuttering and apply the procedure.

17. *Dissociate response-reduction procedures from those that reinforce responses.* You should not deliver reinforcers along with or in proximity with response-reduction procedures. If you do and if it so happens that the reinforcers are stronger than the response reduction procedures, you will have reinforced the undesirable behavior. Some clinicians say "wrong," but immediately smile, touch, or hug the child. These positive responses from the clinician may neutralize the effects of "wrong" or even reinforce the undesirable response.

18. *Minimize the duration of response-reduction procedures.* Time-out should be brief. No response reduction procedure should be applied for too long. If it looks like you have to, you are not using an effective treatment procedure. Maybe you have a wrong or extremely difficult target for the child; maybe you do not have effective reinforcers to increase the desirable behavior; perhaps you are not administering treatment contingencies properly. Analyze your procedures to make them more effective. If you cannot figure it out, talk to your supervisor, but do not continue with the response reduction procedure.

19. *Remove reinforcers that maintain undesirable behaviors.* If you see the child constantly reaching for your bag on the table, do not continue to reprimand the child; instead, remove the bag and keep it out of the child's reach and sight. See what reinforces the undesirable behavior. If it is something that can be eliminated, do so immediately.

20. *Expose the client to more reinforcing consequences than to response-reduction consequences.* Overall, treatment sessions should be much more reinforcing (fun)

than aversive to the child. You should be giving more tokens than you withdraw; you should be praising the child more frequently than you reprimand. Of course, to do this, you should be using procedures that help shape the target behaviors.

Aversive Nature of Response-Reduction Procedures

Response-reduction procedures are aversive not only to clients but also to clinicians. No clinician enjoys applying aversive procedures. Prudent and limited use of response reduction procedures that are only minimally aversive, socially acceptable, and do not involve emotional or physical harm often are necessary in treatment programs. Careless use of aversive procedures can create negative side effects including strong and persistent emotional responses in the clients. See Hegde (1998a) for a more detailed discussion of the negative side effects of response-reduction procedures and ways of minimizing such side effects.

We have argued that in all treatment sessions, the emphasis should be on positive reinforcement procedures. You should design treatment procedures to avoid response-reduction procedures; if this is not possible, the need should be minimal.

Always think of simplifying the desirable target response; find an effective reinforcer for it; target alternative, other, or incompatible responses that will then increase, and will decrease the undesirable behavior. See if extinction will work before you apply procedures that are more aversive. At the end of the session, count the number of positive reinforcers and response-reducing consequences that you delivered. If you have not applied reinforcing consequences more often than the response-reduction consequences, critically evaluate your treatment procedures. Possibly, the reinforcers you have selected are not functional; the target behavior is too difficult for the client; the wrong responses are still somehow getting reinforced; you are not modeling the target responses as often as necessary; and you have not targeted alternative, incompatible, desirable responses for reinforcement. Discuss these and other possibilities with your clinical supervisor. Remember always that frequent use of response-reduction procedures suggests that something is wrong. Your goal is to avoid response-reduction procedures, if possible; this requires the most effective way of structuring your treatment program and use of the most powerful positive reinforcers.

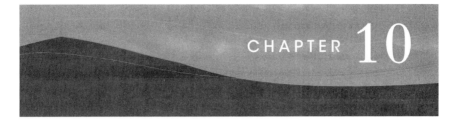

CHAPTER 10

Maintenance of Target Behaviors

Chapter Outline

- Maintenance of Target Behaviors in Natural Settings
- Maintenance Procedures
- Developing Home Treatment Programs
- Follow-up Assessments

You soon will find in your clinical practicum that promoting maintenance of target behaviors in natural settings and over time is a more challenging job than establishing them in the first place. Therefore, you must pay at least as much attention to response maintenance strategies as you do to their establishment strategies. For example, with persons who stutter, you may have to work harder on fluency maintenance than on establishment.

You often will read that generalization is the final goal of treatment. When a child who learns to produce certain phonemes in the clinic fails to produce them at home, you are told that the *correct production did not generalize.* Therefore, you are asked to *program generalization* before you dismiss a client.

A critical look at generalization shows that it should not be the final goal of treatment. **Generalization** is a declining rate of response when untrained stimuli are presented and reinforcers are withheld (Hegde, 1998a). Generalized but *unreinforced* responses are *extinguished.* Therefore, if generalization is the final target, we will have to assume that a declining rate of response is the final goal of treatment. No clinician assumes this. Instead, you are told to have parents and others *reinforce* generalized responses produced at home and other nonclinical settings. This action leads to a contradictory conclusion that generalized responses are reinforced responses. If so, generalization must be redefined as reinforced responses. There is then no difference between treatment and generalization strategies. Therefore, to avoid all these contradictions, we emphasize that generalization is not the final objective of clinical intervention.

Maintenance of Target Behaviors in Natural Settings

The *final treatment goal is maintenance* of target behaviors. The clinically established communicative behaviors must be produced in conversational speech, in the natural environment, and must be sustained over time. Behaviors that generate favorable consequences are likely to be maintained. If the client reliably produces the behaviors in the clinic but not at home and other settings, then we must have people in those settings do some of the things the clinician did to establish those behaviors. We achieve this by designing a maintenance strategy.

A **maintenance strategy** is an extension of treatment to natural settings (Hegde, 1998a). The main task in implementing a maintenance strategy is to teach people in the life of the client to support and sustain target behaviors. A significant part of the strategy also is to teach the client to manage his or her own behaviors. Therefore, the key players in the maintenance strategy are the clients and people who interact with them.

Maintenance Procedures

To promote maintenance, you must *extend treatment to natural settings*, but there is little that is substantially new in the maintenance techniques themselves. What is new about the strategy is that the clinician must train others in contingency management at home and at other nonclinical settings.

Treatment strategy changes the client's behavior, but the maintenance strategy changes the behavior of people around the client. If people in the client's life continue to behave in their usual manner, the client may not maintain the target responses. For example, you may have taught a nonverbal child certain words that the child reliably produces in the clinic. But at home, the child continues to point to things he or she wants and the parents continue to give what the child pointed to. As a result, the newly established words are not produced or maintained at home. To have the child request things with words, the parents have to stop reinforcing the pointing behavior and require and reinforce word productions. Therefore, to implement a maintenance strategy, you should learn to work with parents, spouses, siblings, friends, teachers, and colleagues of the client so that they react differently to the client.

Recall that in Chapter 8, *treatment* in communicative disorders was defined as a *rearrangement of a communicative relationship between the client and his or her listeners*. You, the clinician, were the initial listener in rearranging that communicative relationship. The final listeners are the people surrounding the client. In both cases, listeners help change the behavior of the client. Although you know how to change the client's (speaker's) behavior, other listeners do not. To help them learn the techniques of changing the behavior of their particular speaker (your client) is the heart of maintenance strategy.

By training the people in the client's life to manage the reinforcement contingencies, you will be shifting the target behavior control from yourself to others. You also will be shifting the location of response control from the clinic to at least a few natural settings. The basic idea here is that like treatment, response maintenance also is a management procedure.

In addition to shifting response control to others, you must take a few other steps as well. Maintenance is a consideration even when you select and teach the target behaviors. As the target behaviors are produced more reliably in the clinical setting, you initiate other, more crucial procedures of response maintenance. Therefore, in a comprehensive maintenance strategy, take the following steps (Hegde, 1998a, 2008c).

Step 1. Select Useful Behaviors

As pointed out in Chapter 7, behaviors that are useful to the client are more likely to be produced and maintained in natural settings. Communicative behaviors that serve the needs of the client are likely to receive reinforcement from others. Therefore, by selecting client-specific, meaningful, and useful behaviors, you set the stage for later maintenance strategy.

Step 2. Reinforce Target Responses in Conversational Speech

Phonemes trained only at the word and phrase levels do not tend to be frequently produced in natural settings where connected speech is expected. Certain other target behaviors, for example, skills of fluency and voice qualities, trained only at the word level, may be ineffective when the client speaks continuously in natural settings. Therefore, the target behaviors must always be reinforced in conversational speech in the final stages of treatment.

As early as possible, move treatment to conversational speech level. In the treatment of stuttering and voice disorders, move through the simpler levels of words and phrases as rapidly as you can. Spend more clinical time monitoring and reinforcing the target behaviors in conversational speech than in words or phrases. In the case of articulation disorders, reinforce the correct production of speech sounds in continuous speech. In teaching words to children with language disorders, move to phrases, sentences, and continuous speech as quickly as possible. Do the same in teaching grammatical morphemes, syntactic structures, and pragmatic features.

Step 3. Shift Reinforcement Schedules

A behavior reinforced continuously does not resist extinction as much as the one reinforced intermittently. The longer a behavior resists extinction, the greater the chance that it will come under some reinforcement contingency. This situation then will help maintain the target behavior. Therefore, after having established the target behaviors initially through continuous reinforcement, begin to reinforce on an intermittent schedule.

In gradual steps, move from a FR2 to progressively higher ratios. As you decrease the amount of reinforcement, pay close attention to response rates. You may have to lower the ratio if the response rates decline. In the final stages of treatment, when the target responses are monitored in conversational speech, reinforce only sporadically.

Step 4. Use Social and Conditioned Generalized Reinforcers

Social reinforcers are more prevalent in the natural settings. Therefore, even when you have to use primary reinforcers, pair them with social reinforcers, including verbal praise. If the same kinds of reinforcers are encountered in the clinic and natural settings, the responses are more likely to be maintained.

Besides social reinforcers, use conditioned generalized reinforcers. A token system with a variety of backup reinforcers increases the chances of similar reinforcers being encountered in the natural setting. Also, the family members may be able to implement a similar token system at home to sustain the response rates. The job of the client's family members will be easier if they can use an established system of reinforcement.

Step 5. Spread the Discriminative Stimulus Control

A discriminative stimulus is a stimulus in whose presence a response has been reinforced. As a result, the response is likely in the presence of that stimulus. Any stimulus may acquire the power to evoke a response because of its systematic association with reinforcement.

The discriminative stimulus will not continue to evoke the response for very long, if the response is not reinforced. However, an initial response in the presence of a discriminative stimulus gives the opportunity to reinforce that response to sustain it.

The most important discriminative stimuli are persons, physical stimuli, and physical settings. The clinician is the first discriminative stimulus for the target response. By systematically reinforcing the target response, the clinician comes to exert a strong control over it. Soon, the clinical setting also will come to control the target response.

Some dramatic examples illustrate the power of the clinician and the clinical setting in evoking target responses. For instance, parents often are amazed at the amount of fluency their children who stutter exhibit in front of the clinician and in the treatment room. Anywhere else, however, the children may stutter just as much as they did before treatment. The child who reliably produces words in the treatment room may continue to gesture at home. A woman's hoarseness may all but disappear when she walks into the treatment room. But just as dramatically, her typical hoarse voice may reappear as she leaves the clinic. This disappearance and reappearance of problem behaviors are due to the discriminative stimulus value of the clinician and the treatment room and lack of discriminative stimuli in non-clinical settings.

The task is to spread this discriminative stimulus control exerted almost exclusively by the clinician and the clinical setting to other people in nonclinical settings. When associated with reinforcement, other people and other settings begin to evoke target behaviors. Therefore, to spread the discriminative stimulus value:

Ask the client's family members to sit in the treatment room. If they are associated with treatment and reinforcement, the family members may acquire some power to evoke the target responses at home. Whenever possible, the parents and other members of the family should at least observe the treatment sessions. They should do this not from the unseen side of one-way mirrors, but by sitting in the treatment room. This is done to associate their presence with treatment. At this stage, family members do not reinforce or do anything else. In the latter stages of treatment, ask your friends or others who are strangers to the client to observe treatment sessions. Discuss this with parents and clients before you invite other persons to sessions because it raises the issue of confidentiality. You need the permission of adult clients and parents or guardians of minors.

Move treatment outside the treatment room. The restricted treatment room is useful and often necessary to establish target behaviors because it provides a controlled environment free of distraction. But the room is so different from a client's everyday environment that the client's learning is restricted to its confines. Therefore, when the client begins to produce the target behaviors in conversational speech, move treatment out of the treatment room. Take a walk with the client outside the clinic. Converse with the client and monitor the production of target behaviors in conversational speech.

If the client's response rate drops dramatically when you move out of the treatment room and you find it hard to control the regression, move back into the treatment room and try again later. If the client sustains responses, then progressively move to different situations. Take the client to shopping centers, restaurants, bookstores, toy stores, and other relevant places and have the client talk to people there. Follow the guidelines in carrying out this procedure:

1. **In the beginning, take the client to less-threatening situations.** You may not even ask the client to talk to any strangers the first time you two go outside the clinic. Let the client talk to you in the new environment while you monitor and reinforce the target responses.

2. **Let the client rehearse what he or she will tell a stranger in a new setting.** For example, you might have a client who stutters talk to a bookstore

clerk. What the client plans to tell the clerk should be rehearsed with your help so that he or she can speak slowly and fluently.

3. **The first few times, stay close to the client.** If needed, give a subtle signal to trigger the target response. You may touch the client's shoulder as he or she begins to speak to prompt the correct response. In the case of a man who stutters, for example, the touch may mean that he must slow down his rate.

4. **Take note of correct and incorrect productions.** Give subtle and quick reinforcement. This is important, because the strangers the clients talk to will not reinforce. It is your reinforcement in these new situations that will establish the discriminative stimulus value of those situations and listeners.

5. **Gradually increase the distance between you and your client.** As the client begins to talk to strangers, slowly move away from him or her.

6. **Take the client to progressively more difficult situations.** As the target responses are maintained in each new situation, take the client to a more difficult situation. Reinforce the client in all situations.

Step 6. Teach Others to Evoke and Consequate Target Behaviors

This technique is the heart of maintenance strategy. It must be implemented whether there is initial generalization or not. Treatment will have been extended to the natural environment, if the significant others in the client's life know (a) the exact target behaviors, (b) how to evoke them, and (c) how to enhance them. The target behaviors then have the greatest probability of being maintained.

Take the following steps in teaching others to evoke and administer consequences to target behaviors:

1. **Describe and demonstrate the target behaviors to others.** When you invite the family members and others to observe the treatment sessions, describe the target behaviors being taught. Tell them precisely what the client is expected to do. Do not use jargon. Give simple and direct descriptions. For example, while treating a child who stutters, say, "I want Johnny to talk very slowly. Perhaps as slowly as I am talking now. [Model the target rate.] Johnny should stretch his words like this. [Model a few words by prolonging the syllables.] When Johnny stretches his words, he does not stutter that much. When he practices slower speech without stuttering for a while, he can begin to speak a little faster until his speech will sound okay and he will be speaking more fluently."

   While teaching a set of basic words to a child who has a language delay, tell the parents you are teaching a few words, not a "core vocabulary." When you have to use technical terms (e.g., *present progressive* or *prepositions*), give examples. Show the parents and other members of the family a list of words, phrases, and sentences you teach the child. Give a copy of target behavior lists to parents and others.

In treating voice disorders, contrast the desirable and undesirable voice or resonance qualities. In simple terms, describe the relation between vocal abuse and voice problems. With the help of charts and drawings, show them how the vocal mechanism works and how important it is to maintain appropriate vocal behaviors.

2. **Demonstrate how to evoke target behaviors.** Let family members watch you evoke the target behaviors. They should know how to model the target behaviors for the client. Although they are not expected to shape the behavior or model excessively at home, the parents, spouses, and siblings should suggest the target behavior when the client fails to produce it at home. For instance, the family of a person who stutters should model the correct way of slowing the rate of speech. They should do it by stretching the words and not by pausing between words. The family members of a child with a language delay or articulation problem should know how to quickly and correctly model words, phrases, and sentences under training.

3. **Teach family members the subtle ways of prompting target behaviors.** When the parents begin their work at home, the need to model extensively will not be crucial. The parents most likely will have to prompt the target responses. When prompts do not work, the parents must stop the client, remind the target behavior, and perhaps model as well.

Teach parents to give subtle prompts when a failure to produce the target behavior seems imminent. When family members begin to modify the client's behavior in natural settings, loud and obvious signals are not acceptable to clients. When prompts have to be given in the presence of guests and visitors, the prompts must be so subtle that the others present do not notice them. A subtle and brief hand gesture or even a movement of a finger may be all that is needed to slow down the rate of speech, reduce the vocal pitch, increase vocal intensity, and decrease hoarseness of voice. Similar gestures can be devised to remind the client to open his or her mouth to increase oral resonance or to assume a certain articulatory posture. A person sitting next to the client at the dining table may touch the client to prompt the production of a target response. For each specific target response, devise such a specific, brief signal.

In training the family members to provide such prompts, demonstrate selected unobtrusive signals and teach the client to reliably respond to them in the clinic. Then ask the parents to give those signals frequently at home. Some clients may need a more pronounced stimulus in the beginning. If so, in progressive steps, reduce that obvious stimulus to a brief signal so that only the family and the client will know what has transpired.

During treatment sessions, give the same signal you ask the family members to use at home. When you take the client out of the treatment room to natural settings, experiment with different types of signals, and find out which one works the best for the client. Ask the parents to use the same signal at home.

4. **Teach family members how to create opportunities for the client to produce the target behaviors.** Often, clients who are communicatively handicapped are reluctant to talk even when their problems have been mostly remediated. Persons who stutter or those with hearing loss may talk less in groups just as they did before treatment, although they are now expected to use their newly acquired skills of fluency or oral language. Treated persons with aphasia also may be reluctant to talk in front of other persons. A child who has just learned to say some words may not speak them. Having gotten used to your client's role as a silent partner, the family and friends may not ask the person with a communicative disability to take part in conversation. Therefore, train family members and other persons to include the client in verbal exchanges. If the family members previously spoke for the client, ask them not to do that. For instance, the child who has learned to make requests should be asked to make relevant requests. The wife of a person who stutters should stop ordering for him at restaurants.

5. **Teach how to reinforce target behaviors.** The client's family, teachers, friends, or colleagues should know how to reinforce the target behavior productions at home and in other situations. Point out to parents and others the importance of immediate reinforcement and demonstrate how to provide it. Also tell them it is equally important to stop the client at the earliest sign of a wrong response. Ask them not to wait until a lengthy but wrong response is completed. Show how you do this.

Like prompts that help evoke responses in natural settings, response consequences also should be delivered in a subtle manner. Most clients do not want to be reinforced in front of other persons. A man who stutters does not want his wife to say, "You are very fluent, honey!" in front of formal dinner guests. But reinforcing a stuttering person for speaking fluently in such formal occasions is important. Therefore, a special signal that is not a prompt but a reinforcement may be given discretely. Signals that prompt behaviors are given when the behavior is imminent and signals that suggest approval and praise (reinforcement) are given soon after the target behaviors are produced. If such signals are used often in the company of strangers and acquaintances, and backed up by verbal praise as soon as possible, the signals may act as discriminative stimuli.

Parents and others need not reinforce continuously. By the time maintenance strategies have begun at home, the client will have been reinforced in the clinic on a fairly large intermittent schedule. Therefore, infrequent reinforcement might be effective. Ask family members to increase the frequency of reinforcement only when the correct responses do not seem to be nearly as high as you report for treatment sessions.

6. **Teach how to provide corrective feedback, but only minimally.**
Generally, parents and others should be trained to reinforce more often
than to punish. When wrong responses are produced, it is better to give a
swift prompt than to give a punishing signal. For example, it is better to
prompt a stuttering person who starts with a fast rate to slow down the
rate than to whisper "no!" A hand gesture to slow down is more neutral
than such verbal punishers and may be more effective. Therefore, train family members and others to prompt correct responses when incorrect
responses seem imminent.

7. **Train family members to stop reinforcing inappropriate behaviors.** Family members may continue to reinforce incorrect or inappropriate behaviors. As noted before, a previously nonverbal child may continue
to get reinforced for gestures at home. When it is clear that the child can
use words, parents and others should withhold reinforcers for gestures and
other nonverbal behaviors. Reinforcement should be contingent on newly
learned desirable behaviors.

8. **Assess whether family members and others are prompting and
reinforcing the target behaviors.** Ask them to tape record a sample
conversation or other kinds of exchange and bring it to you. You should
ask for such tape recorded evidence periodically for you to give them feedback on the performance of the family members. If they are making
mistakes, you should catch them as soon as possible and give them corrective instructions. This allows you to collect data on response maintenance
at home.

9. **Train family members to conduct home treatment programs.**
Although you will most often train parents to promote maintenance of
target behaviors you have established in the clinic, you may sometimes ask
family to conduct formal treatment sessions at home. For example, while
working with small children and infants, you often have to train parents to
conduct some portion of treatment at home. Infant language stimulation,
early intervention for stuttering and articulation disorders, and intervention for vocal abuse in young children may require a substantial amount of
parental work. See a subsequent section on developing home management
programs for details.

If parents and spouses can be trained to hold brief and parallel training
sessions at home, responses may be stabilized at home sooner than otherwise
expected. Possibly, parents and spouses who also are therapists even in an
informal or limited sense will better promote response maintenance. If
parents and spouses cannot do this, at least a few minutes of brief informal
sessions at home are highly desirable. When family members agree to do
this, they should set aside a time for speech work at home. They should
tape record each session they hold and submit it to you for your review
and feedback.

Training significant persons in a client's life is perhaps the most challenging and yet the most necessary task in promoting maintenance. You will have to constantly think of new ways of meeting this challenge.

Step 7. Teach the Client Self-Control

We try to control our behaviors with varying degrees of success. But clients who learn to systematically control their behaviors have constant therapists in themselves. Clients who can monitor their behaviors do not depend much on family and friends to sustain their communicative behaviors. Therefore, teaching self-control is an important task in promoting response maintenance.

1. **Teach clients to judge the accuracy of their behaviors.** Ask the child in articulation treatment to say whether his or her productions were correct or not. In a matter of few training trials, most children can make this judgment. Children who are encouraged to make those judgments frequently begin to monitor their behaviors more closely. They stop as soon as they begin to misarticulate a sound.

   Persons getting treatment for stuttering may be asked to judge the occurrence of stutterings, abrupt onset of phonation, a faster than required rate of speech, muscular tension while speaking, and most other target responses. Likewise, they can judge the occurrence of smooth phonation, desired rate, relaxed articulation, and so forth. Speakers who stutter who appreciate the contrast between their stuttered speech and target fluency skills will begin to monitor their speech production. They are likely to stop at the beginning of a stutter. With further training in self-monitoring, they may stop as soon as they feel tension in their speech musculature and start with greater relaxation. When clients use such tactics, the clinician can reduce the amount of response consequation.

2. **Train clients in target behavior charting.** Ask clients who become proficient in recognizing their own correct and incorrect responses to chart their behaviors along with you. Ask them to make a tally mark on a sheet of paper every time they stutter, articulate a phoneme incorrectly, produce an undesirable vocal characteristic, and so forth. Also ask them to tally their correct responses. Many children are eager to do it. Other children may be asked to count their correct and incorrect behaviors by placing different colored plastic chips in two cups placed in front of them.

   When your clients learn to measure their correct and incorrect behaviors in the clinic, ask them to bring data on their performance outside the clinic. Measuring their behaviors in outside situations will help them monitor their target responses more closely. Individuals who stutter may be asked to record the frequency of their dysfluencies in situations when tape-recording their speech is not practical. Adult voice clients also may record the frequency of occurrence of hoarseness or hard glottal attacks and so forth. Small, handheld counters can be used to record the frequency of behaviors.

3. **Teach clients to implant signals that remind them of the target behaviors in their everyday lives.** For instance, clients who stutter or have high-pitched voices may draw arrows pointing downward on small pieces of paper and paste them on telephone receivers, office desks, and other places where they need reminders to reduce the rate of speech or the pitch of their voice.

Train clients to select consequences for their own behaviors. Clients who have been trained to judge the accuracy of their target behaviors and measure them in clinical and nonclinical settings can learn to self-consequate behaviors. Self-administered consequences can be more immediate than those administered by the clinician. A voice or a fluency client may feel subtle tension in the throat that is a signal for stuttering or hoarseness. The clinician may not be able to respond to this without using a biofeedback unit. But if the client can be trained to pause, relax, and try again, such subtle muscular signals of impending incorrect behaviors will be modified before they occur. This is excellent self-control. Some clients can be trained to self-administer time-out. A man who stutters, for example, may be trained to stop speaking for a few seconds each time he stutters. By doing this, he may be able to reduce his stutterings even when no one is monitoring his fluency and stuttering.

Step 8. Teach the Client to Prime Others to Administer Consequences

A common problem with contingency management in everyday life is that family members may not notice the production of correct behaviors or may take them for granted. They may think that their only job is to stop undesirable behaviors. They may not realize that it is more important to encourage the desirable behavior. For instance, parents who are asked to monitor their child's correct and incorrect productions of target phonemes may notice incorrect production more often than correct productions. The child then hears more critical words than encouraging words.

To counter this tendency, train the family to prompt and reinforce as often as they can and punish as minimally as they have to. Still, many people in the client's life may be slow to reinforce. Therefore, teach clients to prime others to reinforce them. **Priming** is a special way of prompting others to reinforce; it is done by those who wish to receive reinforcement. The clinician asks the parent to reinforce their daughter for her correct production of phonemes (Hegde, 1998a). At home, the daughter primes her parents to reinforce her correct productions.

Reinforcement priming is done by drawing other people's attention to one's own behaviors that are expected to be reinforced. Whenever we show off our good behaviors or point out something we did well, we may be priming for reinforcement. We may do it with people who are notorious for ignoring good behaviors in others.

Teach clients to *draw attention to their target behavior productions* and ask the family members to reinforce immediately. Tell the family that you want the client to draw attention. Otherwise, they may think the client is showing off. A girl may let her parents know that she correctly produced a phoneme throughout a segment of conversation. A man who stutters may remind his wife that he has been speaking fluently for several minutes. Or, soon after fluently ordering food in a restaurant, he may draw his wife's attention to his successful but previously troubled performance. A woman with hoarseness may tell her listeners that she has been speaking very softly or very little in an otherwise loud family discussion. A man with aphasia may draw his friend's attention to correct naming of persons or objects.

Vocal emphasis on a target language feature may be another way of drawing attention to it. A boy who has learned to produce the regular plural morpheme slightly emphasizes it in his words, phrases, and sentences. This vocal emphasis may force attention of a parent who may otherwise ignore the production.

Train clients to ask their friends and family to signal with a subtle hint that an undesirable response has been made. A woman with pitch breaks may request her roommate to signal with her finger that pitch breaks occurred. A woman who stutters may ask her husband to stop her whenever she stutters or speaks rapidly.

Step 9. Give Sufficient Treatment

A simple reason why many clients do not maintain target responses is that they have terminated treatment against your advice or you have prematurely dismissed the client from services. There is not much you can do when clients discontinue therapy for reasons unrelated to your effectiveness. The family may move out of the area or run out of resources to continue treatment. But if the treatment was discontinued because they did not see much progress, you have something to think about. You must change or improve your treatment procedures. This is not a maintenance issue because the treatment was not completed. It is a maintenance issue when you prematurely dismiss a client who has been showing good progress.

Clients may be prematurely dismissed because the target responses are produced reliably in the clinical setting. The clinician may not realize that much work still needs to be done. For example, a child who correctly produces phonemes in words may still need help in producing them in conversational speech. A man who has learned to maintain an appropriate vocal pitch in the clinic may still be speaking with his unacceptably high pitch elsewhere. A woman with aphasia may say a few words in the clinic but may not remember any of them after the treatment sessions. But in all such cases, the clinician may dismiss the client from services because the target behaviors are produced at some level of response topography and accuracy in the clinical setting.

When clients are dismissed prematurely, either the target responses have not been trained sufficiently in conversational speech or no maintenance procedures have been implemented. Because maintenance is treatment also, prematurely dismissed clients will not have received sufficient treatment. More importantly, treatment may be insufficient regardless of maintenance procedures. In this case, treatment will not have sufficiently strengthened the target behaviors. Also, maintenance procedures may have been started prematurely. Some clients who make rapid progress in treatment may show shaky but quick generalization, creating an illusion that sufficient treatment was given. Therefore, the clinician must strengthen complex response topographies in the clinic by intermittent reinforcement. Then the treatment should be gradually extended to natural settings.

Step 10. Give Booster Treatment

Some clinicians assert that treatment is not successful unless clients are permanently cured so that they never need our services for the rest of their lives. Any relapse of stuttering in a treated person often is sharply pointed out by critics who claim there is no successful treatment for stuttering. Voice disorders, too, tend to relapse in some cases, and the same argument is made. But a successfully treated disorder may return, and this is not necessarily a negative reflection on the previous success. No successful medical treatment comes with a guarantee that the patient will not catch the same disease again. Similarly, successful treatment of stuttering or any other communicative disorder does not come with a guarantee that clients will be free from the disorder for the rest of their lives. Such a guarantee is not a precondition to judge the effectiveness of a treatment procedure.

Communicative disorders that return after successful treatment suggest that the conditions that created the disorder were confronted again by the person who was treated. We may not fully understand these conditions, or if we did, we may have no control over some or all them. This is a matter for further research.

Meanwhile, the clinician can take pride when a disorder is treated successfully, although there is likelihood of relapse. But a careful clinician plans to take care of this eventuality. Therefore, tell your clients, especially the fluency and voice clients, that they may need additional treatment sometime in the future. Assure them that when the problem emerges again, it can be handled successfully. Caution them, though, that they should contact you at the earliest sign of relapse. A slight increase in dysfluencies, hoarseness or harshness of voice, undesirable pitch, and so forth must be brought to the clinician's attention. The sooner the process of relapse is caught, the faster the progress in resumed treatment.

Treatment resumed for a client after dismissal is called **booster treatment.** The need for booster treatment shows that we have many problems to solve in the maintenance of treatment gains. But until research solves them, we must have a schedule for booster treatment for every client who needs it.

The need for booster treatment is most acute for persons who stutter. Most children and adults successfully treated for stuttering need booster treatment sometime after they are dismissed from original treatment. Fluency is not maintained in many treated individuals not because the original therapy was useless, but because they did not receive booster treatment. Therefore, plan on giving booster treatment to every person treated for stuttering. Although not much data exist, voice disorders due to vocal abuse, too, may relapse because the vocally abusive behaviors may reemerge after a period of absence.

Booster treatment is typically the *same treatment* that was successful initially unless something more powerful has been developed since dismissal. Technical improvements made during the intervening time should be included in booster treatment.

The duration of booster treatment is typically brief. In most cases, a few sessions may be sufficient, especially if the client has returned in the early stage of relapse. If the relapse is substantial, booster treatment may be prolonged.

Some clients need repeated booster treatments spread over a few years. Though discouraging to most clients, if it is explained to them that a few repetitions of treatment is a method of fading out the treatment completely, the clinician is likely to gain their cooperation.

Booster treatment is also an opportunity to *strengthen family members' skills* in monitoring the client's target behaviors. It is possible that the client's target behaviors deteriorated mainly because the family members' monitoring of those behaviors deteriorated.

Booster treatment is interlinked with follow-up assessments discussed in the final section of this chapter. Extension of treatment to the natural environment, coupled with a schedule of follow-up and booster treatment, are the best the current treatment technology can offer to maintain target behaviors across speaking situations and over time.

Developing Home Treatment Programs

Home treatment programs are different from maintenance programs implemented by families. In a home maintenance program, families strengthen behaviors the clinician has already established. *In a home treatment program, the parents may have to establish at least some of the behaviors.* In clinic-based interventions, the primary treatment responsibility rests with the clinician, but in home treatment programs, that responsibility is assigned to family members.

Home treatment programs are especially recommended for *infants at risk for developing communicative disorders.* Among others, infants who show early signs of intellectual disabilities, potential hearing problems, neurologic impairment, language delay, or certain genetic syndromes are candidates for early intervention. Early intervention by professionals may not be practical because of lack of trained personnel, limited clinical facilities, and lack of funds to pay for extended professional help. In such cases, parent training in early intervention may be the only practical course.

Home treatment programs also are needed in cases where *clients receive limited treatment from a professional* with the understanding that the family members will continue some systematic treatment at home. Clients and families who go out of town to consult with a specialist in speech-language pathology and those who cannot continue therapy for any reason are in this category. In such cases, clients of all ages may receive home treatment from their family.

Developing home treatment programs requires more information than can be offered here. You must consult other sources for details (Billeaud, 2003;

McDonald & Gillette, 1986; Odom & Karnes, 1988; Rossetti, 2001). Take note also that research on the effectiveness of home-based communication intervention is limited. Only a few basic principles for developing a home training program are summarized in this section.

The clinician should never simply give a written home program and ask the parents to follow it. Therefore, home training programs should be recommended only after the clinician has:

- Thoroughly assessed a client;

- Developed and tried an intervention program that works;

- Trained the parents in a home treatment program, including objective record-keeping procedures; and

- Developed plans to make herself or himself available to supervise the family members' work, assess the data supplied by them, modify the treatment program, and retrain the family members when necessary.

A thorough *assessment of the infant or the child* should include an evaluation of communicative behaviors or their potential. In the case of infants, the early signs of speech and language are assessed. Such behaviors as attention, social smile, play, social or emotional responses to other people, interaction with other children, general motor development, physical development, babbling and cooing, early speech sound productions, single-word productions, and use of words in social communication are among the several aspects of child development that are assessed. Sensory development, intellectual status, and neurological and physical health of the infant also are assessed by psychologists and medical specialists. Unless a team of specialists has made a complete assessment of the child or infant, it may not be appropriate to recommend an extensive home communication treatment program. Children who need home treatment programs most likely have other disabilities for which different specialists also will develop home treatment programs. For example, programs for motor, sensory, and physical development may be recommended.

The speech-language pathologist must *develop and experiment with a treatment program* with the infant or the child to make sure it works. Because what works with one infant may not necessarily work with another, the clinician must develop a trial period of treatment to establish effective target behaviors and treatment procedures. The clinician should complete a few days or weeks of systematic work before recommending a program for home use. Continuous data recorded during treatment should be used to assess what an infant has learned in treatment.

The trial treatment is also the opportunity to *train parents in the home treatment program*. Parents should take part in all sessions of trial therapy. They should also take part in the selection of target behaviors and in further refining them as treatment continues. They should know how to move on to more complex targets. By initially watching how the clinician uses the procedures and then implementing those procedures in the presence of the clinician, parents learn to teach communicative behaviors. During the trial treatment, the clinician should teach parents how to record a child's responses and in general record-keeping procedures.

Assessment of treatment data and periodic supervision of parents' work at home is essential to avoid mistakes in implementation. Tape-recorded samples of treatment sessions and, preferably, videotaped samples must be evaluated by the clinician. The clinician should promptly review parents' charts and recording sheets to evaluate changes in an infant's behavior. Frequent telephone contact may be necessary to answer parent questions and to offer suggestions based on submitted data. Periodically, the clinician may visit the home and observe the parents. At this time, the clinician may demonstrate new procedures.

When the data show no significant progress under a home treatment program, a *speech-language pathologist should offer formal treatment.* This may have to be done regardless of home progress, if the communicative disabilities warrant systematic, formal, professional help.

Follow-up Assessments

Follow-up is an assessment of response maintenance over time. It is a *conversational probe* of communicative behaviors. Students in clinical practicum often do not work long enough with the same clients to make follow-up assessments. Each semester of clinical practice, you may be assigned different clients. But follow up is an important part of clinical work. Even if you did not have frequent opportunities to practice follow-up assessments, you must know the procedures. You will be making those assessments when you take a professional position.

An individualized follow-up schedule is prepared before a client is dismissed from treatment. How the client has progressed often dictates how soon and how often follow-ups are scheduled. For practical reasons, a client may be dismissed sooner than expected with the understanding that the client will return for an assessment sooner than usual. A strong response rate at a very high level of accuracy maintained in natural settings on repeated measures may suggest that the first follow-up need not be too close to dismissal.

Typically, the first follow-up assessment is scheduled *3 months* after a client is dismissed from services. Assuming that the client has maintained the communicative behaviors, the next assessment may be scheduled after 6 months. If the behaviors are maintained, subsequent assessments may be scheduled in yearly intervals. A *3- to 4-year follow-up* is needed for speakers who received treatment for their stuttering. A similar schedule may be needed for voice clients. Children who receive treatment for articulation disorders probably do not need such a lengthy follow-up. If correct production of articulation is maintained for a year or so, chances of misarticulations returning may not be great. With other clients, such as those with aphasia or progressive neurological and physical diseases, the follow-up assessment schedule is based on the client's health and progress in speech or language treatment.

Timely follow-up assessments help determine the *need for booster treatment.* These assessments must be used to prevent significant deterioration in target behaviors by offering booster treatment at the earliest possible time. Therefore, in a typical follow-up, *take an extended conversational speech sample*. Make it as naturalistic as possible. If time permits, record the sample in a nonclinical setting as well. Take the client out for a walk and engage in conversation. Use a micro tape recorder to record the conversation. Give a test only if it samples connected speech and it gives you some unique data. Because such tests are practically nonexistent, an extended conversational speech sample is your best measure.

In sampling language features, you may have to contrive the conversation or direct it in some specific manner to have the client produce those features. Follow the guidelines given in Appendix G on taking conversational speech samples.

Calculate the *percentage correct response rate* for the speech or language sample. Analyze the sample to derive such quantitative data as the following:

- Percentage dysfluency rate

- Percentage correct production of phonemes

- Percentage correct use of grammatical morphemes and other language features

- Number of words in sentences

- Percentage of speech time a particular voice quality was maintained

- Frequency of pitch breaks per minute of continuous speech

- Percentage of words on which inappropriate nasal resonance was heard

- Percentage of spoken words that were intelligible

- Number of words or syllables spoken per minute

If the follow-up assessment data suggest that the target behaviors are not maintained or have declined in frequency, arrange for immediate booster treatment, which is treatment offered anytime after dismissal for an initial period of treatment. The goal of initial treatment is to establish and strengthen communication skills; the goal of booster treatment is to promote maintenance. Remember, the goal of follow-up is to assess response maintenance and to give timely booster treatment to those who need it.

Even with an established follow-up schedule, the client and the family must be told they should contact you for an assessment or consultation as soon as they notice a response deterioration. If they do not understand this, the clients and the family may wait for a scheduled follow-up to seek booster treatment. A follow-up schedule is valid only when target behaviors do not deteriorate in the interim.

Much clinical research needs to be done on maintenance of clinically established target behaviors in natural settings. If you approach the problem from the standpoint of extending treatment to nonclinical settings, you may have greater success than if you tried to program generalization. Scheduled follow-up and booster treatment and further training of the family members in contingency management during booster sessions are additional features of a sound maintenance strategy.

REFERENCES

American Speech-Language-Hearing Association. (1983, September). Social dialects. *Asha, 27*, 23–24.

American Speech-Language-Hearing Association. (1984, April). Organization and maintenance of records for clinical service delivery. *Asha, 26*, 39.

American Speech-Language-Hearing Association. (1985a, June). Clinical supervision in speech-language pathology. *Asha, 27*, 57–60.

American Speech-Language-Hearing Association. (1985b, June). Clinical management of communicatively handicapped minority language populations. *Asha, 27*, 29–32.

American Speech-Language-Hearing Association. (1989a). *AIDS/HIV: Implications for speech-language pathologists and audiologists.* [Technical Report]. Available from www.asha.org/policy.

American Speech-Language-Hearing Association. (1989b, March). Definitions: Bilingual speech-language pathologists and audiologists. *Asha, 31*, 93.

American Speech-Language-Hearing Association. (1993). [1993 omnibus survey results]. Unpublished report.

American Speech-Language-Hearing Association. (1994a, March). Professional liability and risk management for the audiology and speech-language pathology professions. *Asha, 36* (Suppl. 12), 25–38.

American Speech-Language-Hearing Association. (1994b, January). The protection of rights of people receiving audiology or speech-language pathology services. *Asha, 36*, 60–63.

American Speech-Language-Hearing Association. (1994c). *Clinical recordkeeping in audiology and speech-language pathology.* [Relevant Paper]. Available from www.asha.org/policy.

American Speech-Language-Hearing Association. (1997, Spring). Position statement: Multiskilled personnel. *Asha, 39* (Suppl. 17), 13.

American Speech-Language-Hearing Association. (1997–2008). *Membership and certification handbook, speech-language pathology.* Rockville, MD: Author.

American Speech-Language-Hearing Association. (1998). Students and professionals who speak English with accents and nonstandard dialects: Issues and recommendations. Position statement and technical report. *Asha, 40* (Suppl. 18), 28–31.

American Speech-Language-Hearing Association. (2001a). *Roles and responsibilities of speech-language pathologists with respect to reading and writing in children and adolescents (guidelines).* Rockville, MD: Author.

American Speech-Language-Hearing Association. (2001b). *Roles and responsibilities of speech-language pathologists with respect to reading and writing in children and adolescents (position statement).* Rockville, MD: Author.

American Speech-Language-Hearing Association. (2001c). *Roles and responsibilities of speech-language pathologists with respect to reading and writing in children and adolescents (technical report)*. Rockville, MD: Author.

American Speech-Language-Hearing Association. (2002a). A workload analysis approach for establishing speech–language caseload standards in the schools: Guidelines. *Asha Desk Reference, 3*, 409–418.

American Speech-Language-Hearing Association. (2002b). Knowledge and skills for supervisors of speech-language pathology assistants. *Asha, 22* (Suppl.), 113–118.

American Speech-Language-Hearing Association. (2003a). Code of ethics (revised). *Asha, 23* (Suppl.), 13–15.

American Speech-Language-Hearing Association (2003b). Technical report: American English dialects. *Asha, 23* (Suppl.), 45–46.

American Speech-Language-Hearing Association. (2004a). *Guidelines for the training, use and supervision of speech-language pathology assistants*. [Guidelines]. Available from www.asha.org/policy.

American Speech-Language-Hearing Association. (2004b). *Preferred practice patterns for the profession of speech-language pathology*. [Preferred Practice Patterns]. Available from www.asha.org/policy.

American Speech-Language-Hearing Association. (2007a). *Scope of practice in speech-language pathology*. Rockville, MD: Author.

American Speech-Language-Hearing Association. (2007b). *Childhood apraxia of speech* [Position Statement]. Available from www.asha.org/policy.

American Speech-Language-Hearing Association. (2008a). *Bylaws of the American Speech-Language-Hearing Association (bylaws)*. Rockville, MD: Author.

American Speech-Language-Hearing Association. (2008b). *Clinical supervision in speech-language pathology*. [Technical Report]. Available from www.asha.org/policy.

American Speech-Language-Hearing Association (2008c). *Clinical supervision in speech-language pathology*. [Position Statement]. Available from www.asha.org/policy.

American Speech-Language-Hearing Association (2008d). *Knowledge and skills needed by speech-language pathologists providing clinical supervision*. [Knowledge and Skills]. Available from www.asha.org/policy.

American Speech-Language-Hearing Association Committee on Quality Assurance. (1990, December). Update. AIDS/HIV: Implications for speech-language pathologists and audiologists. *Asha, 32*, 47–48.

Andrews, M. L. (2006). *Manual of voice treatment: Pediatrics to geriatrics* (2nd ed.). Clifton Park, NY: Delmar Cengage Learning.

Battle, D. E. (2002). *Communication disorders in multicultural populations* (3rd ed.). Boston: Butterworth Heinemann.

Bernthal, J. E., Bankson, N. W., & Flipsen, P. (2009). *Articulation and phonological disorders* (6th ed.). Boston: Allyn & Bacon.

Beukleman, D. R., & Miranda, P. (1998). *Augmentative and alternative communication* (2nd ed.). Baltimore: Paul H. Brookes.

Beukleman, D. E., Yorkston, K., & Reichle, J. (Eds.) (2000). *Augmentative and alternative communication for adults with acquired neurogenic disorders*. Baltimore: Paul H. Brookes.

Billeaud, F. P. (2003). *Communication disorders in infants and toddlers: Assessment and intervention* (3rd ed.). St. Louis, MO: Butterworth-Heinemann.

Bloodstein, O. (1995). *A handbook on stuttering*. Clifton Park, NY: Thomson Delmar Learning.

Boone, D. R., McFarlane, S. C., & Von Berg, S. L. (2005). *The voice and voice therapy* (7th ed.). Boston, MA: Allyn and Bacon.

Bourgeois, M. (2005). Dementia. In L. L. LaPointe (Ed.), *Aphasia and related neurogenic language disorders* (3rd ed., pp. 199–213). New York: Thieme.

Brice, A. (2002). *The Hispanic child: speech, language, culture and education*. Boston, MA: Allyn and Bacon.

Brookshire, R. (2007). *An introduction to neurogenic communication disorders* (7th ed.). St. Louis, MO: Mosby-Year Book.

Burke, F. R. (1990). Child abuse: Prevention and intervention. Workshop presented at California State University, Fresno.

California State Department of Education. (1989). Program guidelines for language, speech, and hearing specialists providing designated instruction and services. Sacramento: Author.

Campbell, L. (1994). Clinical practicum and English proficiency. Paper presented at ASHA Conference on Multicultural Literacy in Communicative Disorders. Sea Island, GA.

Carr, E., & Durand, V. M. (1985). Reducing behavioral problems through functional communication training. *Journal of Applied Behavior Analysis, 18*, 111–126.

Case, J. L. (2002). *Clinical management of voice disorders* (4th ed.). Austin, TX: PRO-ED.

Charlop, M. H., Burgio, L. D., Iwata, B. A., & Ivancic, M. T. (1988). Stimulus variation as a means of enhancing punishment effects. *Journal of Applied Behavior Analysis, 21*, 89–95.

Charlop, M. H., Kurtz, P. F., Casey, F. G., & Greenberg, F. (1990). Using aberrant behaviors as reinforcers for autistic children. *Journal of Applied Behavior Analysis, 23*, 163–181.

Cheng, L. L. (1991). *Assessing Asian language performance* (2nd ed.). Oceanside, CA: Academic Communication Associates.

Cheng, L. L. (1995). *Integrating language and learning for inclusion, an Asian-Pacific focus*. San Diego, CA: Singular.

Cheng, L. L. (1998). *Management of communication disorders in multicultural populations*. St. Louis, MO: Mosby.

Chomsky, N., & Halle, M. (1968). *The sound pattern of English*. New York: Harper & Row.

Cole, L. (1992, May). Our multicultural agenda. *Asha, 34*, 38.

Coleman, T. J. (2000). *Clinical management of communication disorders in culturally diverse children*. Boston: Allyn & Bacon.

Collins, M. J. (1991). *Diagnosis and treatment of global aphasia* San Diego, CA: Singular.

Cooper, J. J. (2007). *Applied behavior analysis* (2nd ed.). Upper Saddle River, NJ: Prentice Hall.

Corbin-Lewis, K., Liss, J. M., & Sciortino, K. L. (2005). *Clinical anatomy and physiology of the swallowing mechanism*. Clifton Park, NY: Delmar Cengage Learning.

Crary, M. A., & Groher, M. E. (2003). *Introduction to adult swallowing disorders*. Boston: Butterworth Heinemann.

Cummings, J. L., & Benson, F. D. (1992). *Dementia: A clinical approach.* Newton, MA: Butterworth-Heinemann.

Davis, G. A. (2000). *Aphasiology.* Boston: Allyn & Bacon.

DeFina, A. A. (1992). *Portfolio assessment: Getting started.* New York: Scholastic Professional Books.

Dublinske, S., & Healey, W. C. (1978, March). P.L. 94-142: Questions and answers for the speech-language pathologist and audiologist. *Asha, 20,* 188–205.

Duffy, J. R. (2005). *Motor speech disorders* (2nd ed.). St. Louis, MO: Mosby.

Egel, A. L. (1981). Reinforcer variation: Implications for motivating developmentally disabled children. *Journal of Applied Behavior Analysis, 14,* 345–350.

Elbert, M., & Gierut, J. (1986). *Handbook of clinical phonology: Approaches to assessment and treatment.* San Diego, CA: College-Hill Press.

Emerick, L. L., & Pindzola, R. H. (2007). *Diagnosis and evaluation in speech pathology* (7th ed.). Boston: Pearson, Allyn & Bacon.

Flower, R. (1984). *Delivery of speech-language pathology and audiology services.* Baltimore: Williams & Wilkins.

Forrester, K. (2003). Diagnostic criteria for developmental apraxia of speech used by clinical speech-language pathologists. *American Journal of Speech-Language Pathology, 12,* 376–380.

Freed, D. (2000). *Motor speech disorders: Diagnosis and treatment.* Clifton Park, NY: Thomson Delmar Learning.

Gleason, J. B. (2001). *The development of language* (5th ed.). Boston: Allyn & Bacon.

Glennen, S. L., & DeCoste, D. C. (1997). *Handbook of augmentative and alternative communication.* Clifton Park, NY: Thomson Delmar Learning.

Goldberg, B. (1994, June–July). Managing diversity: Its common sense. *Asha, 36,* 44–48.

Goldstein, B. (Ed.). (2004). *Bilingual language development & disorders in Spanish-English speakers.* Baltimore: Brooks Publishing.

Golper, L. G. (1998). *Sourcebook for medical speech pathology* (2nd ed.). San Diego: Singular.

Groher, M. E. (Ed.) (1997). *Dysphagia: Diagnosis and management.* Boston, MA: Butterworth-Heinemann.

Gutierrez-Clellen, V., & Peña, V. (2001). Dynamic assessment of diverse children: A tutorial. *Language, Speech, and Hearing Services in Schools, 32,* 212–224.

Hall, P. K., Jordan, L. S., & Robin, D. A. (2007). *Developmental apraxia of speech* (2nd ed.). Austin, TX: PRO-ED.

Hamayan, E. V., & Damico, J. S. (Eds.). (1991). *Limiting bias in the assessment of the bilingual child.* Austin, TX: PRO-ED.

Haney, M. R. (2002). Name writing: A window to emergent literacy skills of young children. *Early Childhood Education Journal, 30*(2), 101–105.

Harris, G. A. (1993). American Indian cultures: A lesson in diversity. In D. E. Battle (Ed.), *Communication disorders in multicultural populations* (pp. 78–113). Boston: Andover.

Hegde, M. N. (1998a). *Treatment procedures in communicative disorders* (3rd ed.). Austin, TX: PRO-ED.

Hegde, M. N. (1998b). *Treatment protocols in communicative disorders.* Austin, TX: PRO-ED.

Hegde, M. N. (2003). *Clinical research in communicative disorders: Principles and strategies* (3rd ed.). Austin, TX: PRO-ED.

Hegde, M. N. (2006). *A coursebook on aphasia and other neurogenic language disorders* (3rd ed.). Clifton Park, NY: Delmar Cengage Learning.

Hegde, M. N. (2007). *Treatment protocols for stuttering.* San Diego, CA: Plural Publishing.

Hegde, M. N. (2008a). *Hegde's pocketguide to communication disorders.* Delmar Cengage Learning.

Hegde, M. N. (2008b). *Hegde's pocketguide to assessment in speech-language pathology* (3rd ed.). Clifton Park, NY: Delmar Cengage Learning.

Hegde, M. N. (2008c). *Hegde's pocketguide to treatment in speech-language pathology* (3rd ed.). Clifton Park, NY: Delmar Cengage Learning.

Hegde, M. N. (2010). *A coursebook on scientific and professional writing in speech-language pathology* (4th ed.). Clifton Park, NY: Delmar Cengage Learning.

Hegde, M. N., & Maul, C. A. (2006). *Language disorders in children: An evidence-based approach to assessment and treatment.* Boston, MA: Allyn and Bacon.

Hegde, M. N., & Pomaville, F. (2008). *Assessment of communication disorders in children: Resources and protocols.* San Diego, CA: Plural Publishing.

Helm-Estabrooks, N., & Albert, M. L. (2004). *A manual of aphasia therapy* (2nd ed.). Austin, TX: PRO-ED.

Heymann, D. L. (2004). *Control of communicable diseases in man* (18th ed.). Washington, DC: American Public Health Association.

High, W. M., Sader, A. M., Struchen, M. A., & Hart K. A. (2006). *Rehabilitation for traumatic brain injury.* New York: Oxford University Press.

Iwata, B. (1987). Negative reinforcement in applied behavior analysis: An emerging technology. *Journal of Applied Behavior Analysis, 20,* 361–378.

Iwata, B. A., Pace, G. M., Kalsher, M. J., Cowdery, G. E., & Cataldo, M. F. (1990). Experimental analysis and extinction of self-injurious escape behavior. *Journal of Applied Behavior Analysis, 23,* 11–27.

Justice, L. M. (2006). *Clinical approaches to emergent literacy intervention.* San Diego, CA: Plural Publishing.

Justice, L. M., Chow, S., Capellini, C., Flanigan, K., & Colton, S. (2003). Emergent literacy intervention for vulnerable preschoolers: Relative effects of two approaches. *American Journal of Speech-Language Pathology, 12,* 320–332.

Kamhi, A. G., Pollock, K. E., & Harris, J. L. (Eds.). (1996). *Communication development and disorders in African American children: Research, assessment and intervention.* Baltimore: Paul H. Brooks.

Kayser, H. (1995). *Bilingual speech-language pathology: An Hispanic focus.* San Diego, CA: Singular.

Kayser, H. (2007). *Educationg Latino preschool children.* San Diego, CA: Plural Publishing.

Kelly, B. R., Davis, D., & Hegde, M. N. (1994). *Clinical methods and practicum in audiology.* San Diego, CA: Singular.

Kemp, R. J., Roeser, R. J., Pearson, D. W., & Ballachanda, B. B. (1995). *Infection control for the professions of audiology and speech-language pathology.* Chesterfield, MO: Oaktree Products, Inc.

Knepflar, K. J., & May, A. A. (1989). *Report writing in the field of communication disorders: A handbook for students and clinicians* (2nd ed.). Rockville, MD: National Student Speech-Language-Hearing Association.

Krotcoski, A. M. (1998). Guidelines for using portfolios in assessment and evaluation. *Language, Speech, and Hearing Services in Schools, 29,* 3–10.

LaPointe, L. L. (Ed.). (2005). *Aphasia and related neurogenic language disorders* (2nd ed.). New York: Thieme.

Lawhon, T., & Cobb, J. B. (2002). Routines that build emergent literacy skills in infants, toddlers, and preschoolers. *Early Childhood Education Journal, 30*(2), 113–118.

Leonard, R., & Kendall, K. (2007). *Dysphagia assessment & treatment planning: A team approach* (2nd ed). San Diego, CA: Plural Publishing Inc.

Linder, T. (2008). *Transdisciplinary play-based assessment* (2nd ed). Baltimore: Paul H. Brooks.

Logemann, J. A. (1998). *Evaluation and treatment of swallowing disorders* (2nd ed.). Austin, TX: PRO-ED.

Love, R. J. (2000). *Childhood motor speech disability* (2nd ed.). Boston, MA: Allyn and Bacon.

Lowe, R. J. (1993). *Speech-language pathology and related professions in the schools.* Needham, MA: Allyn & Bacon.

Lubinsky, J. (2003, June 24). Standards-based competency. *The ASHA Leader, 8*(12), 15.

Lynch, C., & Welsh, R. (1993, March). Characteristics of state licensure laws. *Asha, 35,* 130–139.

Mace, C. F., Hock, M., Lalli, J. S., West, B. J., Belfiore, P., Pinter, E., et al. (1988). Behavioral momentum in the treatment of noncompliance. *Journal of Applied Behavior Analysis, 21,* 123–141.

Mahendra, N., & Arkin, S. M. (2003). Effects of four years of exercise, language, and social interventions on Alzheimer discourse. *Journal of Communication Disorders, 36,* 395–422.

Malott, R. W., & Trojan, E. A. (2008). *Principles of behavior* (6th ed.). Upper Saddle River, NJ: Prentice Hall.

Mason, S. A., & Iwata, B. A. (1990). Artifactual effects of sensory-integrative therapy on self-injurious behaviors. *Journal of Applied Behavior Analysis, 23,* 361–370.

McCauley, R. J. (1996). Familiar strangers: Criterion referenced measures in communication disorders. *Language, Speech, and Hearing Services in Schools, 27,* 122–131.

McCormick, L., Loeb, D., & Schiefelbusch, R. L. (2003). *Supporting children with communication difficulties in inclusive settings: School based language intervention* (2nd ed.). Boston: Pearson, Allyn & Bacon.

McCormick, L., & Schiefelbusch, R. L. (1990). *Early language intervention: An introduction* (2nd ed.). Columbus, OH: Merrill.

McDonald, J., & Gillette, Y. (1986). Communicating with persons with severe handicaps: Roles of parents and professionals. *Journal of the Association for the Severely Handicapped, 11,* 225–265.

McLaughlin, S. (2006). *Introduction to language development* (2nd ed.). Clifton Park, NY: Delmar Cengage Learning.

McMillan, M. O., & Willette, S. J. (1988, November). Aseptic technique: A procedure for preventing disease transmission in the practice environment, *Asha, 30,* 35–37.

Mecham, M. J. (1996). *Cerebral palsy* (2nd ed.). Austin, TX: PRO-ED.

Merritt, D. D., & Culatta, B. (1998). *Language intervention in the classroom.* San Diego, CA: Singular.

Meyen, E. L., Vergason, G. A., & Whelan, R. J. (Eds.). (1996). *Strategies for teaching exceptional children in inclusive settings.* Denver, CO: Love.

Moore-Brown, B., & Montgomery, J. (2005). *Making a difference in the era of accountability: Update on NCLB and IDEA 2004.* Eau Claire, WI: Thinking.

Murdoch, B. E., & Theodoros, D. G. (2001). *Traumatic brain injury.* Clifton Park, NY: Delmar Cengage Learning.

Murray, L. L., & Clark, H. M. (2006). *Neurogenic disorders of language: Theory driven clinical practice.* Delmar Cengage Learning.

Myers, P. S. (1999). *Right hemisphere damage.* Clifton Park, NY: Delmar Cengage Learning.

Nelson, N. W. (1993). *Childhood language disorders in context.* New York: Macmillan.

Odom, S., & Karnes, M. (1988). *Early intervention for infants and children with handicaps.* Baltimore: Paul H. Brookes.

Owens, R. E., Jr. (2008). *Language development: An introduction* (6th ed.). Boston: Allyn & Bacon.

Paul, R. (2007). *Language disorders from infancy through adolescence* (3rd ed.). Saint Louis, MO: Mosby.

Paul-Brown, D. (1994, May). Clinical record keeping in audiology and speech-language pathology. *Asha, 36,* 40–42.

Payan, R. (1984). Language assessment for bilingual exceptional children. In L. M. Baca & H. T. Cervantes (Eds.), *The bilingual special education interface.* St. Louis, MO: Times Mirror/Mosby.

Payne, J. C. (1997). *Adult neurogenic language disorders: Assessment and treatment.* San Diego, CA: Singular.

Payne, K. T. (2001). *How to prepare for the Praxis examination in speech pathology* (2nd ed.). San Diego, CA: Singular.

Peña-Brooks, A., & Hegde, M. N. (2007). *Assessment and treatment of articulation and phonological disorders in children* (2nd ed.). Austin, TX: PRO-ED.

Pence, K. L. (2007). *Assessment in emergent literacy.* San Diego, CA: Plural Publishing.

Provencio-Arambula, M., Provencio, D., & Hegde, M. N. (2007a). *Assessment of dysphagia: Resources and protocols in English and Spanish.* San Diego, CA: Plural Publishing.

Provencio-Arambula, M., Provencio, D., & Hegde, M. N. (2007b). *Treatment of dysphagia: Resources and protocols in English and Spanish.* San Diego, CA: Plural Publishing.

Reed, V. (2005). *An introduction to children with language disorders* (3rd ed.). New York: Macmillan.

Romski, M. A., & Sevcik, R. A. (1993). Language learning through augmented means: The process and its products. In A. P. Kaiser & D. B. Gray (Eds.), *Communication and language intervention series: Volume 2. Enhancing children's communication: Research foundations for intervention.* Baltimore, MD: Paul H. Brookes.

Roseberry-McKibbin, C. (2002). *Multicultural students with special language needs: Practical strategies for assessment and intervention* (2nd ed.). Oceanside, CA: Academic Communication Associates.

Roseberry-McKibbin, C., & Hegde, M. N. (2006). *An advanced review of speech-language pathology: Preparation for PRAXIS and comprehensive examination* (2nd ed.). Austin, TX: PRO-ED.

Rossetti, L. (2001). *Communication intervention, Birth to Three*. Clifton Park, NY: Thomson Delmar Learning.

Sands, D., French, N., & Kozleski, E. (2000). *Inclusive education for the 21st century: A new introduction to education*. Albany, NY: Wadsworth.

Screen, R. M., & Anderson, N. B. (1994). *Multicultural perspectives in communication disorders*. San Diego, CA: Singular.

Seymour, C. M., & Nober, E. H. (1998). *Introduction to communication disorders: A multicultural approach*. Boston: Butterworth-Heinemann.

Shekar, S., & Hegde, M. N. (1995). Asian Indians: Their language and culture. In L. L. Cheng (Ed.), *Integrating language and learning for inclusion: An Asian-Pacific focus* (pp. 125–148). San Diego, CA: Singular.

Shekar. S., & Hegde, M. N. (1996). Cultural and linguistic diversity among Asian Indians: A case of Indian English. *Topics in Language Disorders 16*(4), 54–64.

Shraeder, T., Quinn, M., Stockman, I., & Miller, J. (1999). Authentic assessment as an approach to preschool speech-language screening. *American Journal of Speech-Language Pathology, 8*, 195–200.

Silver, J. M., McAllister, T. W., & Yudofsky, S. C. (Eds.) (2005). *Textbook of traumatic brain injury*. Arlington, VA: American Psychiatric Publishing Inc.

Skinner, B. F. (1957). *Verbal behavior*. New York: Appleton-Century-Crofts.

Stockman, I. (1996). The promises and pitfalls of language sample analysis as an assessment tool for linguistic minority children. *Language, Speech, and Hearing Services in Schools, 27*, 355–366.

Terrell, S. L., & Terrell, F. (1993). African-American cultures. In D. E. Battle (Ed.), *Communication disorders in multicultural populations* (pp. 3–37). Stoneham, MA: Andover.

Thompson, C. K. (1988). Articulation disorders in the child with neurogenic pathology. In N. J. Lass, L. V. McReynolds, J. L. Northern, & D. F. Yoder (Eds.), *Handbook of speech-language pathology and audiology* (pp. 548–591). Toronto, Ontario, Canada: Decker.

Tomblin, J. B., Morris, H. L., & Spriestersbach, D. C. (Eds.). (1999). *Diagnosis in speech-language pathology* (2nd ed.). San Diego, CA: Singular.

Trueba, H. T., Cheng, L. L., & Ima, K. (1993). *Myth or reality: Adaptive strategies of Asian Americans in California*. Washington, DC: The Falmer Press.

Trueba, H. T., Jacobs, L., & Kirton, E. (1990). *Cultural conflict and adaptation: The case of Hmong children in American society*. Washington, DC: The Falmer Press.

Van Keulen, J. E., Weddington, G. T., & DeBose, C. E. (1998). *Speech, language, learning, and the African American child*. Needham Heights, MA: Allyn and Bacon.

Vogel, D., & Cannito, M. P. (Eds.). (2001). *Treating disordered speech motor control* (2nd ed.). Austin, TX: PRO-ED.

Westby, C. E. (1994). Multicultural issues. In J. B. Tomblin, H. L. Morris, & D. C. Spriestersbach (Eds.), *Diagnosis in speech-language pathology* (pp. 29–50). San Diego, CA: Singular.

Winokur, S. (1976). *A primer of verbal behavior*. Englewood Cliffs, NJ: Prentice-Hall.

Yavas, M. (Ed.). (1994). *First and second language phonology*. San Diego, CA: Singular.

Yorkston, K. M., Beukelman, D. R., Strand, E. A., & Bell, K. R. (1999). *Management of motor speech disorders in children and adults*. Austin, TX: PRO-ED.

APPENDIX A

Glossary of Educational Abbreviations and Acronyms

The following is a list of acronyms, initials, and abbreviations commonly used in education. Additional or different acronyms and abbreviations may be used at specific school sites. The names of tests, associations, and universities have not been included in this list.

ADA	average daily attendance
ADD	attention deficit disorder
ASD	autism spectrum disorder
BCBA	board certified behavior analyst
BICS	basic interpersonal communication skills
CA	chronological age
CALP	cognitive academic language proficiency
CH	communicatively handicapped
DD	developmentally disabled
DIS	designated instructional service
ED	emotionally disturbed (Department of Education)
EDGAR	Educational Department General Administrative Regulations
EEEA	Equity and Excellence in Education Act
EHA	Education of the Handicapped Act of 1975 (now known as IDEA as amended in 1990)
ESL	English as a second language
FAPE	free appropriate public education
FEP	fluent English proficient
FERPA	Family Education Rights and Privacy Act
FES	fluent English-speaking
HBI	home-based instruction
HI	hearing impaired
IDEA	Individuals with Disabilities Education Act (1990 amendment of EHA changed name to IDEA)
IEP	individualized education program
IFSP	Individualized Family Service Plan
IMC	instructional materials (media) center
LD	learning disability/learning disabled
LEA	local education agency
LEP	limited English-proficient
LES	limited English-speaking
LH	learning handicapped
LRE	least restrictive environment
LSH	language speech and hearing specialist
MA	mental age
MR	mentally retarded
NES	non-English-speaking
OCR	Office for Civil Rights
OH	orthopedically handicapped
OSEP	Office of Special Education Programs, U.S. Department of Education
OSERS	Office of Special Education and Rehabilitative Services
OT	occupational therapy or occupational therapist

PDD	pervasive developmental disorder
PL 94–142	Public Law 94–142, The Education for all Handicapped Children Act of 1975
PL 99–457	The 1986 amendments to the PL 94–142, which included the Early Intervention Program for Infants and Toddlers (Part H, now Part C)
PLP	present levels of performance
PT	physical therapy or physical therapist
RS	resource specialist
RSP	resource specialist program
RtI	response to intervention
SDC	special day class
SEA	state education agency
SED	severely emotionally disturbed
SH	severely handicapped
SST	student study team

Glossary of Medical Abbreviations and Symbols

Recording information in a patient's chart is a common form of communication among professionals in the medical setting. It provides a chronological log of patient services. Many abbreviations, acronyms, and symbols are used in recording data. Although there are universal symbols, initialisms, and abbreviations, some may be unique to a specific hospital. To avoid any misunderstanding, if you are unsure of an abbreviation, acronym, initialism, or symbol, do not use it; instead, write out the entire word or phrase. Following is a list of some of the commonly used abbreviations, acronyms, and symbols. (Abbreviations for measurements, tests, and professional associations have not been included in this list.)

a.c.	before meals
ACU	ambulatory care unit or acute care unit
ACVD	atherosclerotic cardiovascular disease
Al	allergy
Amb	ambulatory
A&O	alert and oriented
Asp	aspirate
ATC	around the clock
b.i.d.	twice a day
b.i.n.	twice a night
$\bar{c}$	with
Ca	cancer
CHF	congestive heart failure
CHI	closed-head injury
CN	cranial nerve
CNS	central nervous system
C/O	complains of
CPD	cardiopulmonary disease
CPT	current procedural terminology
CVA	cerebrovascular accident
DC (D/C)	discontinue or discharge
DNT	did not test
DU	diagnosis unknown
Dx	diagnosis
FIM	functional independence measure
Fx	fracture
h	hour
HCPCS	Healthcare Common Procedure Coding System
HIPAA	Health Insurance Portability and Accountability Act
h.s.	hour of sleep or bedtime
HUC	hospital unit clerk
Hx	history
IAO	immediately after onset
ICD-9-CM	International Classification of Diseases, 9th ed, Clinical Modification
ICU	intensive care unit
Lt. (L)	left
LOS	length of stay
MS	mental status
MVT	motor vehicle accident
NGT	nasogastric tube
NKA	no known allergies
n.p.o.	nothing by mouth
OG	oralgastric tube

p.c.	after meals
PHI	protected health information
p.o.	by mouth
p.r.n.	as necessary
pt.	patient
q.	every
q.d.	every day
q.i.d.	four times a day
RO	renew order
Rt. (R)	right
Rx	prescription or therapy (treatment)
s̄	without
SLP	speech-language pathologist
SNF	skilled nursing facility
Stat.	immediately
TAR	therapy authorization request
TBI	traumatic brain injury
t.i.d.	three times a day
t.i.n.	three times a night
TPR	temperature, pulse, respiration
Tx	therapy (treatment)
WFL	within functional limits
WNL	within normal limits
♀	female
♂	male
↑	above or increase
↓	below or decrease
O	absent or no response
Ø	no or none
?	doubtful or unknown

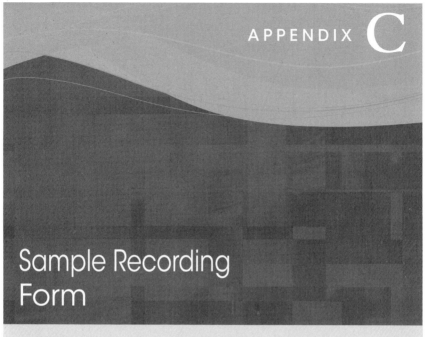

APPENDIX C

Sample Recording Form

What follows is a page of the KASA form. Consult your supervisor for the specific form used in your program.

Knowledge And Skills Acquisition (KASA) Summary Form for Certification in Speech–Language Pathology

The KASA form is intended for use by the certification applicant during the graduate program to track the processes by which the knowledge and skills specified in the 2005 standards for the CCC are being acquired. Each student should review the KASA form at the beginning of graduate study, and update it at intervals throughout the graduate program and at the conclusion of the program.

The student, with input and monitoring of program faculty, must enter a check mark in column B as each of the knowledge and skills is acquired. It is expected that many entries will appear in the coursework and the clinical practicum columns, with some entries, as appropriate, in the "Other" (lab, research, etc.) columns. Please enter the course or practicum number and title and description of other applicable activity.

I. Knowledge Areas

A	B	C	D	E
			How Achieved?	
Standards	Knowledge/ Skill Met? (check)	Course # and Title	Practicum Experiences # and Title	Other (e.g., labs, research) (Include description of activity)
Standard III-A. The applicant must demonstrate knowledge of the principles of:				
• Biological sciences				
• Physical sciences				
• Mathematics				
• Social/Behavioral sciences				
Standard III-B. The applicant must demonstrate knowledge of basic human communication and swallowing processes, including their biological, neurological, acoustic, psychological, developmental, and linguistic and cultural bases				
• Basic Human Communication Processes				
• Biological				
• Neurological				

Code of Ethics of the American Speech-Language-Hearing-Association

(Last Revised January 1, 2003)

Reprinted with permission from *Code of Ethics* [Ethics]. Available from www.asha.org/policy. Copyright 2003 by American Speech-Language Hearing Association. All rights reserved.

Preamble

The preservation of the highest standards of integrity and ethical principles is vital to the responsible discharge of obligations by speech-language pathologists, audiologists, and speech, language, and hearing scientists. This Code of Ethics sets forth the fundamental principles and rules considered essential to this purpose.

Every individual who is (a) a member of the American Speech-Language-Hearing Association, whether certified or not, (b) a nonmember holding the Certificate of Clinical Competence from the Association, (c) an applicant for membership or certification, or (d) a clinical Fellow seeking to fulfill standards for certification shall abide by this Code of Ethics.

Any violation of the spirit and purpose of this Code shall be considered unethical. Failure to specify any particular responsibility or practice in this Code of Ethics shall not be construed as denial of the existence of such responsibilities or practices.

The fundamentals of ethical conduct are described by Principles of Ethics and by Rules of Ethics as they relate to the conduct of research and scholarly activities and responsibility to persons served, the public, and speech-language pathologists, audiologists, and speech, language, and hearing scientists.

Principles of Ethics, aspirational and inspirational in nature, form the underlying moral basis for the Code of Ethics. Individuals shall observe these principles as affirmative obligations under all conditions of professional activity.

Rules of Ethics are specific statements of minimally acceptable professional conduct or of prohibitions and are applicable to all individuals.

Principles of Ethics I

Individuals shall honor their responsibility to hold paramount the welfare of persons they serve professionally or participants in research and scholarly activities and shall treat animals involved in research in a humane manner.

Rules of Ethics

A. Individuals shall provide all services competently.
B. Individuals shall use every resource, including referral when appropriate, to ensure that high-quality service is provided.
C. Individuals shall not discriminate in the delivery of professional services or the conduct of research and scholarly activities on the basis of race or ethnicity, gender, age, religion, national origin, sexual orientation, or disability.
D. Individuals shall not misrepresent the credentials of assistants, technicians, or support personnel and shall inform those they serve professionally of the name and professional credentials of persons providing services.
E. Individuals who hold the Certificates of Clinical Competence shall not delegate tasks that require the unique skills, knowledge, and judgment that are within the scope of their profession to assistants, technicians, support personnel,

students, or any nonprofessionals over whom they have supervisory responsibility. An individual may delegate support services to assistants, technicians, support personnel, students, or any other persons only if those services are adequately supervised by an individual who holds the appropriate Certificate of Clinical Competence.

F. Individuals shall fully inform the persons they serve of the nature and possible effects of services rendered and products dispensed, and they shall inform participants in research about the possible effects of their participation in research conducted.

G. Individuals shall evaluate the effectiveness of services rendered and of products dispensed and shall provide services or dispense products only when benefit can reasonably be expected.

H. Individuals shall not guarantee the results of any treatment or procedure, directly or by implication; however, they may make a reasonable statement of prognosis.

I. Individuals shall not provide clinical services solely by correspondence.

J. Individuals may practice by telecommunication (for example, telehealth/ e-health), where not prohibited by law.

K. Individuals shall adequately maintain and appropriately secure records of professional services rendered, research and scholarly activities conducted, and products dispensed and shall allow access to these records only when authorized or when required by law.

L. Individuals shall not reveal, without authorization, any professional or personal information about identified persons served professionally or identified participants involved in research and scholarly activities unless required by law to do so, or unless doing so is necessary to protect the welfare of the person or of the community or otherwise required by law.

M. Individuals shall not charge for services not rendered, nor shall they misrepresent services rendered, products dispensed, or research and scholarly activities conducted.

N. Individuals shall use persons in research or as subjects of teaching demonstrations only with their informed consent.

O. Individuals whose professional services are adversely affected by substance abuse or other health-related conditions shall seek professional assistance and, where appropriate, withdraw from the affected areas of practice.

Principle of Ethics II

Individuals shall honor their responsibility to achieve and maintain the highest level of professional competence

Rules of Ethics

A. Individuals shall engage in the provision of clinical services only when they hold the appropriate Certificate of Clinical Competence or when they are in the certification process and are supervised by an individual who holds the appropriate Certificate of Clinical Competence.

B. Individuals shall engage in only those aspects of the professions that are within the scope of their competence, considering their level of education, training, and experience.

C. Individuals shall continue their professional development throughout their careers.

D. Individuals shall delegate the provision of clinical services only to: (1) persons who hold the appropriate Certificate of Clinical Competence; (2) persons in the education or certification process who are appropriately supervised by an individual who holds the appropriate Certificate of Clinical Competence; or (3) assistants, technicians, or support personnel who are adequately supervised by an individual who holds the appropriate Certificate of Clinical Competence.

E. Individuals shall not require or permit their professional staff to provide services or conduct research activities that exceed the staff member's competence, level of education, training, and experience.

F. Individuals shall ensure that all equipment used in the provision of services or to conduct research and scholarly activities is in proper working order and is properly calibrated.

Principle of Ethics III

Individuals shall honor their responsibility to the public by promoting public understanding of the professions, by supporting the development of services designed to fulfill the unmet needs of the public, and by providing accurate information in all communications involving any aspect of the professions, including dissemination of research findings and scholarly activities.

Rules of Ethics

A. Individuals shall not misrepresent their credentials, competence, education, training, experience, or scholarly or research contributions.

B. Individuals shall not participate in professional activities that constitute a conflict of interest.

C. Individuals shall refer those served professionally solely on the basis of the interest of those being referred and not on any personal financial interest.

D. Individuals shall not misrepresent diagnostic information, research, services rendered, or products dispensed; neither shall they engage in any scheme to defraud in connection with obtaining payment or reimbursement for such services or products.

E. Individuals' statements to the public shall provide accurate information about the nature and management of communication disorders, about the professions, about professional services, and about research and scholarly activities.

F. Individuals' statements to the public—advertising, announcing, and marketing their professional services, reporting research results, and promoting products—shall adhere to prevailing professional standards and shall not contain misrepresentations.

Principles of Ethics IV

Individuals shall honor their responsibilities to the professions and their relationships with colleagues, students, and members of allied professions. Individuals shall uphold the dignity and autonomy of the professions, maintain harmonious interprofessional and intraprofessional relationships, and accept the professions' self-imposed standards.

Rules of Ethics

A. Individuals shall prohibit anyone under their supervision from engaging in any practice that violates the Code of Ethics.

B. Individuals shall not engage in dishonesty, fraud, deceit, misrepresentation, sexual harassment, or any other form of conduct that adversely reflects on the professions or on the individual's fitness to serve persons professionally.

C. Individuals shall not engage in sexual activities with clients or students over whom they exercise professional authority.

D. Individuals shall assign credit only to those who have contributed to a publication, presentation, or product. Credit shall be assigned in proportion to the contribution and only with the contributor's consent.

E. Individuals shall reference the source when using other persons' ideas, research, presentations, or products in written, oral, or any other media presentation or summary.

F. Individuals' statements to colleagues about professional services, research results, and products shall adhere to prevailing professional standards and shall contain no misrepresentations.

G. Individuals shall not provide professional services without exercising independent professional judgment, regardless of referral source or prescription.

H. Individuals shall not discriminate in their relationships with colleagues, students, and members of allied professions on the basis of race or ethnicity, gender, age, religion, national origin, sexual orientation, or disability.

I. Individuals who have reason to believe that the Code of Ethics has been violated shall inform the Board of Ethics.

J. Individuals shall comply fully with the policies of the Board of Ethics in its consideration and adjudication of complaints of violations of the Code of Ethics.

Sample Clinical Interview

The following is a sample interview with parents of a 5-year-old child who stutters. Note the kinds of questions asked and the types of information sought by the clinician. Also, note how the clinician answered many questions the parents had about stuttering, its causes, and treatment.

Interviewing the Parents of a Child Who Stutters

Clinician: When did you first think that there may be something wrong with Brian's speech?

Mrs. Thomas: About a month ago, on a Sunday morning, I noticed that Brian was repeating a lot. I remember asking him what he wanted to eat for lunch that day. Brian started to say something like "I want a hot dog for lunch," but he had a lot of trouble saying it.

Clinician: What exactly did he do?

Mrs. Thomas: Well, he started like "I-I-I-I-I wa-wa-wa-want a hot d-d-d-d-dog, Mom." He was trying too hard to say it. I could see a lot of struggle to get it out.

Clinician: You had not heard that kind of problem in Brian's speech before?

Mr. Thomas: My wife has not heard it, but I have. About two months ago, when I was reading a story to him, he wanted to interrupt me to ask a question about the story. I don't remember what exactly he said at that time, but I remember him repeating a lot. Periodically I have heard him repeat a bit too much, but I thought it may be a passing thing. I remember him asking me once, "What t-t-t-time is it Dad?"

Clinician: Have you seen an increase in repetitions?

Mr. Thomas: I think so. During the last month or so, his speech problems have increased. He is repeating more and getting stuck more often. Now it takes him longer to get out of a block. And that, too, only after some struggle.

Clinician: What do you mean by a block?

Mrs. Thomas: His mouth and face look like he is trying hard to say something, but nothing comes out. His lips are quivering, mouth is sometimes open, at other times tightly shut. You can see the struggle to say something, but he is not saying anything. This is what scares me the most.

Clinician: Did anything unusual happen around the time you first noticed his repetitions or more recently when you noticed an increase in them?

Mr. Thomas: No, not really. Things have been pretty routine at home.

Clinician: Has he been sick lately?

Mrs. Thomas: No, Brian has always been a healthy boy.

Clinician: What about your health when you were carrying Brian?

Mrs. Thomas: I was fine during pregnancy and the delivery was normal. The baby was healthy. We did not notice any problem until this stuttering came about.

Clinician: What about his speech and language development? Was there any reason to be concerned?

Mrs. Thomas: No. In fact, Brian began to speak earlier than my other son Chad, who is 4 years older than him. We thought he was quite advanced in his speech. He usually talked a lot and learned new words fast.

Clinician: So everything has been normal until you began to notice his stuttering.

Mr. Thomas: We may have missed something, but that is our impression.

Clinician: I want to go back to Brian's stuttering. You said that he repeats a lot. Does he prolong a sound? Have you heard him say something like "I want sssssome ssssoup, please?" I prolonged the *es* sound in both the words. Does he prolong sounds like that?

Mrs. Thomas: Oh, yes. He does it all the time. This morning, while eating a new kind of cereal, he said, "It is rad, Mom," but he prolonged the *a* sound. It was more like "raaaad."

Clinician: Does Brian repeat words and phrases? Does he say "I-I-I want it or let-let-let me do it or he-was he-was he-was coming" and things like that?

Mr. Thomas: Yes, we have heard him do that. Sometimes he repeats a word or a bunch of words many times before he moves on to the next word. Yesterday I heard him say to his brother "Why are you-why are you-why are you-why are you do-do-doing it?"

Clinician: Does he use what we call interjections like *uh* or *um* or *er*? As you know, most speakers have them, but I wonder how much Brian interjects.

Mrs. Thomas: I think he interjects a lot. In fact, Brian drives me up the wall with his *uh*s and *um*s. He starts a lot of sentences with *um*s. This morning he said "Um-um-um what am I-I-I g-g-g-going to have um-um-um-um for breakfast, Mom?" Sometimes he keeps going with *um*s.

Clinician: What about interjected words like *well*, *OK*, and phrases like *you know*, *I mean*, and *you see*?

Mrs. Thomas: He uses them some of the time. We hear more *um*s and *uh*s than what you just described.

Clinician: Does Brian show any facial grimaces when he stutters? Some people who stutter blink their eyes, wrinkle their noses and foreheads, purse their lips, wring their hands, swing their arms, and move their legs. Does Brian do any of these?

Mrs. Thomas: Yes, he does a few of those. I have seen him blink his eyes and wrinkle his nose and forehead. His hands and feet also move when he stutters. His mouth is distorted when he has a bad block. He also looks away from you when he stutters.

Clinician: Does Brian stutter all the time or only some of the time?

Mr. Thomas: His stuttering varies. One day we may hear just a few problems and the next day he may stutter on most of the words he speaks. He may be quite fluent in the morning but struggling to say his name in the afternoon. I find this puzzling. Is this true of other children who stutter, too?

Clinician: Yes, it is. A basic characteristic of stuttering is that it varies across time and speaking situations. Stuttering may be more when speaking on complex or unfamiliar topics. Dialogues in which one must take quick turns to talk and be silent also are difficult for stutterers. People who stutter are more fluent while talking aloud to themselves or when they are speaking in monologue. Stuttering also varies depending on the kinds of persons those who stutter face. Persons who stutter may be very fluent talking to pets and babies. Many adult stutterers talk to their subordinates with increased fluency but when they confront their bosses, fluency may break down abruptly. Does Brian stutter more with some people and less with others?

Mr. Thomas: He is more fluent with his younger sister Michelle, who is 3 years old. He has the most trouble with me, somewhat less with his mother. I would say his stuttering is about average when he talks to his older brother.

Mrs. Thomas: But his worst stuttering comes out when he talks to a stranger or in a new place. I took him to Chad's school the other day. One of the teachers there talked to Brian, who blocked on every word he tried to say. The poor kid couldn't say his name. It was a heartbreaking scene for me. Also, his stuttering is worst when he talks to some of the kids in the neighborhood.

Clinician: Many folks who stutter avoid certain words. Older children and adults use substitutes for difficult words. Do you know of any words that Brian avoids saying?

Mrs. Thomas: I think I do. The other day Brian wouldn't say *John*, who is a friend of Chad. Brian kept saying "Your friend called" but wouldn't say who it was. When Chad asked about four times "Who was it?," Brian finally said "J-J-J-John" and stuttered very badly on it. Of late, I have not heard him say "Hi" to people because he can't get it out. Another puzzling thing about his problem is that he can sing songs and not have a trace of trouble. Is this also typical?

Clinician: Yes, it is! Most persons who stutter have no trouble singing.

Mr. Thomas: It's amazing! Though Brian has certain words on which he stutters frequently, he can say those very same words fluently. I suppose this is also characteristic of stuttering.

Clinician: That is also true. Stuttering on words is a matter of probability. Stuttering is more probable on some words than on other words. But even the words on which the stuttering probability is the highest may be, on occasion, spoken fluently. Therefore, it is not a question of not being able to say the words. As you know very well, Brian can say every word that he stutters on. He knows exactly what to say, he just cannot say it smoothly and easily.

Mrs. Thomas: That makes sense.

Clinician: I want to talk a little bit about the family history. Is there a history of speech disorders in the family? Are you aware of a speech problem on either side of the family?

Mr. Thomas: When I was a kid, I used to stutter. I do not believe that my father ever stuttered, but an uncle of mine did.

Clinician: Do you know when you began to stutter and how severe it was?

Mr. Thomas: I am not sure, but I think I began to stutter when I was about 4. I think it was pretty bad, because I still remember having a lot of trouble in grade school. I remember the painful teasing and the frustration of getting blocked in front of the class and things like that.

Clinician: Did you receive treatment? Do you remember what it was?

Mr. Thomas: I did go to a speech therapist, but not very regularly. I can't remember much about what she did with me.

Clinician: When did your stuttering disappear, if it has? So far, you have not stuttered here.

Mr. Thomas: I do not stutter any more. I think my stuttering was at its peak during my years in intermediate school. High school was different. I began to be more fluent, although I was not taking speech therapy at that time. The problem became less noticeable when I started college, and stuttering disappeared in subsequent years. Is this common?

Clinician: To some degree. Persons who stutter may recover from it at any age, although recovery is more common in preschool children. Also, children who begin to stutter after age 7 also have a better chance of recovery. Children whose stuttering persists through the ages of 5 and 6 are likely to be chronic stutterers. During the early childhood years, girls who begin to stutter recover more often than boys of the same age. Roughly, some 30 percent of stutterers recover from it without much professional help. We call this spontaneous recovery. Mrs. Thomas, how about on your side of the family?

Mrs. Thomas: I do not believe there was any stuttering in my side of the family. I can't be sure, though. I did read in a newspaper article that stuttering runs in the family. Is this true?

Clinician: To a certain extent, stuttering tends to run in the family. The blood relatives of a person who stutters have a greater chance of stuttering, compared to the blood relatives of persons who do not stutter. We call this the familial incidence of stuttering. But the higher familial incidence also is related to the sex ratio. You know that there are more male stutterers than female stutterers.

Mrs. Thomas: Yes, I have wondered about that. I have seen only one woman who stuttered in my life, but many male stutterers. But how does it relate to the familial incidence?

Clinician: The familial incidence is related to the sex of one or more persons labeled as stuttering found in the family. If a male stutterer is found in a family, the familial incidence for that family may be higher, compared to the incidence in the general population. However, if a female stutterer is found in a family, the familial incidence may be the highest. This means that although females are less likely to stutter, a female who stutters poses the maximum risk to the members of her family. In fact, the brothers and sons of a female who stutters run a very high risk of developing stuttering. Sisters and daughters of a male or female who stutters do not run that much of a risk. Of all the people, the sons of stuttering mothers run the greatest risk of developing stuttering.

Mr. Thomas: Does it mean that stuttering is hereditary?

Clinician: Some experts believe that stuttering is genetically transmitted, although the exact mechanism of transmission is not known. However, we must remember that all stutterers do not have relatives who stutter. Therefore, we cannot conclude that stuttering is inherited in all cases. Most experts believe that both heredity and environment play a role in the development of stuttering.

Mrs. Thomas: If it is inherited, is it more difficult to treat?

Clinician: No, there are no data that suggest that. Research has shown that almost all individuals who stutter improve with treatment and many improve to a significant extent. Early treatment of stuttering is especially effective and I am glad that you brought Brian in this early.

Mr. Thomas: Well, that is good news for Brian and for us!

Examples of Dysfluency Types and Calculation of Dysfluency Rates

There is some variability in scoring different forms of dysfluency types. Some clinicians measure only *stutterings* and not specific types of dysfluencies. What follows is a general list of dysfluencies and their examples. Consult your clinical supervisor about the measurement of *dysfluencies* or *stuttering*.

Dysfluency Types	Examples

REPETITIONS:

Part-word repetitions	"What *t-t-t* time is it?"
Whole-word repetitions	"*What-what-what* are you doing?"
Phrase repetitions	"I want to-I want to-I want to do it."

PROLONGATIONS:

| Sound/syllable prolongations | "*Lllllet* me do it." |
| Silent prolongations | A struggling attempt to say a word when there is no sound. |

INTERJECTIONS:

Sound/syllable interjections	"*Um . . . Um* I had a problem this morning."
Whole-word interjections	"I had a *well* problem this morning."
Phrase interjections	"I had a *you know* problem this morning."

SILENT PAUSES:

| A silent duration within speech | "I was going to the *[pause]* store." considered abnormal |

BROKEN WORDS:

| A silent pause within words | "It was won*[pause]*derful." |

INCOMPLETE PHRASES:

| Grammatically incomplete utterances | "I don't *know how to* . . . Let us go, guys." |

REVISIONS:

| Changed words, ideas | "I thought I will write a letter, card." |

How to Calculate Percent Dysfluency Rates

Measure the frequency of all types of dysfluencies exhibited in a sample. Count the number of words spoken in the sample. Calculate the percent dysfluency rate as shown.

$$\frac{\text{Number of words spoken}}{\text{Number of dysfluencies}} \times 100$$

Types of Dysfluency	Frequency
Part-word repetitions	19
Whole-word repetitions	12
Phrase repetitions	22
Silent prolongations	34
Sound prolongations	26
Sound/syllable interjections	21
Word interjections	13
Phrase interjections	16
Broken words	10
Silent pauses	17
Incomplete phrases	9
Revisions	2
Total of all types	**201**
Number of words spoken	978
Percentage dysfluency rate	**20.5**

Note: Some clinicians calculate the *percent dysfluency rate* based on the number of *syllables spoken* (versus the number of *words spoken*, as illustrated). Follow your clinic supervisor's direction. Understand, however, that a dysfluency rate based on *syllables spoken* inflates the fluency estimate because, in a given speech sample, there are more syllables than words; this reduces the percent dysfluency rate. We recommend a dysfluency rate based on *words spoken* because it is a more accurate reflection of the amount of fluency and dysfluency a speaker produces.

Obtaining and Analyzing Conversational Speech Samples

The conversational speech sample provides data essential to the evaluation of your client's articulation, fluency, voice, and language. The information offered suggests guidelines for obtaining and analyzing conversational speech samples of children and adults.

Obtaining Speech Samples

1. **Obtain a representative sample of your client's speech.** Obtain a minimum of 100 utterances. An extended sample of 300 to 500 utterances is preferred. It is necessary to sample conversation in a variety of environments with different individuals. Ask clients to submit a taped sample of their speech at home, work, or school. Tell them that while taping, they should be doing most of the talking. With young children or children with severely limited speech and language, you may need to sample speech over several sessions. If you are unable to adequately sample a child's speech, ask the parent to maintain a record of the child's speech for one week. If the child is reluctant to talk with you, obtain a sample of the child's speech while he or she talks with the parent. Schedule another session in which you may evoke speech from the child. Explain to the parent that you want him or her to talk with the child as he or she normally would while you are out of the room. Record the conversation.

2. **Videotape the sample, if possible.** With video, you will be able to review nonverbal behaviors. In addition to speech, you will be able to note eye contact, gestures, attention to tasks, and so on. You also may observe if your change in posture or position affects the client's communicative behaviors.

3. **Audiotape the sample.** Do this even if you are video recording. Attach a small clip-on microphone to your client's collar if he or she will be sitting in the same place throughout the sample. (This usually results in better quality recording of the client's voice.) Have a paper and pen available to note any relevant nonverbal behaviors.

4. **Check your recording equipment.** Before beginning your session, make sure your equipment is operating correctly. Check batteries, electrical plugs and outlets, and tapes. Turn equipment on before beginning your sample.

5. **Have a variety of materials available.** Different children, adolescents, and adults have different interests. Have various types and sizes of toys available to children (e.g., large and small blocks, trucks, and dolls). Have different types of pictures available (e.g., pictures of sports activities, children playing, and people crying, laughing, and yelling).

6. **Have materials that are culturally and linguistically appropriate for the child.** Know the cultural background of the child before you select the stimulus materials. Follow the guidelines specified in Chapter 6.

7. **Engage adults and adolescents in conversation.** You usually do not need to use stimulus materials for such clients. Often the interview will allow you to obtain one conversational sample. Later you can ask the client

to speak on the phone, talk with the administrative assistant, or speak with another clinician. You occasionally may need to use such stimulus materials as pictures with adolescents.

8. **Try to engage children in conversation before introducing books and toys.** Many children will talk to the clinician if they are given the chance. Do not bring out toys and books until after you first have tried to engage the child in a conversation. Talk with a child about least-favorite and favorite school activities, cartoons, movies, vacations, friends, pets, teachers, birthdays and other special occasions, and so forth. Discuss likes and dislikes about siblings and events that make them happy, mad, or sad. (If a child's speech is unintelligible, you may have to use props to try and understand his or her speech.)

9. **Avoid using books.** Unless you plan to have a client retell a story, do not use books. Children want to look at the pictures or read the books, rather than describe what is happening in the pictures.

10. **Keep questions to a minimum.** Use such open-ended statements as "Tell me about your classes" and "What shows do you watch on Saturday morning?" Avoid asking such closed-ended questions as "Are you taking a math class?" or "Is your birthday coming soon?"

11. **Tell something about yourself.** For example, if you know a child has a sister, talk about your sister first: "My sister really made me upset yesterday. She wouldn't let me watch the TV show that I wanted to watch." Talk about a recent movie you know the child has seen. Talk about an interesting scene in the movie to stimulate talking on the child's part.

12. **Allow children to direct the conversation.** You may present a subject or activity and the child may have a completely different idea of what he or she wants to discuss. Follow the child's lead in beginning communications. You can always direct the conversation later to sample additional language structures.

13. **Give opportunities for the client to exhibit different language structures.** Direct the conversation to allow the client to talk about past, present, and future occurrences. Sample the use of pronouns, declaratives, negation, interrogatives, and so on.

14. **Allow pauses in the conversation.** Do not worry if there are periods of silence in your client interaction. Allow your clients plenty of time to respond to questions. Give them time to continue the conversation.

15. **Relax and have fun with children.** Children like such absurdities as boxes that "talk," balls that bounce to the moon, and puppets that have squeaky voices.

Analyzing Speech Samples

1. **Transcribe the conversational speech sample as soon as possible.** Allow sufficient time to record all necessary information.

2. **Transcribe the sample using Standard English orthography.** It is unnecessary to transcribe an entire sample phonetically. Transcribe unintelligible utterances and misarticulated words phonetically.

3. **Note the context in which speech is produced.** Include in your transcription events preceding each of the client's utterances. For example, if you showed a picture, asked a question, discussed an event, or performed an action, include this as part of your transcription: Clinician: bounced the ball. Client: "Pretty ball."

4. **Include in your analysis mean length of utterance and syntactic, morphologic, semantic, and pragmatic use.** As much as possible, give percentage of occurrences. Describe how many production opportunities (obligatory contexts) were present for a particular feature and in how many of those opportunities the feature was used correctly. For instance, a child may have had 20 opportunities to produce the regular plural morpheme but may have produced it correctly in only 10 of them. This means the child's correct production of the regular plural morpheme is 50%. Try to give such quantitative data for language structures of interest.

5. **Analyze voice characteristics** including pitch, rate, and intensity. These may be statements of clinical judgments unless a disorder is noted.

6. **Analyze fluency.** Describe all dysfluency forms and calculate total percentage of dysfluencies.

7. **Compute speech intelligibility.** Overall speech intelligibility may be computed using the total conversational speech sample, rather than sample for language analysis. Some language analysis programs exclude unintelligible utterances from the analysis. Note if any articulation errors produced at the conversation level are different from or in addition to those noted in single word productions.

8. **Save the conversational speech analysis** to compare with later samples.

Sample Probe
Recording Sheet

The following is an example of a probe recording sheet that demonstrates the probe procedure in which the trained (T) and untrained (U) responses (preposition on in phrases) are alternated to find out the percent correct probe response rate. For additional information on probes, see Hegde (1998a).

Client: Les Likely

Clinician: Mimi Doit

Age: 8

Date: [specify]

Disorder: Language

Session No. 7

Target Behavior: Preposition
  "on" in phrases

Reinforcement: Verbal; for
  the trained responses only

Target Behaviors	**Scoring**
1. Juice on table (T)	+
2. Pillow on sofa (U)	+
3. Dog on floor (T)	+
4. Man on horse (U)	−
5. Woman on bike (T)	+
6. Boy on skateboard (U)	+
7. Girl on roof (T)	−
8. Cookie on counter (U)	+
9. Pot on stove (T)	+
10. Pen on desk (U)	−
11. Clock on wall (T)	+
12. Ball on chair (U)	+
13. Teddy on bed (T)	+
14. Book on shelf (U)	+
15. Hat on head (T)	+
16. Baby on shoulders (U)	+
17. Spot on shirt (T)	+
18. Wrinkle on face (U)	−
19. Cat on tree (T)	+
20. Bird on tree (U)	+

Note: (+) = Correct   (−) = Incorrect
Percentage Correct Probe Response Rate: 70

In this example, 10 trained exemplars were intermixed with 10 untrained exemplars. Responses given to trained exemplars were reinforced and those given to untrained exemplars were not. In calculating the percentage correct probe response rate, responses given to only the untrained exemplars are considered. The client's responses to 7 of the 10 untrained exemplars were correct, yielding a 70% correct probe response rate for the production of preposition *on* in phrases.

Sample Treatment Plan

Treatment plans provide a comprehensive program of treatment, from the beginning of treatment to dismissal. Treatment plans are developed before beginning treatment and can be modified, if necessary, as treatment progresses. Following is a sample of a treatment plan. For additional discussion and examples of treatment plans, see Hegde (1998a, 2006).

University Speech and Hearing Clinic Treatment Plan

Name: Sal Uda
Address: 312 N. South #111
City: Martinsville, 64812
Telephone: XXX-XXXX
School: Preschool

Date of Birth: [specify]
File no.: 900111-3
Diagnosis: Articulation
Semesters in Therapy: 1
Date of Report: [specify]

Background Information

Sal Uda, a four-year-old male, began his first semester of speech treatment at the University Speech and Hearing Clinic on [date]. Sal's speech and language were evaluated on [date]. The evaluation revealed an articulation disorder characterized by substitutions, omissions, and reduced intelligibility. See his folder for a diagnostic report. Treatment was recommended to train correct production of misarticulated phonemes to increase speech intelligibility.

Based on inconsistent production during assessment, the production of the following phonemes was selected for the initial treatment: /p/, /m/, /s/, /k/, and /g/. Production of each phoneme was baserated with 20 stimulus words administered on modeled and evoked discrete trials. Sal's correct production of the target phonemes on modeled and evoked baserate trials was as follows:

/p/	:	15%
/m/	:	10%
/s/	:	22%
/k/	:	18%
/g/	:	14%

Treatment was begun after obtaining the baserates. The following general treatment procedures will be used during the semester. The procedures will be modified as suggested by Sal's performance data. These changes will be described in the final summary report.

Treatment Procedure

Training for each target phoneme will begin at the word level. When Sal's probe response rate at the word level meets a 90% correct criterion, training will be initiated on two-word phrases. A similar probe criterion will be used to shift training to sentences and then to conversational speech.

Intermixed probes on which trained and untrained words, phrases, or sentences are alternated will be administered every time Sal meets a tentative training criterion of 90% correct response rate on a block of 20 evoked training trials. Sal will be trained to meet this criterion at each level of response topography (words, phrases, sentences).

Initially, the clinician will provide stimulus pictures, but Sal will be required to find at least five pictures in magazines or draw two pictures representing the target sound and bring them to the clinic sessions. After he correctly produces the target sound on five consecutive trials, he will paste the pictures in a book to be used for both clinic and home practice.

Training will begin at each level with discrete trials and modeling. The clinician will show Sal a picture, ask a question ("What is this?"), and model the response (word or phrase). Sal will then be required to imitate the clinician's production. When Sal correctly imitates the target sound on five consecutive trials, modeling will be discontinued. The clinician will show Sal a picture and ask "What is this?" to evoke a response.

At the modeled and evoked word levels, verbal reinforcement will be administered on an FR1 schedule for correct productions. At the phrase and sentence levels, an FR4 will be used. At the conversational level, verbal reinforcement will be delivered on an approximate VR5 schedule. All incorrect productions at each level will immediately be interrupted by saying "stop."

Modeling will be reintroduced if Sal gives two to four incorrect responses on the evoked trials. Shaping with manual guidance will be used as necessary.

All productions will be charted by the clinician. Sal also will chart productions with an X under the "happy face" or X under the "sad face." At the end of each session, Sal will assist the clinician in recording his progress on a graph.

It is expected that different target sounds will reach the training criterion at different times. Therefore, the clinician expects to train several sounds at different response topographies in each session. Some sounds may be trained at the word level, while others may be trained at the phrase or even sentence level. When the initially selected target sounds meet the criterion of 90% correct probe rate in conversational speech in the clinic, new target sounds will be baserated and trained.

Maintenance Program

After Sal produces the target sound with 90% accuracy at the evoked word level, his mother will be asked to participate in treatment. Initially, she will observe the treatment procedure, and then she will present stimulus items and chart correct and incorrect productions. She will be trained to immediately reinforce the correct productions, stopping Sal at the earliest sign of an inaccurate production.

After Sal's mother identifies correct and incorrect responses with at least 90% accuracy in the clinic session, she will be trained to work with him at home. The mother will begin with such structured activities as reciting from a list or "reading" from the book he is developing in treatment. Assignments will progress to monitoring and recording speech during dinner and phone conversations with Sal's grandmother. She will be trained to prompt and then praise the correct productions in conversational speech. Sal, the clinician, and Sal's mother will review tape-recorded home assignments. The mother will be given feedback on the procedures implemented at home.

When Sal produces the target sound with 90% accuracy in conversation in the sessions, he will be taken out of the clinic to practice correct productions in nonclinic situations. The clinician will take Sal for a walk on campus and talk with him. Subsequently, he may be taken to the campus bookstore, library, cafeteria, and other places. Eventually, his speech may be monitored informally in shopping centers and restaurants.

When Sal's speech is 98% intelligible and he produces most of his speech sounds at least 90% correct, he may be dismissed from treatment. A follow-up visit will be scheduled for 6 months after dismissal. Based on the initial follow-up results, booster treatment, treatment for persistent errors, or additional follow-ups will be planned.

_____

Marla Model, Student Clinician

_____

Barbara Sierra, M.S., CCC/SLP
Clinical Supervisor

Sample Lesson Plan

L esson plans describe what the clinician intends to do in a treatment session. Lesson plans may be brief or detailed depending on the site and your supervisor. In all cases, lesson plans should give enough information so your supervisor can understand and evaluate them. For various kinds of treatment and lesson plans, see Hegde (2010).

University Speech and Hearing Clinic Lesson Plan

Client: Erik Sounds
Clinician: Julie Matters
Date: [specify]

Date of birth: [specify]
Supervisor: Wendy Marks

Objective: Production of initial /l/ with 90% accuracy at the word level in nonimitated training trials.

Procedures: I will present pictures of words representing /l/ in the initial position. In the beginning, I will model the correct productions. When Erik imitates at 90% accuracy in at least 10 trials, I will skip modeling and ask him to name the pictures. I will reinforce each correct production with verbal praise. I will stop Erik every time he begins to produce an incorrect response by saying "no" or "stop." Toward the end of the session, Erik will begin to plot his progress on chart.

Results:

Objective: Correct production of /f/ in conversational speech with 95% accuracy in all word positions.

Procedures: I will ask Erik to talk about the baseball game he is going to next week. If he has difficulty thinking of things to say, I will prompt him with pictures of baseball games. I will reinforce his correct production on an FR5 schedule. I will react to his incorrect production as described before. I will ask him to self-correct all incorrect /f/ productions in conversational speech.

Results:

Sample Diagnostic Report

The formats and contents of diagnostic reports vary depending on the professional setting and disorders. For a variety of examples of diagnostic reports, see Hegde (1998a, 2010) and Hegde and Pomaville (2008).

University Speech and Hearing Clinic Diagnostic Report

NAME: Susan Murmer
BIRTHDATE: [specify]
AGE: 21
ADDRESS: 44 W. Wilson
CITY: Lothar
TELEPHONE: 000-0000
REFERRED BY: Dr. Marie Meyr

DATE OF EVALUATION: [specify]
DIAGNOSIS: Voice Disorder
EXAMINER: Dawn Goode
SUPERVISOR: Faye Kremtolf
INFORMANT: Self
OCCUPATION: Student
FILE NO: 98032-51

Statement of Problem

Susan Murmer, a 21-year-old female, was seen for a speech and language evaluation at the University Speech and Hearing Clinic on [date]. Susan was referred to the university clinic by Dr. Marie Meyr, an otolaryngologist. Susan reported difficulty speaking for long periods of time. Susan said that Dr. Meyr had diagnosed vocal nodules.

Background Information

Susan's medical history was unremarkable, with the exception of the recent diagnosis of vocal nodules. In a report dated [specify], Dr. Meyr stated the presence of "bilateral vocal nodules in the classic position." Dr. Meyr recommended surgical intervention for removal of the nodules; however, Susan chose not to follow the recommendations. Subsequently, Dr. Meyr recommended voice evaluation and treatment at the University Speech and Hearing Clinic.

Susan reported that she majored in economics and was active on a livestock judging team. She stated that judging took place from October to April, during which time she practiced 3 to 4 hours daily. On judging days, Susan was required to use her voice almost continually for 7 hours. She reported that she must use a louder than normal intensity level during judging. According to Susan, her voice did not interfere with her ability to communicate with others; however, she was concerned about the sound of her voice and how quickly her voice fatigued. She reported that in [date], while yelling, she experienced a sharp pain in the laryngeal area. This experience had frightened her and she sought medical help.

Susan further reported that her voice sounds much better in the mornings and on days when she does not speak much. But often, by evening her voice is hoarse and tired.

Observation and Assessment Results

Oral Peripheral Examination: An oral peripheral examination revealed relatively symmetrical facial features and adequate labial and lingual movement. Palatal structures were within normal limits. Adequate velopharyngeal functions were noted. The soft palate elevated symmetrically on phonation of /a/. Velopharyngeal closure was acoustically judged to be within normal limits. Normal muscular function was demonstrated during rapid articulatory movement.

Hearing: A pure tone audiometric screening was performed at 15 dB HTL for the frequencies 500, 1000, 2000, and 4000 Hz. Bilateral responses were obtained for all frequencies.

Articulation: Articulation was evaluated during Susan's spontaneous speech and reading of the "Rainbow Passage." Speech was 100% intelligible. No articulation errors were noted.

Language: An analysis of a 100–utterance language sample did not reveal any deviations. The mean length of utterance was 7.5 words and 8.0 morphemes. All language structures were correctly used.

Fluency: The conversational speech sample was used to assess fluency and dysfluencies. Susan's dysfluency rate was 3% and consisted mainly of syllable and word interjections. Her rate and types of dysfluencies were not of clinical significance.

Voice: A conversational speech sample of 250 words was obtained to evaluate overall vocal quality. Vocal quality was characterized by inappropriately loud intensity, hoarseness, low pitch, and pitch breaks. Frequent hard glottal attacks and throat clearing were observed throughout the assessment session.

Susan spoke in a loud voice during the evaluation. Sound level meter measurements revealed speech consistently exceeding 60 dB. When asked to lower her intensity, Susan did so for four or five words, then gradually increased her intensity. Susan said that she used a loud voice in other environments. She stated that her roommate had told her not to bother to use the telephone because her voice was so loud she didn't need one.

Chest and clavicular breathing were observed throughout the assessment. Maximum duration of phonation and breath support were measured by having Susan prolong the phoneme /a/. Susan exhibited the ability to sustain /a/ for 5, 7, and 6 seconds over three separate trials, well below the optimal level of 16 seconds. Three separate trials were used to measure Susan's ability to sustain the cognates /s/ and /z/. The average ratio for these trials was 0.70, which was below the expected level of 1.0 for normal speakers. A reading sample also revealed inefficient breath support. In reading, 80% of Susan's phrases deteriorated into glottal fry or hoarseness by the second word of the phrase.

Habitual pitch was measured using the Visi-Pitch™. Habitual pitch during conversational speech was 196 Hz, with a pitch range of 57.8 Hz to 988 Hz. The higher frequencies were noted during pitch breaks. Variable pitch and frequent pitch breaks were noted during spontaneous speech. Optimal pitch was determined to be 262 Hz. Susan could increase her pitch using feedback from the Visi-Pitch. When pitch was raised, hoarseness was eliminated until pitch again decreased.

Rate, resonance, and inflection were evaluated during conversation. These vocal parameters were considered normal.

Summary of Findings

Susan Murmer's otolaryngologist has diagnosed bilateral vocal nodules. The current voice assessment suggests a history of vocal abuse, and that her voice is inappropriately loud and characterized by hoarseness, low pitch, and frequent pitch breaks. Susan exhibited inefficient breath support during phonation and employed several vocally abusive speech behaviors.

Recommendations

It is recommended that Susan Murmer receive speech-language pathology services for treatment of her voice disorder, a minimum of two sessions per week. Treatment should focus on eliminating vocally abusive behaviors, increasing breath support, and increasing pitch. It is also recommended that Susan return to her otolaryngologist for a follow-up visit after 3 months of voice treatment at this clinic.

_____

Dawn Goode, Student Clinician

_____

Faye Kremtolf, M.A., CCC/SLP
Clinical Supervisor

Discrete Trial Treatment Procedure and Recording Form

Discrete trials are often needed in the initial stages of treatment. They are most useful in teaching articulation and language targets.

Discrete Trial Treatment Procedure

In the discrete trial treatment procedure, you may use two to six training stimuli at any one time. The following example shows how to train the present progressive *ing* using modeling and six exemplars (training stimuli). Skip modeling according to the criteria described in the text. See Hegde (1998a) for details.

1. Place the stimulus picture in front of the client. For example, place the picture of a *boy running* in front of the client.

2. Ask a question designed to evoke the correct response. Ask "What is the boy doing?"

3. Immediately model the correct response. "Say, the boy is running."

4. Wait a few seconds for the client to respond.

5. If the response is correct, immediately reinforce the client. If the response is incorrect (the present progressive omitted), say "No" and use other response reduction procedures (response cost, time-out).

6. Record the response on your recording sheet.

7. Pull the stimulus picture away from the client to mark the end of the trial.

8. Start the next trial by again placing the picture in front of the client.

Discrete Trial Treatment Recording Sheet

In the following example, the clinician trained a person with aphasia in naming five photographs or pictures and recorded the responses on the recording sheet. On discrete trials, modeling was introduced then withdrawn as shown.

Client: Wendy Nullnem   Clinician: Arnold Chatters
Age: 65   Date: [specify]
Disorder: Aphasia   Session No. 5
Target Behavior: Naming   Reinforcement: Continuous/Verbal

Target Reponses				**Blocks of 10 Training Trials**							
	1	2	3	4	5	6	7	8	9	10	% Correct
1. "Tom"	m+	–	+	–	–	+	–	+	+	+	—
(Husband)	+	+	e–	–	m+	+	e+	+	+	+	m71% / e83%
2. "Jenny"	m+	+	–	+	–	+	+	+	+	+	—
(Daughter)	e–	–	m+	+	e+	+	+	–	+	+	m83% / e62%
3. "Cup"	m–	+	–	+	–	+	+	+	–	+	—
	+	+	+	+	e+	–	+	+	–	+	m71% / e66%
4. "Water"	m+	+	–	+	+	–	+	+	+	+	—
	+	e–	–	m+	+	+	+	e+	+	+	m86% / e60%
5. "Phone"	m–	+	+	+	+	+	e–	–	m+	+	—
	e–	+	–	+	+	–	+	+	+	+	m85% / e58%

Note: (+) = Correct response   (–) = Incorrect or no response
        m = Modeled trial   e = Evoked trial, no modeling
        Total Number of Trials: _____
        Total % Correct Responses: _____

Daily Progress Notes

Progress notes are recorded after each treatment session to document client progress. Following is a sample of progress notes using "SOAP notes" (subjective, objective, assessment, plan).

City Hospital Speech-Language Pathology and Audiology Department

Name of patient:
Date of birth:
Clinician(s)

Date	Progress Notes	Initials
9/23/09	John appeared alert today. He greeted	
	the clinician with a smile. The client responded to	
	20 yes/no questions with 70% accuracy. He	
	produced simple CV words @ the imitation	
	level with 80% accuracy. John demonstrated	
	progress in both treatment tasks today.	
	Response to yes/no questions ↑ 60% to 70%	
	(in 20 trials). Imitative productions ↑ from	
	75% to 80% for CV words. Continue	
	current activities.	
		LPG SP11111

Date	Progress Notes	Initials
9/24/09	John greeted the clinician with a smile, but	
	appeared tired – his eyes closed occasionally	
	during the 30-minute session. Client responded	
	to yes/no questions with 70%. Imitative tasks for	
	CV words was 60%. John demonstrated ↓ in	
	both tasks today. As noted, he seemed tired.	
	This was discussed with nurse who repeated that	
	John had not slept well. Rec. continue current	
	activities, but reevaluate if John's behavior or health	
	change.	
		LPG SP11111

Sample Progress Report

Progress reports summarize services offered to a client. They usually contain information on the client's background, treatment objectives and procedures, results or the outcome to date, and recommendations. The formats of progress reports vary depending on professional settings, disorders, and the professional or the agency that receives them. For a variety of progress reports, see Hegde (1998a, 2010).

Speech and Hearing Center
Speech-Language Progress Report

[Date]

Richard Smith, M.D.
3030 E. Fairview Ave., #24
Oceanview, CA 93711

PATIENT: John North
DOB: [specify]
PERIOD COVERED: From: To:
NUMBER OF SESSIONS ATTENDED:
LENGTH OF SESSIONS:

Dear Dr. Smith:

John North, a 3-year, 3-month-old boy was seen for a speech and language evaluation on [date]. The evaluation revealed significantly delayed speech and language with verbal apraxia. At that time, John was basically nonverbal with the exception of a few single syllable word approximations. He had less than 15 functional words. As a result of the evaluation, John was enrolled in speech-language treatment. He received treatment approximately twice a week from [dates].

Summary of Treatment

Goal 1: Production of the following sounds with at least 90% accuracy in conversational speech in the clinic and home setting: /p/, /b/, /m/, /n/, /t/, /d/, /k/, /g/, and /s/.

Treatment: Treatment began at the phoneme level for each sound and progressed to the word, phrase, and conversation level after a criteria of 95% accuracy was met at each level. Tactile, auditory, and visual stimulation initially were used to train sound production. Verbal praise and token gain and loss were used during treatment.

Progress: This goal has been met.

Goal 2: Production of the following language features in continuous speech during structured treatment activities with 90% accuracy: present progressive, regular plural morphemes, possessives, regular past tense inflections, and prepositions.

Treatment: John was presented with stimulus pictures representing each word in the phrase. The clinician modeled each phrase and John was required to touch each card as he imitated the clinician (e.g., *boy is jumping*). John was praised for his correct productions. Incorrect productions were interrupted and the clinician modeled the correct production.

Progress: John met the goal for the following structures: present progressive, plurals, possessives, and the prepositions "in," "on," and "under." John continues to work on the regular past tense.

Impressions and Recommendations

John has made excellent progress in his speech and language treatment sessions. His willingness to try to interact with others and the reinforcement of successful communication have had a positive effect on his behavior and social development. Excellent parental support and participation from his mother has encouraged carryover into other environments. John is now able to communicate using a larger vocabulary of single words and simple sentences of two to three words. It is recommended that John continue to receive speech-language services two times per week. Treatment will emphasize the following:

1. Continued training on the regular past tense

2. Production of the following sounds: /f/, /w/, /y/, /ʃ/, and /l/

3. Increased mean length of utterance

4. Parent training to work with John at home

I hope this information is helpful. Please contact me if you have questions.

Yours sincerely,

Susan Frances, M.A., CCC-SLP
Speech-Language Pathologist

Sample Final Summary

The final summary is written at the end of a treatment period (such as at the end of a semester). It provides information on the client's treatment, progress, and recommendations for continuing treatment. The format and contents of final summaries vary depending on the professional setting, the disorder, and the professional or the agency that receives them. For a variety of final summaries, see Hegde (1998a, 2010).

University Speech and Hearing Clinic Final Summary

Client: John J. John
Address: 444 E. Southdrive
City: Grayson
Telephone: 000-0000
Occupation: Student
Period Covered:
From: To:
Clinic Schedule
Sessions per week: 2
Number of clinic visits: 22

Birthdate: [specify]
Clinic File No.: 910077
Diagnosis: Stuttering
Semesters in Clinic: 1
Date of Report: [specify]

Length of sessions: 1 hour
Total clinic hours: 22 hours

Status at the Beginning of Treatment

John J. John, a 25-year-old male, began his first semester of treatment at the University Speech and Hearing Clinic. John reported that he stuttered. He said it interfered with his part-time job as a store clerk and that people occasionally made fun of his speech. He reported that he had received speech therapy when he was 9 or 10 years old, but that he always continued to stutter.

Two conversational speech samples were analyzed before beginning treatment. Language, voice, and articulation were subjectively evaluated and judged to be normal. The first speech sample, obtained in the clinic, contained 1,400 words with a dysfluency rate of 18%. The second sample was recorded by John when he talked with his wife at home. This sample revealed a dysfluency rate of 16%. Both samples contained part-word repetitions, whole word repetitions, interjections of words and phrases, pauses, and prolongations. A complete diagnostic report dated [specify] is placed in the folder.

Summary of Treatment

Treatment involved training fluent speech through the use of a management of airflow, easy vocal onset, and reduced rate of speech through vowel prolongation. A detailed treatment program written for John may be found in the folder.

Initially, each of the fluency skills was trained separately. John was asked to inhale a larger than usual amount of air, immediately exhale a small amount of air through his mouth, and begin saying the word in a soft and easy manner. He was asked to prolong the vowels and speak at a reduced rate. This process usually resulted in stutter-free speech.

Stutter-free speech was trained starting with words and phrases. In gradual steps, treatment progressed to controlled sentences and conversational speech. In all treatment sessions, the criterion of fluency required of John was 98% or better. Both dysfluencies and errors in fluency skills (e.g., failure to inhale or exhale, abrupt phonatory onset, rapid rate) were measured in all sessions. When John maintained at least 98% fluent speech at any level of training for either a block of 50 utterances (phrases, sentences) or for a duration of 10 minutes or more, the training was moved to the next level of response topography. If John's dysfluency rate increased when moved to a higher level of training, he was returned to the lower level.

At the earliest sign of an incorrect response or a dysfluency, John was asked to "Stop." In the initial stages, he was told what went wrong. For example, the clinician said: "You forgot to breathe in"; "You did not breathe out"; "You were about to stutter"; and so forth. Later on, he was asked simply to "Stop." Correct productions of target behaviors resulting in stutter-free speech were verbally reinforced at the end of the response chain. Initially, a continuous schedule was used; gradually, the amount of reinforcement was reduced to an approximate VR5 schedule at the conversation level.

John was trained to chart the correct use of target behaviors and all dysfluencies. After John demonstrated accurate monitoring of responses and 98% fluency at each level, home assignments were given for that level. John's wife observed four sessions in which she was trained to monitor his fluent speech by stopping and reinforcing him as the clinician did. John and his wife were recommended to practice the skills of fluency for at least 20 minutes each day. John's wife was asked also to monitor his speech in most speaking situations.

To promote maintenance, the clinician accompanied John to the campus bookstore and cafeteria where he talked to other persons. The clinician monitored John's speech by giving subtle hints to prompt the target responses and provided verbal reinforcement whenever practical. Various probes were taken to document changes in his dysfluency rate.

Results

By the end of the semester, John's dysfluency rate in conversational speech with the clinician at the clinic was 98%. However, a 10-minute conversational speech sample recorded at his home with his wife showed a fluency rate of 94%. A probe of his speech with his boss at work showed a fluency rate of 92%.

Recommendations

It is recommended that John continue treatment for his stuttering. The treatment next semester should emphasize maintenance of fluency in home, office, and other settings.

_____

Dana Monroe, Student Clinician

_____

Greg Hallstoni, M.S., CCC/SLP
Clinical Supervisor

Sample Referral Letters

S peech-language pathologists write many kinds of referral letters to other professionals. Three common kinds are illustrated on the following pages. See Hegde (1998a, 2010) for additional examples.

Sample Referral Letter 1

The following sample illustrates the kind of letter a speech-language pathologist might write to another professional to acknowledge the referral of a client for speech-language services.

[date]

John Jones, M.D.
228 N. Way, Suite 101
Bloomington, CO 78123

Dear Dr. Jones:

Thank you for referring Sal Uda to our Clinic. He was seen for a speech and language evaluation on [date]. Sal was accompanied to the evaluation by his mother who expressed concern over her son's lack of speech intelligibility.

Results of the assessment revealed a severe articulation disorder, with multiple sound substitutions and omissions. Receptive language was age appropriate; however, expressive language was delayed. Sal was cooperative during the evaluation and easily stimulable for the sounds he misarticulated and omitted.

I recommended that Sal begin treatment for his speech and language disorder. He will be seen two times per week for one hour each visit.

Enclosed is a copy of Sal's speech and language evaluation report. If you have any questions, please contact me at 555-5555.

Sincerely,

Dorothy Ozzz, M.A., CCC/SLP
Speech-Language Pathologist

Sample Referral Letter 2

The following sample illustrates the kind of letter one speech-language pathologist might write to another to make a referral.

[date]

Donna Jones, M.S.
Speech-Language Pathologist
Melvin Communication Clinic
Melvin, Alaska

Dear Ms. Jones:

Robert Fine, a 67-year-old man who suffered a stroke nearly four months ago, was diagnosed with apraxia and aphasia, characterized by moderate auditory comprehension and severe verbal expression deficits. At the time of assessment, his conversational speech consisted primarily of several automatic phrases.

Robert has received treatment at our clinic for the past three months. He has demonstrated significant progress. He is able to express himself in 6- to 7-word utterances. He accurately uses many language structures including nouns, various verb tenses, modifiers, plurals, possessives, and some prepositional phrases.

Although Robert has made good progress, he needs continued treatment to stabilize his conversational speech skills in home, community, and social situations. Because he is moving to your town, I am referring him to your clinic. Robert is highly motivated to continue treatment. He would be an excellent candidate for your treatment program. I hope you will consider accepting Robert as a client. If you have questions, please contact me at 888-8888.

Sincerely,

Georgia Shurr, M.S., CCC/SLP

Sample Referral Letter 3

The following sample illustrates the kind of letter a speech-language pathologist might write to a physician (or another professional) to refer a client.

[date]

Jean Jayne, M.D.
333 W. Hills, Suite 101
Beverly, NM 20111

Dear Dr. Jayne:

I saw Jerry Blank in my office for a voice evaluation on [date]. He requested an evaluation because he felt that his voice was "too deep." During the evaluation he reported chronic hoarseness and occasional pain in the laryngeal area.

During the voice evaluation, Jerry exhibited a harsh, breathy voice with frequent pitch breaks. He had difficulty sustaining phonation. His intensity sometimes became inaudible toward the end of phrases.

I recommended that Jerry have a laryngeal evaluation. He reported that you were his otolaryngologist and that he would be making an appointment with you. According to Jerry's request, I have enclosed a copy of his voice evaluation.

If you have questions, please contact me.

Sincerely,

Micron MacGregor, M.S., CCC/SLP
Speech-Language Pathologist

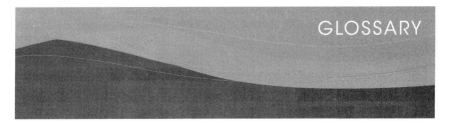

American Speech-Language-Hearing Association (ASHA)—The national professional organization representing speech-language pathologists and audiologists.

Antecedents—Events that occur before responses; clinically, all kinds of treatment stimuli, including pictures and clinician's modeling.

Aspiration—Entry of food and liquid into the airway; a symptom of dysphagia.

Assessment—Clinical procedures implemented to understand a client's communicative problem and his or her personal and family history, along with existing and nonexisting communicative skills; includes measurement of communicative skills and related behaviors.

Automatic reinforcers—Reinforcing sensory consequences of responses.

Aversive stimuli—Events that people work hard to avoid or move away from.

Avoidance—A behavior that prevents the occurrence of an aversive event and hence gets reinforced.

Avoidance conditioning—Teaching behaviors that terminate, reduce, or avoid aversive events.

Backup reinforcers—Events, objects, and opportunities that clients gain access to by exchanging tokens they have earned in treatment sessions.

Baselines—Pretreatment target skill measures that help demonstrate improvement under treatment.

Bedside evaluation—A quick and subjective evaluation of a patient; in speech-language pathology, it is often an evaluation of a patient's swallowing, memory, orientation, and so forth.

Behavioral momentum—Rapidly evoking a high-probability response and immediately commanding a low-probability response to reduce noncompliance or to increase the low-probability behaviors.

Benchmarks—Used synonymously with objectives to outline steps and outcomes necessary to obtain a long-term goal.

Block scheduling—A service scheduling method found in public schools; students in specific schools receive services for only a predetermined period of time (e.g., only for 6 weeks, 4 to 5 days each week); clinicians then move on to serve children in another block; contrasted with intermittent scheduling.

Booster treatment—Treatment given any time after the client was dismissed from the original treatment to maintain responses.

Cardiologist—A physician with specialized training in cardiovascular diseases.

Certificate of Clinical Competence (CCC)—Awarded by the American Speech-Language-Hearing Association to speech-language pathologists and audiologists who have met certain standards.

Childhood apraxia of speech—Disorders of articulation thought to be due to a central speech motor planning and programming deficit in the absence of speech muscle impairment; both articulation and prosodic problems may characterize the disorder.

Client-specific approach—A method of selecting target behaviors that are relevant and useful for the individual client; contrasted with normative approach.

Clinical Fellowship—A period of paid or voluntary professional work done beyond the master's degree under supervision; required by ASHA to award its certificates of clinical competence.

Cluttering—A disorder of fluency characterized by an excessively fast rate of speech negatively affecting speech intelligibility.

Collaborative instruction model—A model in which the speech-language pathologist and classroom teacher coordinate their lessons and work together to provide students with appropriate learning opportunities.

Compensatory treatment—Teaching the production of certain skills in atypical manners, in spite of neurophysiological limitations that cannot be eliminated.

Conditioned generalized reinforcers—Tokens, money, and other reinforcers that are effective in a wide range of conditions because their effects do not depend on a specific state of need (as food does).

Conditioned reinforcers—Social consequences that reinforce behaviors because of past learning experiences; the same as secondary reinforcers.

Consecutive interpreting—An individual talks, pauses, and then the interpreter translates.

Consultative model—The speech-language pathologist works with the client's family, teachers, or other professionals to address the needs of the client.

Contingency—An interdependent relation between events that help teach and sustain skills; the dependent relation between stimuli, responses, and their consequences.

Contingency priming—Prompting others to reinforce one's own behaviors.

Continuing education units (CEUs)—ASHA and licensing agency requirements that stipulate a certain number of annual hours of attendance at approved educational experiences (e.g., lectures, courses, conferences, seminars) to keep current in the profession.

Continuous schedule—A schedule in which all responses are reinforced.

Controlled evidence—Data that show that a particular treatment, not some other factor, was responsible for the positive changes in the client's behavior.

Corrective feedback—Response-contingent presentation or withdrawal of a stimulus that reduces the frequency of that response.

Council for Clinical Certification (CFCC)—Sets the standards for and awards the Certificate of Clinical Competence.

Council on Academic Accreditation in Audiology and Speech-Language Pathology (CAA)—Accredits university training programs that meet ASHA standards.

Credential—A document that indicates that certain competencies have been met and authorizes the individual holding the credential to provide services according to its parameters.

Designated instructional services (DIS)—A term used in the schools to describe certain special education services, including speech-language pathology and audiology.

Diagnosis—A determination of the nature of a disorder and its causes, if possible.

Diagnostic report—Provides comprehensive information on a client's pretreatment status.

Dietitian—A professional with training in nutrition and diet.

Differential reinforcement—Use of reinforcement techniques to increase certain behaviors while at the same time certain other behaviors decrease as a side effect.

Differential reinforcement of alternative behavior (DRA)—Reinforcing a specified desirable behavior that serves the same function as the one to be reduced.

Differential reinforcement of incompatible behavior (DRI)—Reinforcing a desirable behavior that is not compatible with an undesirable behavior targeted for reduction.

Differential reinforcement of low rates of responding (DRL)—Reinforcing progressively lower frequencies of an undesirable behavior to shape it down.

Differential reinforcement of other behavior (DRO)—Reinforcing many unspecified but desirable behaviors while not reinforcing a specified but undesirable behavior targeted for reduction.

Direct response reduction strategy—Reducing behaviors by placing a contingency on them. Contrasted with indirect response reduction strategy.

Discharge report—A report written at the time clients are dismissed from treatment.

Discrete trials—Successive opportunities for producing responses that are clearly separated by brief durations of time.

Discrimination—A behavioral process of establishing different (and appropriate) responses to different stimuli.

Dysarthrias—Motor speech disorders caused by damage to the central or peripheral nervous system that affect (among other systems) speech-related muscles.

Dysphagia—Swallowing disorders due to various diseases, trauma, or injury that negatively affect normal swallow of food and liquid.

Effectiveness (of treatment)—Assurance that treatment, not some other factor, was responsible for the positive changes documented in a treatment research study.

Electronic Data Interchange (EDI)—Any electronic transaction that happens between a provider and an agency such as a hospital or third-party payer.

Emergent literacy—Certain skills related to reading and writing that preschoolers exhibit; include such basic skills as recognizing the letters of the alphabet, printing the letters, naming the letters, sight reading of words, and so forth.

Escape—A behavior that reduces or terminates an aversive event (such as moving away from a dangerous situation) and hence becomes more frequent under similar circumstances. See also avoidance.

Escape extinction—Blocking an escape response (such as a child's attempt at leaving the treatment room) to prevent negative reinforcement for it.

Ethnocultural generality—Applicability of treatment procedures across clients of varied ethnocultural backgrounds.

Ethnographic interview—An interview that is directed by the responses a family member provides and that focuses on the client and his or her interactions within the family.

Evoked trial—A structured opportunity to produce a response when the clinician does not model but asks questions or provides other more naturalistic stimuli.

Exclusion time-out (TO)—Response-contingent exclusion of a person from a reinforcing environment; the typical effect is response reduction. See also nonexclusion time-out and time-out.

Exemplar—A response that illustrates a target behavior; all individual target responses the clinician teaches a client.

Experiment—A controlled condition in which a treatment is applied, withheld, reapplied, and so forth to show that the treatment is effective.

Experimental group—The group that receives treatment and hence shows changes. See also control group.

Extinction—The procedure of terminating reinforcers for responses to be reduced; the same as ignoring.

Extinction burst—An initial and temporary increase in responses when reinforcers are withdrawn.

Fading—A method of reducing the controlling power of a stimulus while still maintaining the response.

Fixed interval (FI) schedule—An intermittent schedule of reinforcement in which an invariable time duration separates opportunities to earn reinforcers.

Fixed-ratio (FR) schedule—An intermittent schedule of reinforcement in which a certain number of responses are required to earn a reinforcer.

Follow-up—Probe or assessment of response maintenance subsequent to dismissal from treatment.

Functional equivalence training—Reinforcing desirable behaviors that serve the same function as the undesirable behaviors.

Functional independence measures (FIMS)—Patient objectives used in medical settings, written with the emphasis on a patient's ability to perform functional tasks (e.g., tell when he or she is ill) with as little assistance as possible.

Functional outcome—Generalized, broader, and socially and personally meaningful effects of treatment; an overall improvement in communication between clients, their families, and their caregivers.

Generality (of treatment)—The applicability of a treatment procedure in a wide range of situations involving other clients and clinicians.

Generalization—A declining rate of unreinforced response in the presence of untrained stimuli.

Group design strategy—Methods in which treatment effects are demonstrated by treating individuals in one group and not treating individuals in another group. See also single-subject strategy.

Health Insurance Portability and Accountability Act (HIPAA)—A law passed by the U.S. Congress in 1996 to improve the effectiveness and efficiency of health care and protect client confidentiality.

Heterogeneous grouping—A practice used in the schools of grouping together students who exhibit different disorders.

High-probability behaviors—Frequently exhibited behaviors that reinforce less-frequently exhibited behaviors.

Homogeneous grouping—A method used in the schools of grouping together students with similar disorders.

Imitation—Learning in which responses take the same form as their stimuli; modeling provides the stimuli.

Implied consent—Approval given without a specific statement of authorization. For example, it may not be necessary for a secretary to obtain written authorization before accessing a client's record, because reviewing client records is typically a part of a secretary's duties.

Improvement—Documented positive changes in a client's behavior under treatment; no guarantee that the treatment was effective.

Incompatible behaviors—Behaviors that cannot be produced simultaneously.

Indirect response reduction strategy—Reducing certain behaviors by increasing other behaviors; indirect because no contingency is placed on behaviors to be decreased.

Individual education programs (IEPs)—Education programs for children with disabilities or special needs.

Individualized family service plans (IFSPs)—Plans developed for infants and toddlers and their family members.

Informative feedback—Information on the performance levels that reinforce behaviors.

Inherent consent in the private interests of the client—Permission to release information assumed when release of information is in the best interest of the client.

Initial response—The first, simplified component of a target response used in shaping.

Instructions—Verbal stimuli that gain control over other persons' actions.

Interfering behaviors—Behaviors that interrupt the treatment process.

Intermediate responses—Responses other than the initial and final that are used in shaping.

Intermittent reinforcement—Reinforcing only some responses or responses produced with some delay between reinforcers.

Intermittent scheduling—A method of scheduling services in public schools; services are offered each week to all students in all schools; contrasted with block scheduling.

Intermixed probes—Procedures of assessing generalized production by alternating trained and untrained stimulus items. See also probes and pure probes.

Isolation time-out (TO)—Response-contingent removal of a person from a reinforcing environment and placing him or her in a nonreinforcing environment; the typical effect is the reduction in that response.

The Joint Commission—formerly known as Joint Commission on Accreditation of Healthcare Organizations (JCAHO); a regulatory agency that sets standards for patient care and accredits many hospitals.

Knowledge and Skill Acquisition (KASA) Form—A format approved and required by the American Speech-Language-Hearing Association to document students' progress in meeting its academic and clinical requirements to enter the profession of speech-language pathology or audiology.

Laryngectomee—Individuals who have had their larynx surgically removed, often because of such diseases as cancer.

Laryngectomy—The surgical procedure of removing the diseased or badly damaged larynx.

Lesson plans—Written statements used in school settings to describe treatment planned for one or a few sessions.

License—A state-issued document that allows a qualified person to offer clinical (or other kinds of) services to the public. Unlike the ASHA's certificate of clinical competence, a license has the authority of a state law.

Literacy skills—Traditional reading and writing skills, contrasted with *emergent literacy skills*.

Maintenance strategy—Extension of treatment to natural settings.

Manual guidance—Physical guidance provided to shape a response.

Mode (of responses)—Manner or method of a response; imitation, oral reading, and conversational speech are different response modes.

Modeled trial—An opportunity to imitate a target response when the clinician models it.

Modeling—The clinician's production of the target response the client is expected to learn; used to teach imitation.

Multidisciplinary team—A group of professionals (and family members) who work together within their respective scopes of practice to determine and provide optimal patient management.

National Examination in Speech-Language Pathology and Audiology (NESPA)—A national test designed to assess academic and clinical knowledge deemed essential to practice the professions of speech-language pathology or audiology; part of the Praxis series of tests administered by the Educational Testing Service; required to earn the ASHA Certificate of Clinical Competence and most state licensure.

National Student Speech-Language-Hearing Association (NSSLHA)—Student organization of the American Speech-Language-Hearing Association.

Natural environment—A term used by the federal government to describe a typical location where nondisabled children can be found.

Negative reinforcers—Aversive events that are removed, reduced, postponed, or prevented; responses that do these increase in frequency. See also reinforcers and positive reinforcers.

Neurologist—A physician with specialized training in function and disorders of the nervous system.

Nonexclusion time-out (TO)—Response contingent arrangement of a brief duration of time in which all interaction is terminated; the typical effect is response education. See also exclusion time-out and time-out.

Normative strategy—A method of selecting target behaviors for clients based on age-based norms.

Norms—Averaged (mean) performance of a typical group of persons on a selected test or measure.

Omission training—Reinforcing a person for not exhibiting a certain behavior; the same as DRO.

Operational definitions—Scientific definitions that describe how what is defined is measured. See also constituent definitions.

Orofacial examination—An assessment of the structural and functional integrity of orofacial structures; also known as oral-peripheral examination.

Orthodontist—A dentist with specialized training in dental occlusion.

Otolaryngologist—A physician specializing in evaluation and treatment of disorders of the ear, nose, and throat.

Partial modeling—Withdrawing modeling in gradual steps.

Pediatrician—A physician specializing in the medical care of children.

Physiatrist—A physician trained in rehabilitative medicine.

Positive reinforcers—Events that, when presented immediately after a response is made, increase the future probability of that response. See also reinforcers and negative reinforcers.

Post-reinforcement pause—A period of no response after one receives a reinforcer.

Posttests—Measures of behaviors established after completing an experimental teaching program. See also pretests.

Preferred practice—Desirable professional activities and practices; often recommended by such professional organizations as ASHA.

Premorbid—A client's state before an incident resulting in a disorder.

Pretests—Measures of behaviors established before starting an experimental teaching program. See also posttests.

Primary reinforcers—Unconditioned reinforcers (e.g., food) whose effects do not depend on past learning.

Probes—Procedures to assess generalized production of responses. See also intermixed probes and pure probes.

Procedures (of treatment)—Technical operations the clinician performs to effect changes in the client behaviors; behaviors of clinicians.

Professional liability—Legal and ethical vulnerability to charges of malpractice; often covered by an insurance policy.

Progress reports—Report written to summarize a client's treatment and its results.

Prompts—Special stimuli that increase the probability of a response; prompts may be verbal or nonverbal.

Protected health information (PHI)—A term used to describe any health information that is created or received by the health care provider and can or does identify the individual.

Punishment—Procedures of reducing a behavior by response-contingent presentation or withdrawal of stimuli; the same as corrective feedback.

Pure probes—Procedures for assessing generalized production with only untrained stimulus items. See also probes and intermixed probes.

Random assignment—A method of assigning randomly selected subjects to either the experimental or the control group without bias.

Random procedure—A method of selecting subjects from a large population without bias; each subject in the population has the same chance of being selected.

Reinforce—Strengthen, increase.

Reinforcement—A method of selecting and strengthening behaviors of individuals by arranging consequences under specific stimulus conditions.

Reinforcement withdrawal—Taking reinforcers away to decrease a response (e.g., response cost and time-out).

Reinforcers—Events that follow behaviors and thereby increase the future probability of those behaviors. See also positive and negative reinforcers.

Reliability—Consistency with which the same event is repeatedly measured.

Replication—Conducting repeated research to show that a given procedure works with different clients, in different settings, and when used by different clinicians.

Response class—A group of responses created by the same or similar contingencies; functionally but not necessarily structurally similar responses.

Response cost—Response-contingent withdrawal of reinforcers that decreases those responses.

Sample—A smaller number of individuals selected from a larger population. See also population.

Satiation—Temporary termination of a drive or need because it has been satisfied.

Schedules of reinforcement—Different patterns of reinforcement that generate different patterns of responses.

Scope of practice—Professional activities that are approved by the virtue training, awarded license, or earned certification and credentials. Professionals cannot perform activities that are outside the scope of practice.

Secondary reinforcers—Conditioned reinforcers whose effects depend on past learning (e.g., verbal praise).

Self-control—A behavior that monitors other behaviors of the same person.

Shaping—A method of teaching nonexistent responses that are not even imitated. The responses are simplified and taught in an ascending sequence. Also known as successive approximations.

Simultaneous interpreting—The interpreter translates as the individual talks.

Single-subject strategy—Methods of demonstrating treatment effects by showing contrasts between conditions of no treatment, treatment, withdrawal of treatment, and other control procedures when all subjects are treated. See also group design strategy.

SOAP notes—Frequently utilized means of communicating patient progress among professionals in hospitals through notations in the patients' charts; acronym for subjective, objective, assessment, plan.

Social reinforcers—A variety of conditioned reinforcers that include verbal praise.

Speech-Language Pathology Assistants (SLPAs)—Those who have an associate's degree and restricted coursework and practical experience in speech-language pathology; may work only under the supervision of a speech-language pathologist who holds an ASHA's certificate of clinical competence and state license where applicable.

Stuttering—A disorder of fluency characterized by excessive amounts of dysfluencies or excessive duration of dysfluencies both often associated with such additional features as muscular tension, avoidance of speaking situation, and negative emotions associated with speech and speaking situations.

Swallowing disorders—The same as dysphagia.

Targets behavior—Behavior a client is taught.

Telepractice—Provision of services via technology.

Terminal response—The final response targeted in shaping.

Time-out (TO)—A period of contingently nonreinforcement-imposed response; the typical effect is reduced rate of that response. See also exclusion time-out and nonexclusion time-out.

Tokens—Objects that are earned during treatment and exchanged later for backup reinforcers.

Topography—The form or shape of behaviors; how behaviors sound, feel, or appear.

Transdisciplinary team—Different professionals and paraprofessionals who, with proper training, may provide some services for another team member.

Treatment—In communicative disorders, it is the management of contingent relations between antecedents, responses, and consequences; it is a rearrangement of communicative relationships between a speaker and his or her listener.

Treatment plan—A report that describes short- and long-term goals and the procedures used to obtain those goals.

Trial—A structured opportunity to produce a response.

Universal Healthcare Precautions—Common procedures that help prevent or minimize the chances of potential infections while working with patients and clients.

Validity—The degree to which a measuring instrument measures what it purports to measure.

Variable interval (VI) schedule—An intermittent reinforcement schedule in which the time duration between reinforcers is varied around an average.

Variable-ratio (VR) schedule—An intermittent reinforcement schedule in which the number of responses needed to earn a reinforcer is varied around an average.

Verbal stimulus generalization—Production of unreinforced responses when untrained verbal stimuli are presented.

Videofluorographic evaluation—An objective procedure in which the client's swallowing mechanism is recorded on a video.

INDEX